MASTER
MEDICINE

Psychiatry

Commissioning Editor: Michael Parkinson
Project Development Manager: Barbara Simmons
Project Manager: Frances Affleck
Designers: Judith Wright, George Ajayi

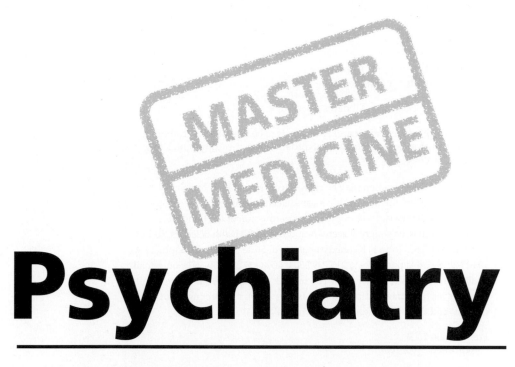

Psychiatry

A clinical core text for integrated curricula with self-assessment

ELSPETH GUTHRIE

MSc MD MBChB MRCPsych
Professor of Psychological Medicine and Medical
Psychotherapy
School of Psychiatry and Behavioural Sciences
University of Manchester

SHÔN LEWIS

MD FRCPsych
Professor of Adult Psychiatry
University of Manchester

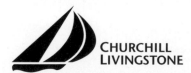

CHURCHILL
LIVINGSTONE

EDINBURGH LONDON NEW YORK PHILADELPHIA SYDNEY TORONTO 2002

CHURCHILL LIVINGSTONE
An imprint of Elsevier Limited

First edition 2002
   Reprinted 2006, 2007

ISBN 978 0443 062766

British Library Cataloguing in Publication Data
A catalogue record for this book is available from the British Library

Library of Congress Cataloging in Publication Data
A catalog record for this book is available from the Library of Congress

Note
Medical knowledge is constantly changing. As new information becomes available, changes in treatment, procedures, equipment and the use of drugs become necessary. The authors and the publishers have taken care to ensure that the information given in this text is accurate and up to date. However, readers are strongly advised to confirm that the information, especially with regard to drug usage, complies with the latest legislation and standards of practice.

The
publisher's
policy is to use
**paper manufactured
from sustainable forests**

Printed in China

Acknowledgements

We would like to thank the following: Dr Jayne Byrne, for providing the photograph of the lewy body for the chapter on Psychiatry of Older Adults and for giving helpful advice; Dr Bob Baldwin who also gave helpful advice on the same chapter; Dr Cathy Shaw for useful comments on several chapters.

Contents

Using this book

Philosophy of the book

'What do I need to know about psychiatry? What are the basic skills I need to learn? How much psychiatry should a newly qualified doctor know in order to provide the best treatment and care for patients in the general hospital setting?' This book aims to help you with these and other similar questions.

In this book, essential information is presented in a concise and ordered fashion. We have focused upon areas of psychiatry that the medical student needs to know in order to qualify as a doctor, and the kind of psychiatric problems that are most common in a general hospital and primary care setting. Thus, there are two chapters devoted to psychiatric problems in the general hospital and, where relevant, many chapters have specific sections on psychiatric problems in primary care. In comparison with other psychiatric undergraduate textbooks, we have chosen not to have specific chapters on Forensic Psychiatry or Learning Disabilities, as newly qualified doctors are unlikely to require detailed knowledge of these areas, although we have included some basic information in other relevant chapters in the book. This book should provide you with sufficient information to pass finals and be of use to you in your early years as a doctor, if you do not specialise in psychiatry.

It is impossible to draw boundaries around medical knowledge and learning as this is a continuous process which should continue throughout your medical career. With this in mind, we have included web addresses of useful websites in as many topic areas as possible, that you may wish to search for more detailed information.

The aims of this introductory chapter are:

- to help plan your learning
- to show you how to use this book to increase your understanding as well as knowledge
- to help you determine the relevant skills you will need to acquire
- to realise how self-assessment can make learning easier and more enjoyable.

Layout and contents

The main part of the text describes topics considered to be of 'core' importance to the major subject areas. Within each chapter, essential information is presented in a set order with clear learning objectives and details of what you need to know. Where relevant, key facts about psychiatry in the primary care setting are presented. It is recognised that at the level of an undergraduate or newly qualified doctor a detailed understanding is not required; instead the ability to set out principles is all that is expected.

In the final section of each chapter, there are opportunities for you to check your knowledge and understanding. This self-assessment is in the form of multiple choice questions, patient management problems and, where relevant, objective structured clinical examination (OSCE) stations. All of these are centred around common clinical problems which are important in judging your performance as a doctor. It is impossible to learn clinical skills from a book; these can only be acquired in a clinical setting or clinical skills laboratory. We have, however, provided basic guidance about important psychiatric skills, and the OSCE stations should help guide you as to the kinds of psychiatric skills that may be tested in a final examination.

Using this book

If you are using this book as part of your exam preparations, we suggest that your first task should be to map out on a sheet of paper three lists dividing the major subjects (corresponding to the chapter headings) into your strong, reasonable and weak areas. This will give you a rough outline of your revision schedule, which you must then fit in with the time available. Do not read passively. It is important to use the self-assessment questions to check your current level of knowledge and skills that you will need to work on in a clinical setting.

It is a good idea to discuss topics and problems with colleagues and friends; the areas which you understand least well will soon become apparent when you try to explain them to someone else. Many medical schools in the UK have adopted a format of problem-based learning (PBL). If you are a member of a PBL group, it is often helpful to choose a topic or area that you are least familiar with to present to the group, rather than an area you know well. You are unlikely to learn anything new if you do the latter.

Developing your skills in a clinical setting

Some students are wary of psychiatry and fearful of psychiatric patients, mistakenly thinking that psychiatric patients are dangerous. The media re-inforce this stereotype, and even within the medical profession, psychiatry and psychiatrists can be stigmatised. As the doctors of tomorrow, you are in a key position to change peoples' attitudes towards mental illness, and to foster a more informed and humane approach. One of the most important things to learn from this book is that most patients with mental health problems are not treated by psychiatrists and are never admitted to in-patient psychiatric wards. Most patients are treated either by general practitioners in the community or by physicians in the general hospital setting. Depression and anxiety are the most common kinds of psychiatric problems and, as a junior doctor, you should be familiar with detecting and treating these conditions, when they occur in patients in the general hospital or community setting.

There are many skills in psychiatry, such as carrying out a mental state examination or the assessment of a patient's cognitive state, which you can practise with patients, who are not under the care of psychiatrists, but who are being treated by their general practitioners or hospital physicians.

When you are actually attached to a psychiatric firm, it is important to see and practise interviewing as many patients as possible. It is very good experience to do psychiatry 'on-call' as you will see how patients, who are very highly aroused or acutely psychotic, can be treated and managed by skilled staff in a sympathetic and competent manner. If you shadow the psychiatry SHO on-call, you will be given ample opportunities to take histories from patients who present to the emergency department with mental health problems.

Approaching the examinations

The discipline of learning is closely linked to preparation for examinations. Many of us opt for a process of superficial learning that is directed towards retention of facts and recall under exam conditions because full understanding is often not required. It is much better if you try to acquire a deeper knowledge and understanding, combining the necessity of passing examinations with longer term needs.

First, you need to know how you will be examined. What form does the clinical examination take? Will you be examined on a long case, or OSCE-style 5–10 minute stations? If you are sitting a written examination, what are the length and types of questions? How many must you answer and how much choice will you have?

Now you have to choose what sources you are going to use for your learning and revision. Textbooks come in different forms. At one extreme, there is the large reference book. This type should be avoided at this stage of revision and only used for reference, when answers to questions cannot be found in smaller books. At the other end of the spectrum is the condensed 'lecture note' format, which often relies heavily on lists. Facts of this nature on their own are difficult to remember if they are not supported by understanding. In the middle of the range are the medium-sized textbooks. These are often of the most use whether you are approaching final university examinations or the first part of the professional examinations. The best advice is to choose one of several medium-sized books on offer on the basis of which you find the most readable. The best approach is to combine your own notes, textbooks and past examination papers as a framework for your preparation.

Armed with information about the format of the exams, a rough syllabus, your own lecture notes and some books that you feel comfortable in using, your next step is to map out the time available for preparation. Include time to practise your clinical skills, either in a clinical situation, or the skills laboratory at your hospital. Do not leave this until the last minute, as you may find it difficult to access patients or skills labs as the examination draws near. Allow time for breaks and work steadily, not cramming. If you do attempt to cram, you have to realise that only a certain amount of information can be retained in your short-term memory, so as you cram up on one subject, another that you have previously learnt, will be lost. Cramming simply retains facts. If the examination requires understanding then you will be in trouble.

It is often a good idea to begin by outlining the topics to be covered and then attempting to summarise your knowledge about each in note form. In this way your existing knowledge will be activated and any gaps will become apparent. Self-assessment also helps determine the time to be allocated to each subject or examination.

The main types of examination

Multiple choice questions

Unless very sophisticated, multiple choice questions test your recall of information. The aim is to gain the maximum marks from the knowledge that you can remember. The stem statement must be read with great care highlighting the 'little' words such as *only*, *rarely*, *usually*, *never* and *always*. Overlooking negatives, such as *not*, *unusual* and *unsuccessful* often causes marks to be lost. *May occur* has an entirely different connotation to *characteristic*. The latter may mean a feature which should be there and the absence of which would make you question the correctness of the diagnosis.

Remember to check the marking method before starting. Most multiple choice papers employ a negative system in which marks are lost for incorrect answers. The temptation is to adopt a cautious approach, answering a relatively small number of questions. However, this can lead to problems, as we all make simple mistakes or even disagree vehemently with the answer in the computer. Caution may lead you to answer too few questions to obtain a pass after the marks have been deducted for incorrect answers.

Short notes

Short notes are not negatively marked. Predetermined marks are given for each important key fact. Nothing is gained for style or for superfluous information. The aim is to set out your knowledge in an ordered concise manner. Do not devote too much time to a single question thereby neglecting the rest, and remember to limit your answer to the question that has been set.

Essays

Similar comments apply to essays. The examiner will have a list of key facts for which he/she can award marks. A small proportion of marks can also be awarded for the style of the essay. It is important, therefore, to stick to the topic in the question and to develop a logical argument or theme. All questions should be given equal weight. A brilliant answer in one essay will not compensate for not attempting another because time runs out.

Objective structured clinical examinations

Although clinical examinations are not the main focus of this book, many examples of objective structured clinical examination (OSCE) stations have been included. By using a predetermined structured marking regime, OSCE stations help to standardise clinical examinations. Most medical schools run OSCEs which have a mixed format. Psychiatry stations may be included with other specialties, which means the candidate has to have command of a wide range of skills, and be able to switch between different subjects very easily. This mimics clinical practice, particularly in a primary care situation, but it can be quite stressful for candidates. Most OSCEs consist of a large number of stations. The higher the number of individual stations, the higher the reliability of the examination, as variance is minimised. It is very important, therefore, to perform well on as many stations as possible. A bad performance on one or two stations is unlikely to impact on your overall performance, but

candidates can sometimes become discouraged or demoralised if they feel they have done badly on a particular station. It is very important to focus only on the station you are doing, and to forget about the other stations.

OSCE stations should test clinical skills rather than knowledge. In psychiatry, the key skills for an undergraduate to learn are; to take a history (psychiatric history, alcohol history, sexual history etc); perform a mental state examination; perform a cognitive state examination; assess suicidal risk; prescribe antidepressants; explain a particular psychiatric condition to a patient; and be able to diagnose common psychiatric conditions.

The best (and only) preparation for an OSCE is to practise clinical skills. Do not think, because you have done something once or twice, that you have mastered the skill. Even with very basic skills, such as taking blood, it is very easy to differentiate students who know what to do, but have only carried out the procedure once or twice, from students who have done it many, many times. The same is true in psychiatry, and a lack of clinical experience is easily exposed in an OSCE.

Vivas

The viva examination can be a nerve-wracking experience. You are normally faced with two examiners. Your main aim during the viva should be to control the examiners' questioning so they constantly ask you about things you know. Despite what is often said, you can prepare for this kind of examination. Questions are liable to take one of a small number of forms centered around subjects that cannot be examined in a traditional clinical examination.

During a viva there are certain techniques which help in making a favourable impression. When discussing patient management, it is better to say 'I would do this' rather than 'I have read this'. Try to strike a balance between saying too little and too much. Try not to go off the topic. Aim to keep your answers short and to the point. It is worthwhile pausing for a few seconds to collect your thoughts before launching into an answer. Do not be afraid to say 'I don't know'; most examiners will want to change tack to see what you do know about.

Conclusions

You should amend the framework for using this book according to your own needs and the examinations you are facing. Whatever approach you adopt your aim should be for an understanding of the principles involved rather than rote learning of a large number of poorly connected facts.

At undergraduate level, most universities pass the vast majority of medical students. The final examinations are to test whether students are fit and safe to practise and enter the pre-registration year. Examiners are looking for evidence of basic competence, a basic knowledge of common medical conditions and an appropriate professional attitude. Good luck.

1 Signs and symptoms of mental illness

Overview

This first chapter is concerned with the major signs and symptoms of mental illness. As with other branches of medicine, a symptom is a problem of which a patient complains, whereas a sign is an abnormality that is detected by observation and examination. The two can be similar: a patient can complain of breathlessness and appear breathless. Equally, a patient can complain of hearing voices (symptom) and appear to be responding to voices by shouting at the television (sign).

The most common signs and symptoms of mental illness are discussed below. They are usually categorized according to whether they involve abnormalities of behaviour, mood, speech or thoughts, perceptions and cognitive processes. Neurological signs are sometimes a feature of certain mental illnesses and are included in this chapter, where relevant.

Learning objectives

You should:

- be able to recognize and describe abnormal behaviour and abnormal mood states associated with mental illness

- be aware of the importance of social and familial norms, when determining abnormality

- appreciate the significance of different types of mood state in relation to different forms of mental illness.

1.1 Abnormalities of behaviour and mood

Behaviour

Most psychiatric conditions involve some pervasive change in the person's normal behaviour. Different societies tolerate different kinds of behaviour, and when assessing social behaviour, it is most important to establish whether the subject's behaviour is out of keeping with his/her normal behaviour and/or out of keeping with his/her social/cultural background.

Rate of behaviour
Behaviour can be slowed down in depressive illnesses (*retardation*) or speeded up in hypomania.

Distractibility
A subject may be unable to concentrate and constantly be fidgeting or moving around the room.

Social inappropriateness
A subject may break normal social conventions (e.g. stand on a table, invade personal space).

Dress
A subject may dress in a bizarre or unusual manner (e.g. may have stripped naked or have covered himself/herself in plastic bin bags).

Sexual appropriateness
A subject may masturbate in public or behave in a sexually provocative manner.

Response to internal experiences
A subject may talk to the television or the fire hydrant because he/she is responding to delusional or hallucinatory experiences.

Spontaneous movements
A coarse *tremor* is common in anxiety. *Choreiform* movements are characterized by abrupt jerking movements, which sometimes also have a writhing quality. In Huntington's disease, the face, upper trunk and arms are most affected by coarse jerky movements. Snorting and

sniffing are often also present. A *tic* is a rapid, involuntary, recurrent, non-rhythmic motor movement (or vocalization) that is usually reminiscent of an expressive movement such as blinking, shoulder-shrugging or neck-jerking. Vocal tics include throat-clearing, barking, sniffing and hissing. Tics can be simple or complex. A *stereotypy* is a repetitive non-goal-directed action that is carried out in a uniform way. A *mannerism* is a repetitive non-goal-directed motor action such as an unusual hand movement when shaking hands or some other form of unusual greeting. *Echopraxia* is the copying of a movement performed by someone else. *Grasp reflex* is the involuntary grasping of a person's fingers or object when placed in the palm of the subject's hand. It is present in the newborn infant but is a sign of organic brain disturbance in the adult.

Unusual postures

Subjects with schizophrenia sometimes assume bizarre and unusual postures, which they maintain for hours or days at a time (*catatonia*). Patients can lie with their head a few inches off a pillow or assume the position of crucifixion. In some patients, there is a feeling of plastic resistance as their body is moved, and they can be placed in peculiar postures, which they then maintain. This is called *waxy flexibility*. Such states are relatively rare these days, owing to the development of more powerful, and effective pharmacological treatments.

Obsessional rituals

Obsessional rituals are repetitive, purposeful behaviours that subjects carry out in relation to obsessional thoughts, impulses or ruminations (see below). The behaviours are carried out to reduce anxiety, which is caused by obsessional concerns. The rituals often consist of checking, cleaning, counting or dressing behaviours.

Mood

Altered emotional states are common in psychiatric disorder. It is normal and appropriate for most people to experience a range of emotions in relation to life events, including happiness, sadness, irritability, fear, anger and anxiety. The question of abnormality of mood or affect arises when the mood state seems either extreme or prolonged.

Depression

Depression is a lowering of mood, characterized by extreme feelings of sadness, emptiness, emotional pain and isolation. The mood state is usually persistent and pervasive. It is accompanied by associated changes in behaviour and thoughts. The individual may withdraw socially, becomes disinterested in normal activity and feels pessimistic about the future. He/she views himself/herself and others in a negative way, and in extreme states delusional beliefs may develop (see below).

Elation

Elation is an abnormal elevation of mood, characterized by feelings of great energy, happiness, excitement and power. It occurs in hypomania and drug-induced states. The subject often feels irritable and frustrated as he/she is surrounded by others who do not share his/her enthusiasm or vivacity. It is also accompanied by changes in behaviour and thoughts. The individual is very distractible, moving from one idea to another. His/her thought processes are speeded up, resulting in pressure of speech and flight of ideas (see below). Grandiose delusions can also develop (see below).

Anxiety

Anxiety is a subjective sense of internal tension, which is often associated with intrusive thoughts or worries (see below). It is accompanied by autonomic arousal, such as tachycardia, sweating, dry mouth, pale skin, etc. A *phobia* is a specific state of anxiety associated with the fear of a particular object (e.g. spider or travelling on buses).

Incongruity of mood

Sometimes a subject's mood is inappropriate to the social circumstances. This occurs in most normal people on occasions (for example one may be overcome with uncontrollable giggles at a funeral, despite frantic attempts to control oneself). In psychiatric conditions, however, there is no awareness of the inappropriateness of the mood, or any attempt to control it.

Labile affect

Lability of affect is an exaggerated emotional responsiveness most often seen in organic states. Subjects will find themselves bursting into tears when talking about relatively trivial events. They do not feel sad but cannot control their emotional responses. It is often an indication of organic brain damage.

Flattening of affect

Flattening of affect is not the same as depression, which is a lowering of affect. Flattening of affect is a blunting of emotional responsiveness so that individuals cannot experience normal variations in mood. They appear rather fatuous or unconcerned. Blunting of affect occurs in chronic schizophrenia and certain organic states, particularly frontal lobe problems.

1.2 Abnormalities of thought and speech

Learning objectives

You should:

- be able to recognize and identify major abnormalities in speech and thought associated with mental illness
- be able to identify thought processes characterized by flight of ideas and loosening of associations
- know which abnormalities of thought are associated with schizophrenia
- understand the difference between obsessional ideas and delusions.

Disorders of speech and thought can be classified according to problems with the stream, form and type of belief or speech content. Often disorders of speech reflect problems that the patient has with thinking. The two, however, are not always synonymous, and disorders of speech and thought are usually assessed separately.

Stream

Speech or thought can be speeded up in drug-induced states or mania, and slowed down in depression. In severe depression, speech can become retarded or completely stop. *Circumstantiality* is characterized by the inclusion of trivial and unnecessary details in speech, which create confusion or boredom in the listener. The speech, however, is goal directed (i.e. the person eventually gets to the point) and normal in its grammatical form.

Form

The order of thought can be disrupted in a variety of ways. *Perseveration* is the repetition of the same sequence of thought, shown by either the repetition of words or phrases, or the repetition of some specific behaviour. If the subject is asked a question, the last few words of the question may be repeated over and over again. Perseveration is common in organic states, particularly generalized brain disorders. *Verbal stereotypies* are repetitive words or phrases, often shouted by the subject, which have no specific relevance to the current situation. *Flight of ideas* is a disorder of the form of thought that often coincides with an increase in the speed of thoughts (pressure of speech) and is most common in mania (Box 1). Ideas follow each other rapidly and the

---

Box 1
Example of flight of ideas

I love you my darling, you are beautiful, you are the one, you are the one, the red light is on, so I'll carry on! . . . . I love you . . . . you are beautiful . . . you are the sun . . . . let's have fun . . . funtastic . . . . plastic . . . . drastic. . . . fun in the sun . . . . umh . . . . yum yum . . . . hee hee . . . . I love you . . . . . .

---

subject shifts from one topic to another. Changes of thought can be triggered by rhyme (*clang association*) or assonance or alliteration. Equally new thoughts can be triggered by external experiences as the subject's attention drifts from one topic to another, but usually there is some connection between them. It is very difficult to interrupt the subject or to interject into the conversation, which is usually completely one-sided.

Loosening of associations is characterized by a problem with the logical order of thought. The continuity of the subject's speech is disrupted and incoherent. No logic in the order of speech can be discerned, unlike in flight of ideas. This kind of speech pattern occurs most often in schizophrenia. In a mild form, it is very difficult to detect reliably, but the interviewer is left with a profound sense of confusion and unease. What the subject says does not quite make sense, but specific abnormalities are difficult to identify. In a more severe form, the patient's conversation is unconnected and impossible to follow (Box 2). It may be filled with *neologisms* (made-up words) or peculiar phrases.

Type of belief

There are three main particular types of abnormal belief that occur in psychiatric disorders. They are worry, obsessional thoughts and delusions.

Worry

Worry is a normal human experience and is a predominantly verbal, conceptual activity aimed at problem solving. It is concerned with future events where there is uncertainty of outcome and usually occurs as a chain of thoughts that have a negative affective content. Worries tend to be realistic, are hard to dismiss, are distracting and are associated with a compulsion to act upon them. Normal worry may, therefore, provide an important func-

---

Box 2
Example of loosening of associations

Interviewer What have you been doing today?
Patient It's a botty stop . . . . . I'm going to stick up my botty with a total botty fart form of man fart.

tion in motivating people to solve dilemmas or problems. Excessive worry or problematic worrying, however, becomes disabling and counter-productive. Problematic worries, in comparison with normal worries, are more intense and uncontrollable. They are more likely to concern ideas about illness, health or injury, and such concerns result in distress and dysfunction.

Obsessional thoughts

Obsessional thoughts have been described as intrusive thoughts that the subject actively resists but cannot get rid of, although he/she realizes they are senseless, stupid or unnecessarily unpleasant. Most ordinary people have experienced some form of obsessional phenomena, the most common form being an unwanted tune that one tries to forget but keeps coming into one's mind over and over again. *Obsessional ruminations* are complex sequences of thoughts or ideas with the same qualities (Box 3). Unlike worries, the subject recognizes that the thoughts or concerns are unrealistic and actively tries to push them from his/her mind. The content is usually distressing, and common concerns include thoughts about disease or contamination, sex, religion and aggression.

Delusions

A delusion is a false belief that the subject holds with total conviction and that is out of keeping with his/her social, educational and cultural background. Delusions used to be regarded as being unshakeable and unamenable to rational argument. New psychological treatments have recently been developed which suggest that delusional beliefs, in certain patients, can be modified by intense, structured psychological techniques. However, for the purposes of diagnosis, delusions are generally resistant to most attempts to challenge them. Delusions are usually false and of a rather fantastic nature. They do not, however, have to be false, rather the reasoning behind the development of the belief has to

be false. As an example, a man believed his wife was having several affairs with other men, because he could hear the men hiding in the roof space of the house. He believed the men must be midgets, as the roof space was very small. This man's wife was not being unfaithful to him, but even if she had been, the beliefs he held would still be delusional because their basis was without rational foundation. They developed from auditory hallucinations, which were secondary to the man's alcoholism. Delusions can comprise single beliefs or complex belief systems in which many people and organizations are involved.

Primary delusions Primary delusions occur independent of any other psychiatric phenomena, when the subject develops a sudden new (often bizarre) meaning. There are two kinds of primary delusional experience: *delusional perception* and an *autochthonous delusion*. A delusional perception is a misinterpretation of a normal perceptual experience that suddenly develops special significance for the subject. For example, a subject may see a red sailing boat on the water and suddenly realize that this means that his wife is the devil's child and is going to kill him. An autochthonous delusion is one that arises 'out of the blue' without any cue or specific trigger. Primary delusions occur most commonly in schizophrenia. Sometimes they will be preceded by a change in the subject's mood, which is not consistent with an affective disorder. The subject may feel strange and perplexed and have a sense of dread or foreboding that something awful is about to happen. Out of this strange feeling, which is termed a *delusional mood*, the delusion then emerges. For example, a woman began to feel very uneasy and strange. She began to feel that the air was different and alive with electricity. When she went outside, everything seemed strange. She began to feel very frightened. She then realized that her neighbour had been killed and eaten by reptiles, and had been replaced by them. They were building a machine to kill everyone on the estate where she lived. They were going to take her over and make her work for them as a slave.

Secondary delusions Secondary delusions occur as a consequence of some other psychiatric phenomena, usually an abnormal mood (either severe depressive disorder or hypomania) or hallucinations. Secondary delusions that arise from the subject's abnormal mood state are usually *mood congruent* (i.e. in keeping with the mood state). Patients with very severe depressive disorders can develop *delusions of guilt* or worthlessness, poverty, disease (*hypochondriacal delusions*) or nihilism (extreme beliefs re the destruction of the world or the imminent death of the subject). They do not develop delusions about being the richest person in the world, the most sexually attractive person in the world or being able to fly. Those kinds of belief, which are called grandiose delusions, occur secondary

---

> **Box 3**
> Example of obsessional ruminations and rituals
>
> A 37-year-old woman developed the idea that she had been irradiated following the Chernobyl disaster. She recognized that the risk was in reality very small, but she could not stop thinking about it. She worried about going out as she thought the levels of irradiation would be higher outside. She also began to think that she would receive more radiation when she walked under door frames. To protect herself from this, every time she walked through a doorway, she tapped her head three times and turned round. She realized this was silly but could not stop herself from doing it and became extremely anxious if she did not do it.

to an elevated mood state. *Delusions of reference* are most common in schizophrenia and are beliefs that people, authority figures or organizations have special significance for the subject. The subject may believe that the television is referring to her or that the prime minister or the Queen is referring to her. They often arise secondary to auditory hallucinations. *Persecutory delusions* also occur commonly in schizophrenia and involve ideas that the subject is in danger from others who are trying to follow or harm him/her.

Delusions concerning the control of thoughts. Certain patients develop specific abnormal ideas about the control of their thoughts. They may believe that thoughts are being placed in their mind which are not their own (*thought insertion*), or that thoughts are being taken out of their mind (*thought withdrawal*). They can also believe that their thoughts are not private and that others know what they are thinking (*thought broadcasting*). Usually, the subject tries to make sense of these experiences by elaborating some causal explanation, often involving telepathy, a machine that controls their mind, or satellite broadcasting. These beliefs are most common in schizophrenia.

Delusions concerning the control of the body. These ideas are sometimes called *passivity experiences* as the subject can feel like a passive creature being manipulated by some outside force or power. The subject feels controlled by an external agency, which makes him/her have certain thoughts or impulses or perform certain actions. For example, a man believed that he had been kidnapped, while in Ireland, by students (persecutory delusion) who had cut out his heart and replaced it with a transmitter. He now felt he was being controlled by the National Computing Centre, which was sending signals to the machine in his chest, making him walk with his left arm behind his head (passivity experience). These beliefs are characteristic of schizophrenia. Table 1 summarizes the key questions that should be addressed in relation to the assessment of a patient's delusional experience. Overvalued ideas are abnormal beliefs which are not held with the conviction of a delusion. Ideas of reference are a common example, where the person has the impression that the television is referring to him, but is not wholly convinced.

1.3 Abnormalities of perception

Learning objectives

You should:

- be able to recognize and identify abnormalities of perception associated with mental illness

- be able to differentiate an illusion from a hallucination.

Table 1 Key aspects of delusional experience that should be assessed

Dimensions of delusional experience	Methods of assessment
Primacy of the belief	1. How did the belief arise? 2. Is the belief secondary to or consistent with the subject's mood? 3. Is the subject experiencing any other abnormal phenomena. If so, could the belief be secondary to these phenomena?
Conviction of the belief	1. How strongly does the patient believe the delusion? 2. Has the patient acted on his/her beliefs (i.e. if he believes he is going to be boiled alive by his neighbours, has he tried to run away)? 3. How does the patient explain why his/her family or close others do not share his/her belief? 4. How convinced does the patient remain of his belief even when presented with evidence to the contrary?
Organization of the belief	1. How detailed is the belief? 2. How many false beliefs does the patient have? 3. Are they connected?
Bizarreness of the belief	1. How implausible is the belief? 2. How understandable is the belief? 3. Does it derive from ordinary live experience?
Extension	1. How many people does the belief involve? 2. Did the belief start in relation to one organization or person and then develop on to involve others?
Special characteristics	1. Does the belief involve ideas about control of thoughts? 2. Does the belief involve ideas about the control of the body?
Dangerousness of the belief	1. How dangerous is the belief? 2. Is the patient at risk of harm to himself/herself or others on account of the belief?

Altered perception can occur in any of the sensory modalities. There are a wide range of different experiences that have been described. Table 1.2 lists the most common signs and symptoms associated with different psychiatric disorders.

Changes in intensity

Colours can seem brighter than usual in drug-induced states. Ordinary noises can take on the quality of piercing and shattering sounds in anxiety disorders or post-traumatic states. Perceptions can have a diminution of intensity; for example, pain or sensation can be reduced in hysteria or neurological disorders.

Changes in quality

A normal wind can be experienced as a storm in delirium or prior to an epileptic fit. Visual images can become imbued with rich combinations of unnatural colour in drug-induced states (e.g. mescalin).

Abnormal characteristics

Sometimes objects can appear normal in intensity or quality but perception can be imbued with an emotional quality that alters perceptual experience. In *derealization*, individuals feel cut off and alienated from the perceptual world. Objects appear distant or strange. In *depersonalization*, the individual himself/herself feels odd or unusual, detached and distant from the world. Both states can occur in many different psychiatric conditions, including drug-induced states, anxiety disorders, temporal lobe epilepsy and schizophrenia.

Illusions

Illusions are transpositions or distortions of real perceptions. They arise, therefore, from real experience. A patient who talks to his drip stand as if it is a policeman is having an illusory experience. Illusions can occur in most psychiatric conditions and are also commonly experienced by ordinary people at some time in their lives. Illusions are more likely to occur if sensation is impaired in some way (e.g. visibility is reduced because it is dark), the conscious level is reduced (e.g. delirium), one is inattentive or there is a heightened sense of emotional arousal. *Pareidolia* is the term used to describe a particular kind of illusory experience characterized by seeing a multitude of vivid faces, creatures or other forms. These usually arise from a background source that has irregular outlines or markings, such as the sky, a fire or a wall.

Hallucinations

Hallucinations are false perceptions that are not distortions of real perceptions but arise de novo and occur simultaneously with and alongside real perceptions, in external space. Hallucinations can occur in any modality but the most common are auditory and visual hallucinations. Hallucinations have the quality of a real perception and hence subjects react to them as if they are real. It is very unusual, however, to experience hallucinations in different modalities, related to the same experience, at the same time. An individual may hear a dog barking or see a dog sitting in front of him/her. It is very unusual for an individual to see the dog and hear it barking at the same time.

Auditory hallucinations
Auditory hallucinations can consist of strange noises, tunes, whistling, gun shots, sounds of machines, animal noises and human voices. All are perceived and experienced as real. Voices can be experienced as either talking to the person (second person; Box 4) or talking about him/her (third person; Box 5). Individuals can also hear their own thoughts spoken aloud (*echo de la pensée*; thought sonorization) or a running commentary on their actions. Third person auditory hallucinations, hearing one's own thoughts aloud or a running commentary occur particularly in schizophrenia.

Visual hallucinations
Visual hallucinations can be simple, such as a flash of light, or complex, such as an image of an animal or person. They can occur in many different kinds of mental disorder but are particularly associated with organic states and drug-induced conditions.

Tactile hallucinations
Tactile hallucinations are relatively uncommon. Individuals can experience light sensations, or prickles

---

Box 4
Example of second person auditory hallucinations

'Lie down now', 'sit down you stupid bastard' 'you're disgusting' 'you should be shot' 'you're an animal and you should be shot like an animal'

Box 5
Example of third person auditory hallucinations

'do you know him?' 'he's really crazy, he sleeps with dogs' 'yes, I can smell him . . . you can smell he's been with dogs, he even looks like a dog' 'he can't hide . . . he's trying to hide . . . ' 'he can't escape what he's done . . . we all know what he's done . . . ' 'he's crazy' 'he's a mad dog . . . mad dog . . . filthy mad dog'

Table 2 Major signs and symptoms associated with different forms of mental illness

	Schizophrenia	Severe depressive disorders	Hypomania and mania	Delirium
Behaviour	Bizarre behaviour May avoid eye contact or make intense eye contact Responses to hallucinations Poor self care Parkinsonism (drug side-effects)	Retarded Socially withdrawn Avoidance of eye contact Decreased facial expressions	Distractible, socially disinhibited Abnormal liveliness of movement, singing Inappropriate sexual behaviour	Agitation Distractible Confused Fluctuating level of consciousness Drowsy
Affect	Incongruous; can also be fearful, elated or low	Low	Elation, irritability	Fearful
Speech and thoughts	Loosening of associations Persecutory delusions Ideas of reference Delusions of thought control Delusions of body control Poverty of thought	Slow speech Suicidal ideation Hopelessness Delusions of poverty, hypochondriacal delusions, nihilistic delusions	Pressure Flight of ideas Grandiose delusions	Slurred or rambling incoherent speech Persecutory delusions
Perception	Second person auditory hallucinations Third person auditory hallucinations, running commentary	Second person auditory hallucinations	Second person auditory hallucinations	Second person auditory hallucinations Visual hallucinations Illusions

on their skin, electrical or sexual sensations. In certain organic states, individuals can have a very unpleasant experience of insects or small creatures crawling under the skin: so-called *formication*.

Hallucinations of taste and smell
Hallucinations of either smell or taste are also uncommon in psychiatric disorders, although strange smells are often experienced in the prodromal phase of temporal lobe epilepsy.

Pseudo-hallucinations
Many patients describe unusual or abnormal perceptual experiences that do not have the quality of either an illusory or hallucinatory experience. Images may be seen, or voices heard 'in the mind' as opposed to being experienced in external space. Such phenomena are termed pseudo-hallucinations, and they usually lack the clarity of a true hallucination. They can occur in most psychiatric disorders including anxiety states and personality disorders, as well as in schizophrenia.

Hypnagogic and hypnopompic hallucinations
Hypnagogic and hypnopompic hallucinations are special types of hallucination that occur in relation to sleep. Hypnagogic hallucinations occur when people are falling asleep and hypnopompic when people are waking from sleep. They are different from dream states in that the individual does not feel a sense of participation as he/she does in a dream. The most common form is auditory.

Autoscopic hallucinations
Autoscopic hallucinations are an unusual and distressing experience where the individual sees himself or herself, i.e. sees his/her double. This can occur in normal subjects if they are very tired or in an emotionally charged state; however, it is most commonly associated with organic states, particularly disorders of the parietal lobe. *Negative autoscopy* is the experience of looking in the mirror and not being able to see one's image.

1.4 Cognitive deficits

Learning objectives

You should:

- understand the normal processes involved in memory
- understand the nature of basic cognitive processes and the regions they relate to in the brain
- be able to assess immediate short- and long-term memory
- be able to assess orientation
- be able to recognize dyspraxias and dysphasias

The process of laying down normal memory can be divided into three components. First, an event has to be noted (*registration*); second, it is held in short-term (*working*) memory; third, it is stored in long-term memory. *Encoding* is the process by which information is transformed into a stored, mental representation. *Retrieval* is the process of bringing the stored memory back into consciousness.

Recent theories suggest that, for long-term storage, memory is encoded as a combination of descriptions which vary in the level of detail they contain. If something interesting or distinctive happens, an event will be tagged with a specific descriptor. The ease with which events are remembered depends partly upon how many distinctive cues were encoded when the episode occurred. Retrieval is characterized as a process in which some information about a target memory is used to construct a description of the memory and this description is used in attempts to recover fragments of information. Experiences are retrieved by accessing the knowledge structure used to encode the event.

Memory retrieval is also affected by mood. Depressed patients find it more difficult to recall positive memories in relation to cues than non-depressed subjects.

Short-term memory
Short-term or working memory is memory over seconds and minutes. It has a limited capacity which is surprisingly constant. Healthy people can retain about 7 items in short-term memory. These items will drop out of short-term memory unless *rehearsal* takes place. Key areas of the brain involved in short-term memory are the frontal cortex and the medial temporal cortex including hippocampus. Lesions to these areas frequently result in memory deficits. Verbal short-term memory, such as memory for words and phrases, is performed in the left hemisphere. Non-verbal memory, such as memory for designs, is performed in the right hemisphere.

Long-term memory
One of the most important aspects of memory is *autobiographical* or *episodic memory*. This consists of remembered events that are of personal significance. These events are the building blocks from which an individual's identity is constructed. Autobiographical memory has an important role in the creation and maintenance of a self-history and self-concept. People's memories of their own personal history are organized in terms of lifetime periods (e.g. schooldays, time at college), so-called extended-event time lines. Certain groups of patients

with psychiatric disorder (e.g. those with depressive disorders) have difficulty in retrieving specific autobiographical memories. It has been suggested that this *over-general memory recall* may impede people's ability to think of constructive solutions to problems that they face. Semantic memory relates to long-term memory for words, grammar and ideas and is located in the frontal cortex. Procedural memory relates to the performance of learned skills.

Amnesia

Amnesia is the name given to memory deficits. *Antrograde amnesia* is the name given to on-going deficits of new learning. This occurs after head injury, in dementias and delirium, and in Korsakoff's syndrome. Long-term memory is intact, but the ability to encode information from short-term into long-term memory is disrupted, resulting in a continuing memory deficit from the time of the initial problem. *Retrograde amnesia* is a disruption of long-term memory which is seen in more severe head injuries and dementias. The duration of antrograde and retrograde amnesia is a good indicator of the severity of head injury.

Dysphasia

Dysphasia is the disruption of speech by an organic lesion and can be found after head injury or stroke or in advanced dementia. In *expressive dysphasia* (also called non-fluent dysphasia) the patient is unable to produce many words or none at all. It is usually due to lesion in broca's area in the left frontotemporal cortex. *Receptive dysphasia* (also called fluent dysphasia) involves the person being able to talk at normal rate but with words used wrongly and in a jumbled order. It is caused by a lesion in Wernicke's area in the left temporal lobe.

Dyspraxia

Visuospatial skills, such as the ability to draw or copy figures and locate objects including parts of the body in space, are largely right parietal lobe functions. Lesions in this area including in dementia will lead to dyspraxias where the person is unable to draw or copy accurately. Linked to this is the inability to find one's way about an environment, a common feature of dementia. *Right left disorientation* may also be linked.

Orientation

Disorientation for time, where the patient cannot state the day or date, is often seen early in organic states including dementia and delirium. Disorientation for place, such that the person is unaware of where he/she is, is seen in more severe organic states. Disorientation for person, such that the patient is unaware who he/she is, is rare and is seen only in advanced dementia.

Frontal lobe deficits

The frontal cortex occupies 40% of the cerebral cortex. It houses the most advanced cognitive functions, those to do with abstract thinking, reasoning, social behaviour and planning. Frontal lobe deficits are often subtle and lead to changes in personality, ability to problem solve or think in a common sense fashion.

Attention and concentration

Many different labels have been used to describe different aspects of attention. *Selective attention* refers to the ability to focus on a critical target stimuli while ignoring other extraneous stimuli. If an individual's selective attention is impaired, he/she will be *distractible*, shifting attention from one target to another in a disorganized fashion. *Sustained attention* refers to the maintenance of attention over time. Other aspects of attention involve the extent to which attention is self-directed and organized, and the amount of effort that is invested in the process (i.e. the 'intensive' aspect of attention).

In clinical settings, the term *attention* is usually used to describe selective attention (i.e. the ability to focus on a specific task) while *concentration* refers to the ability to maintain attention over time (i.e. sustained attention).

Insight

Insight is difficult to define and measure, but it is the degree to which the patient recognizes that he/she has a mental illness. It involves being able to recognize abnormal mental processes, attribute them to mental illness and understand treatment is required.

Self-assessment: questions

Multiple choice questions

1. Hallucinations
   a. Have a subjective quality of being real
   b. Are located in internal space
   c. Are never tactile
   d. Arise from external objects
   e. Are always a sign of mental illness

2. A delusion is:
   a. A false belief
   b. In keeping with the individual's cultural background
   c. Always untrue
   d. Usually amenable to reason
   e. Never acted upon

3. An obsessional rumination:
   a. Is a complex idea
   b. Is recognized by the sufferer to be silly or out of proportion
   c. Is not actively resisted
   d. Can be followed by the development of rituals
   e. Is usually acted upon

4. The following signs are characteristic of schizophrenia:
   a. Second person auditory hallucinations
   b. Primary delusion
   c. Visual hallucinations
   d. Delusions of thought control
   e. Lability of mood

5. A mannerism:
   a. Is the same as a stereotypy
   b. Is purposeful
   c. Only occurs in mental illness
   d. Is only carried out on one occasion
   e. Only occurs in men

Case history questions

History 1

A 24-year-old woman is brought to the Emergency Department by her brother. He says that she has been behaving strangely for the last 2 days. She has appeared very frightened and agitated. She has been hiding in the house and has been especially frightened of the cooker. She has told her brother that the devil is in the cooker and is going to take her to hell. She has been shouting at the cooker and saying, 'no. . .no. . .leave me alone . . . '. She is frightened of the television and has thrown it out of the window. She has been covering her ears and shouting 'shut up' 'shut up'. He has also heard her scream, 'I won't do it'.

When she is assessed by a psychiatrist, she is clearly very frightened. She is crouched in a corner of the room mumbling to herself. She keeps saying, 'he's coming, he's coming . . . and when he comes . . . I die'.

Her brother says that she is not religious and the family hold no particularly strong religious beliefs.

1. Is this woman's behaviour normal?
2. What abnormal signs of mental illness is she showing?

History 2

A 48-year-old woman with multiple sclerosis is referred to a psychiatrist by her neurologist. She is in the advanced stages of the disease and is confined to a wheel chair. She is looked after by her husband, who is a devoted and kind carer. She has started to believe that her food is being poisoned and as a consequence has stopped eating. She initially thought her neighbours were poisoning her food but now believes it is her husband. She still accepts water from him. She believes her clothes have been stolen by her neighbours, who come into the house at night time. She hears them walking about. She has also seen the neighbour's dog, which she says sits outside her window in the evening. Her neighbours do not have a dog and none of her clothes are missing, according to her husband. She also sees a policeman frequently at night time in the bathroom and is re-assured that he is keeping an eye on her. He always stands behind the door, where her husband says there is usually a dressing gown hanging up. She has been feeling very low over the last 5–6 months, since her mother died. She is unable to enjoy anything and has stopped reading (one of her previous pleasures). She is frequently tearful and is particularly low in the mornings. Her cognitive function has slowly been deteriorating over the last 3 years.

1. Describe the abnormal perceptions that this woman is experiencing
2. Describe the abnormal beliefs
3. Are her beliefs primary or secondary?
4. What are the possible underlying diagnoses?

History 3

> A 24-year-old man, called Jo, is admitted to hospital. The psychiatrist elicits the following experiences.
>
> 1. He hears voices in his mind that tell him he has special powers
> 2. He believes the psychiatrist can read his mind
> 3. He tells the psychiatrist there is a loudspeaker in his room that says things like, 'Jo is sitting on his bed, now he's getting up, he's going to clean his teeth'
> 4. He tells the psychiatrist that he hears other people talking about him. He has heard his mother and his sister discussing him and they both think he is wasting his life and is a lazy bastard
> 5. He believes the staff are hiding his mother and sister on the ward and does not believe them when they tell him that his mother died 5 years ago and his sister lives in Australia.

1. What are the different phenomena described in 1–5 above?

Self-assessment: answers

Multiple choice answers

1. a. **True.** Hallucinations are perceived as being real by the individual who experiences them.
   b. **False.** Hallucinations are located in external space.
   c. **False.** They can be in any modality.
   d. **False.** They arise spontaneously de novo.
   e. **False.** Hallucinations can be experienced by well individuals, although this is relatively rare.

2. a. **True.** A delusion is a false belief.
   b. **False.** It is out of keeping with the individual's cultural background.
   c. **False.** It can be true, but the basis upon which the individual has come to hold the belief will be unreasonable and illogical.
   d. **False.** It is held with conviction.
   e. **False.** Individuals can act upon their delusions.

3. a. **True.** A rumination is a complex or systemized obsessional thought.
   b. **True.** The sufferer recognizes the idea is silly or irrational.
   c. **False.** The sufferer usually resists the thought and tries to put it out of mind.
   d. **True.** Repetitive behaviours may develop to reduce anxiety concerning the obsessional belief.
   e. **False.** Obsessional thoughts are rarely acted upon.

4. a. **False.** Third person auditory hallucinations are characteristic of schizophrenia.
   b. **True.** Primary delusions are suggestive of schizophrenia.
   c. **False.** Visual hallucinations occur in many conditions including schizophrenia but are more characteristic of organic brain disorders.
   d. **True.** Delusions of thought control, including thought insertion, withdrawal and broadcasting are suggestive of schizophrenia.
   e. **False.** Lability of mood is most common in organic mental states.

5. a. **False.** A stereotypy is a repetitive movement that is not purposeful.
   b. **True.** A mannerism is purposeful.
   c. **False.** Adolescents frequently adopt a variety of mannerisms.
   d. **False.** It is repetitive.
   e. **False.** It occurs in both males and females.

Case history answers

History 1

1. Her behaviour is abnormal because it is out of keeping with her own family and social background. Sometimes when individuals present with religious ideas, it is difficult to determine whether or not their ideas are actually abnormal, although they may seem unusual or strange.
2. This lady shows the following signs of mental illness. Her behaviour is abnormal: she is agitated, she has thrown the television out of the window and has been talking to the cooker. Her mood is fearful. She appears to be responding to auditory hallucinations, although it is difficult to determine whether they are second or third person. She has a persecutory delusion involving the devil, whom she believes is trying to take her to hell.

History 2

1. She is experiencing visual hallucinations of a dog, which predominantly occur at night time. She is also experiencing illusions of a policeman, which also occur at night time. She may also be experiencing non-specific auditory hallucinations, as she appears to hear strange noises at night time, which she attributes to her neighbours.
2. She has a persecutory delusion that she is being poisoned by her husband and a delusion that her clothes have been stolen.
3. Her beliefs are secondary to the abnormal perceptual experiences. Her lowered mood may also be an important factor.
4. Visual hallucinations and illusions are suggestive of an organic disorder. The symptoms are worse at night time, which is consistent with a fluctuating level of consciousness. Her cognitive function has been deteriorating for over 3 years because of her multiple sclerosis. She is also suffering from a depressive disorder, which may be exacerbating her symptoms.

History 3

1. Pseudo-hallucinations. The voices are not located in external space, so they are pseudo-hallucinations and have no specific significance.

2. Thought broadcasting. He believes the psychiatrist can read his mind and, therefore, knows what he is thinking.
3. Running commentary. This is a special form of third person auditory hallucinations.
4. Third person auditory hallucinations. His mother and sister are having a conversation about him.
5. Paranoid delusion secondary to his auditory hallucinations. The term paranoid means a delusion that refers to the self.

2 Psychiatric assessment

Overview

This chapter describes the skills of history taking in patients with mental illness. It describes how to perform a Mental State Examination and the Mini Mental State Examination. It provides you with a template for how to make sense of psychiatric histories and describes how to perform a risk assessment. It includes guidance about personal safety, which should be read carefully. It also briefly describes how services for the mentally ill are organized in England and Wales. Finally, it covers important issues about stigma and prejudice in relation to mental illness.

2.1 Core history-taking skills

Learning objectives

You should:

- be familiar with the structure and format of the psychiatric history
- be able to take a psychiatric history.

As with other branches of medicine, the student doctor should begin taking a history by formally introducing himself/herself to the patient, showing some formal identification and seeking permission from the patient to take a history. The student doctor should explain that he/she would like to take notes, and again seek permission from the patient to do this.

Some students are nervous about taking histories from patients with psychiatric problems. A common fear is that the patient may be aggressive or threatening. This, however, is extremely unlikely, as most patients who suffer from mental ill health are not violent. Some patients, however, may be tired or very depressed, and they may be unable to concentrate for long periods of time. The history may have to be taken in instalments over a few days. Patients who are treated in the community or in an inpatient setting may have a fixed programme of daily activities, which should not be interrupted. In such cases, it is best to make an appointment with the patient and negotiate a mutually convenient time to meet.

The main history-taking skills are summarized in Box 6. As with a general medical history, it is important to start with open questions and then move to more closed questions to elicit specific details. *Open questions* are non-specific, for example 'can you tell me how you've been feeling recently?', or 'can you tell me about some of the problems you've been experiencing recently?'. They encourage the patient to describe problems or difficulties in his/her own words. They enable a great deal of information to be obtained by the use of relatively few questions, which can make the interview procedure more efficient and less time consuming. *Closed questions* usually give the patient a fixed choice with two or three alternatives, (e.g. would you say that your mood is about the same as last week, better than last week or

---

Box 6
History-taking skills

1. Formal introduction
2. Explanation of nature and purpose of interview
3. Elicit consent
4. Use of open questions moving to closed for specific details
5. Use of facilitatory statements
6. Pick up cues (either verbal or non-verbal) when appropriate
7. Maintain control of interview using empathic statements and refocusing techniques

worse than last week?). They should be used sparingly, as they are time consuming and, if used a lot, can make the interviewer appear pedantic and unempathic.

If the patient is finding it difficult to describe his/her experiences, it can be helpful to respond by making encouraging noises, or nods, or making understanding statements (e.g. 'that sounds difficult', 'that must have been hard for you'). This is called *facilitation*, and it is an extremely useful technique to learn as it encourages patients to talk in depth about difficulties. It helps the psychiatrist to assess the severity of mood state or abnormal psychological experiences.

Cue-based responses are also helpful in eliciting information about mood. The interviewer can pick up on the patient's non-verbal or verbal cues. Non-verbal cues relate to the patient's body language, which may be indicative of a particular mood state (e.g. anxiety, depression or anger). Verbal cues relate to the language or tone of voice that the patient uses in conversation, which may be suggestive of some underlying mood state. If the interviewer chooses to make a cue-based response, it is best to couch it in a tentative manner, so that the patient can choose either to accept or reject it, without this damaging the overall interviewer –patient relationship (e.g. although you say you're coping, ... when you were talking about your son, just now, I noticed your eyes fill with tears . . . and I'm not sure . . . but I wondered whether you still feel very upset).

As well as being able to elicit information from the patient, and encourage the patient to talk freely, it is also important to be able to control the interview. The purpose of history-taking is to collect specific information in a logical and systematized way to enable the doctor to make a diagnosis and formulate the problem. On some occasions, particularly if the interviewee is very garrulous or circumstantial, the doctor may have to interrupt and be more directive, without appearing rude or insensitive. This is best done in the following manner: acknowledge what the patient has been talking about, explain that this has been helpful, explain that you need to ask about other parts of his/her life and ask the patient's permission to do this. Box 7 gives two examples of how to *re-focus* an interview.

It can also be helpful to summarize information, to check with the patient that the details are correct. For example, 'let me just check if I may, that I've understood you correctly . . . you've been feeling worse this last week, your mood has been low all the time, you've not been sleeping well, waking at 4.00 a.m. most nights, you've lost interest in eating and you've not seen anyone all week'. This kind of summary helps the doctor to check that he/she has understood things correctly, and it is usually perceived by the patient as being very empathic. It can also provide the basis for moving on to

---

Box 7
How to re-focus an interview

Example 1   Moving to a different part of the history

Patient   And it were a good school, we all enjoyed it, we had a great laugh with some of the teachers . . I remember there was one . . . what was her name . . . Ms Glover . . . yes she was a great teacher . . . she used to do impressions of the prime minister . . . and other important people . . .

Interviewer   Yes, it sounds as if you had a really good time at school, and I think I've got a good picture of what it was like. I need to ask you about some other areas of your life. If that's OK. I wonder if we could move on to after you left school, and to talk about some of the jobs you've done.

Patient   Yes . . . well I was a joiner for most of my life . . . . .

Example 2   Moving back to focus on further details of the presenting complaint

Patient   He just doesn't understand, I keep trying to tell him, but he won't listen . . . the other week he went out . . . I didn't know where he was going, what time he would be back, nothing . . . he turns up at 2.00 a.m. in the morning, wouldn't say where he's been, smelling of drink . . . (this is the third example the patient has given of her husband's unreasonable behaviour).

Interviewer   Well, I think I'm getting a picture of some of the difficulties you're facing and the problems between you and your husband. I wonder, however, if we could just go back to talking about how you've actually been feeling . . . as I didn't quite get a picture of how long you've feeling low and just how bad it's been at times. It's quite important for me to be clear about this . . . is this OK?

---

enquire about more sensitive issues, such as, in the above example, the doctor could move on to asking about suicidal ideation.

Towards the end of the interview, the student/doctor should give the patient some indication that the interview is drawing to a close. This can be done by telling the patient that there a few minutes left, and that there are one or two points that you would like to clarify. Time must always be allowed for the patient to voice any queries and for these queries to be answered. It is best to ask, 'before we finish . . . is there anything you would like to ask me?'. If the patient asks a question that you cannot answer, for example about treatment, it is important to tell the patient that you will pass on his/her concerns to the appropriate person (e.g. registrar). It is important that you do pass on these concerns, as patients will sometimes tell medical students or relatively junior doctors about worries that they have not revealed to other members of staff. At the very end of the interview, it is important to thank the patient for his/her time and cooperation.

Format of a psychiatric history

Presenting complaint and history of presenting complaint

The main purpose of the first part of the psychiatric history is to establish the nature of the psychiatric condition. It should start with the presenting complaint and the history of the presenting complaint. It is helpful to focus upon the patient's main symptom before moving on to associated symptoms. If the patient's main symptom is depression, a full history of the depression should be elicited before moving on to enquire about other symptoms associated with depression, such as poor concentration or sleep loss. A useful analogy is to think about taking a history of chest pain. If a patient presents with chest pain, it is usual to establish the nature of the pain, its quality, severity, consistency, duration, radiation, relieving and exacerbating factors. It would be unusual to ask about ankle swelling before one had a clear history of the pain itself. Students, however, often ask one or two questions about depression and then move on to other symptoms without establishing a clear picture of the nature and severity of the mood state itself.

Only after a clear account of the main symptom has been obtained should the interviewer move on to associated symptoms. Basic knowledge about the different psychiatric syndromes is required to be able to check whether specific symptoms that may be expected in a certain condition are present.

After the symptomatology has been established, it is usual to enquire whether there were any changes in the patient's circumstances prior to the onset of the disorder. Some people themselves will identify an important event that may have precipitated their illness; others may have experienced such an event but not made a connection between the event and the later onset of their illness.

Past psychiatric history

It is logical to enquire about previous episodes of illness, after one has discussed the patient's current problems. All contacts with psychiatric services should be recorded including details of the nature of the illness and the kinds of treatment that the patient received. Treatment of psychological illness in primary care should also be recorded.

It is helpful to establish with the patient whether the current illness is similar to previous episodes or whether there are significant differences either in the severity or nature of the condition.

Family history

A history of psychiatric and medical illness in the patient's nearest relatives should be elicited. Any deaths should be recorded and how the patient dealt with those deaths should be described. The degree of contact with surviving relatives should be noted and the quality of patient's relationships with parental figures, when a child, should be described. Relationships with siblings should also be briefly described.

Personal history

The main purpose of taking a detailed personal history is to try to identify factors that may have made the patient vulnerable to developing a psychiatric illness, or may make the illness difficult to treat.

The personal history is divided into the following categories.

Early development. The date of birth and any obstetric complications prior to or during delivery should be noted. Factors indicating any developmental delay should be recorded (e.g. late milestones). Any childhood illnesses, particularly meningitis or encephalitis, or brain or head injuries should be noted. Other illnesses, such as diabetes, which may have resulted in long separations from parents because of admissions to hospital, should be noted.

Home and environment. It is important to gain some of impression of the patient's childhood experiences and the general level of support and love provided within the family. It is particularly important to elicit whether there is any evidence of parental neglect or childhood physical or sexual abuse (see section 2.6).

School. Academic achievement should be noted and the age at leaving school. Relationships with peers and teachers (authority figures) should be briefly described. Was the patient able to make and maintain friendships when he/she was a child? In particular, it is important to know whether there is any history of bullying or being bullied at school, truanting or other aberrant behaviour.

Occupation. The types of job held and duration of employment should be recorded. Reasons for leaving jobs should be elicited. If the patient is currently employed, details of the type of work, stresses, gains from work and relationshisp with colleagues at work should be elicited. If the patient is not working, it is important to establish why.

Sexual relationships and long-term partnerships. Brief details about the experiences of puberty and adolesence should be noted. Sexual orientation should be established. Details of any long-term relationships or marriages should be recorded. It is important to get some idea of the duration of the relationships, their quality and reasons for ending. If the patient is currently in a close relationship, it is helpful to understand the degree of support the patient receives from his/her partner and any difficulties or stresses in the relationship. Any difficulties or problems with sexual performance, either in the current relationship or with previous partners, should be noted.

Children. The age and gender of each of the patient's children should be recorded, and details given of their social circumstances (e.g. they may not live with the patient). Any difficulties (e.g. behavioural problems or physical illness) should be noted. If the patient is female, details of all pregnancies and any miscarriages or abortions should be noted. Any evidence of puerperal illness should be noted.

Social circumstances. Any problems or difficulties with housing should be elicited and any financial pressures.

Forensic history. Details of problems with the police, prison sentences or civil actions should be recorded. It is also important to establish whether the patient has any history of violence and, if so, whether it was related to psychiatric illness.

Premorbid personality. The patient should be asked about his/her usual temperament and ways of managing stress. Is there evidence that the patient is a worrier or is someone who never expresses his/her emotions? Is the patient prone to mood swings or overly sensitive? Certain types of personality predispose to the later development of psychiatric disorder. If a patient is suffering from depression, you should try to establish whether there is evidence of premorbid depressive, anxious or obsessional-compulsive traits. In schizophrenia, you should look for evidence of a premorbid schizoid personality.

Medical history. Any current medical conditions should be noted and previous operations or serious medical conditions recorded.

History of alcohol and illicit substances used. Details of patient's average weekly alcohol consumption should be recorded. If there is evidence of alcohol abuse, then a full alcohol history should be taken. Details of this are given in Chapter 8. Any illicit drug use should be recorded.

History from an informant

It is always important to obtain a corroborating history from one of the patient's close relatives, provided the patient gives consent. Although some patients are good judges of their own character, an accurate picture of the patient's premorbid personality is often obtained from relatives. Other important pieces of information, which the patient may have concealed (e.g. suicidal thoughts), may come to light.

Medication

Known allergies should be recorded together with the patient's current medication.

Other information

Further information about different kinds of psychological assessment are given in the following chapters; sexual history, Chapter 9; alcohol history, Chapter 8; history of somatic problems, Chapter 12; assessment of the elderly person with psychiatric problems, Chapter 13; assessment of the young person with psychiatric problems, Chapter 14.

Two examples of history taking are given that illustrate some of the particular skills involved. In the first example (Box 8), a student takes a history of the presenting complaint from a patient who has been suffering from depression. In this example, the student (Tom) demonstrates the core skills of communicating with a patient who is depressed. These are summarized in

---

Box 8
History-taking of a presenting complaint

Subject: depression
Patient: middle-aged female
Focus: presenting complaint and history of presenting complaint
Preparation: check with a member of the medical and nursing staff that it is alright to interview the patient alone. Inform staff where the interview will take place.

Student   (*Makes eye contact and smiles.*) Good morning, my name is Tom. I am a fourth year medical student. You are Mrs Peters?
Patient   Yes.
Student   I wonder, would you mind if I talked to you for a few minutes, about some of the difficulties you've been having recently. I'd like to take a history, it's rather like the interview you will already have had from Dr Davies. (*Asks permission, explains purpose of interview*)
Patient   No that's OK love.
Student   Thank you. Could we move to the visitors room, which is empty, as it's more private. (*Obtains consent*)

Patient   Yes (They move to the visitors room. Tom ensures they are seated in comfortable chairs, without a desk, slightly at an angle to each other. His chair is closest to the door.) (*Ensures appropriate setting*)
Student   Could I ask what your full name is and your date of birth? (*Establishes identity*)
Patient   Margaret Peters, 22.02.58.
Student   Do you mind if I take some notes. (*Asks permission to take notes*)
Patient   No.
Student   Before you came into hospital, were you working, outside the home?
Patient   Yes. I was a home help. Twenty hours a week.
Student   Right. Could you tell me a little about what brought you into hospital? (*Open question*)
Patient   Well . . . . . . I don't know where to start. I lost my husband last year. He was killed in a car crash.
Student   Oh dear . . . . . . that must have been awful. (*Understanding statement*)

Box 8 (*contd*)

Patient Yes . . . . . . yes it was. So sudden . . . . you know. He'd had his breakfast as usual, went to work and the next thing I knew was a policewoman coming to the door. She was very nice. I knew from the look on her face something awful had happened. I thought it was my father, but then she told me it was Danny. Another car had lost control and gone straight into his car. She said he must have been killed instantly.

Student A great shock for you. (*Understanding statement.*)

Patient Terrible, terrible. I was numb for weeks. I didn't feel upset. Everything just felt like a blur. I just got on with things, the funeral, sorting out his things, all the forms and things . . . . . . I just did everything . . . . my daughter said I was like a robot . . . . .

Student You felt detached from things? (*Clarification*)

Patient Yes, I didn't feel anything at all . . . . it was so strange.

Student Roughly how long did that last for? (*More specific question*)

Patient Oh, it must have a few months.

Student Er can be you a bit more specific . . . er 1 or 2 months, or 3 or 4, or longer than that? (*Closed question*)

Patient Six months. Then about 6 months after his death, I just began to feel awful . . . . not crying . . not upset . . . . . but this terrible feeling of dread inside me . . . . . . whenever I had to do anything . . . . I didn't want to see people . . . . talk to people . . . . I just wanted to hide away . . . . . . be left alone . . . . . I felt so empty inside . . . .

Student Empty . . . . . it sounds as if you felt very low. (*Picks up verbal cue of empty*)

Patient I was very low . . . . . it was like I'd come to the end . . . . . everything had stopped. I didn't eat . . . . . I didn't care about anything.

Student It sounds as if you felt down most of the time? (*Clarifies whether mood state was persistently lowered, does not pick up cues re eating and social withdrawal at this stage but makes a note to return to them after all the details of mood have been recorded.*)

Patient Yes, I couldn't get myself out of it. Even if my daughter came round . . . . . she couldn't make me feel better. (*Student notes that her mood did not respond to social cues*)

Student Did your mood ever brighten . . . . . during the day . . . . or if you went out? Did it vary? (*More specific question*)

Patient No.

Student And it sounds as if you really were very low? (*Tries to establish the severity of the mood state*)

Patient Yes, I've never felt as bad . . . .

Student Have you ever felt worse?

Patient No.

Student And roughly for how long did you feel like this? (*More specific question*)

Patient Oh, until I came into hospital . . . . until they gave me that electrical treatment?

Student That must be about 6 months.

Patient Yes.

Student I wonder when you felt as low as you did, what thoughts were going through your mind? (*Having established details re mood, the student now goes on to elicit associated thoughts: he should be looking for associated negative cognitions and suicidal ideation.*)

Patient Umh well I kept thinking . . . . . kicking myself for not saying good bye to him. He left in a hurry and we'd had a bit of a tiff the night before . . . nothing serious . . . but I'd not kissed him goodnight and didn't kiss him before he left for work . . . . . (*eyes fill with tears*) . . . . . I just wish I'd not been such a cow . . . . so stupid and mean . . . . . and I know it's silly but I began to think I was a really terrible person . . .

Student I know this is distressing (*acknowledges non-verbal cue – patient's tearfulness*), can you tell me a little more about that . . . . . . it sounds very painful . . ?

Patient I felt I was evil and a bad person . . . I thought I should be put down . . . . that I didn't deserve to live . . . . I began to think everything was my fault . . . . . I thought cos I'd not kissed him somehow I'd caused the accident . . . . . it was my fault . . . . . other things were my fault as well . . . . . I began to think I was responsible for the trains not running and for other accidents on the road. (*Abnormal negative cognitions that are also false beliefs*).

Student How strongly did you believe those things? (*Tries to establish whether the false beliefs were delusional, i.e. held with unshakeable conviction*)

Patient I did believe them . . . . . . I did . . . . . it was a state of mind I got into . . . . . I can't explain it . . . .

Student And er . . . . . given how you felt . . . . . . you were very down . . . . . . you felt you were to blame for many things . . . . I wonder did you ever have thoughts of harming yourself . . . . . (*Asks about suicidal ideas . . . . . does so in context*)

Patient No . . . . . . I never did . . . . I never thought about killing myself if that's what you mean?

Student OK that's fine. Now you mentioned that you weren't eating? (*Now goes on to elicit associated symptoms of depression*)

Patient No . . . . I didn't cook and I didn't want to eat. I lost about 2 stone in weight. I just didn't care. I didn't wash my clothes, or brush my hair towards the end . . . . I just didn't care. (*Elicits weight loss of 2 stone and self-neglect and poor personal hygiene*)

Student And your sleep, what was that like. (*Open question*)

Patient Terrible. I'd lie awake at night. Listen to the trains in the night, maybe that's why I began to worry about the trains and think everything with the trains was my fault. I'd get up and go back to bed, but I'd often be up until about 3.00 a.m. and then fall asleep but only for a couple of hours, then I'd be awake again. I'd be up with the birds. (*Initial insomnia and early morning wakening*)

Student You also mentioned earlier that you lost interest in going out. (*Picks up information patient had given student earlier in the interview*)

Patient Yes . . . I didn't want to see anyone . . . . not even my daughter.

Student And was that a change for you?

Patient Oh yes, love. I've got lots of friends and I love going out and I love my job and looking after my old ladies.

Student So you lost interest in work as well.

Patient Oh yes. I stopped going to work . . . in the summer.

Student That's about 4 months before you came into hospital? (*Clarification*)

Box 8 (contd)

Patient Yes.
Student Your concentration . . . what was that like?
(*Open question*)
Patient How do you mean?
Student Well could you read the paper or follow a programme on TV. (*Close question.*)
Patient No I couldn't do anything . . . I just used to sit in a chair . . . . . I couldn't remember anything either . . . my mind was like a sieve . . . .
Student So just if I could recap . . . . . . very sadly your husband died about a year ago . . . . . . it was a terrible shock for you . . . . . you felt numb (patient nods) . . . . for about six months . . . . . . coped well with things . . . but you weren't right . . . . . then began to feel very low . . . you felt to blame for things . . . . . . and you stopped eating well, you lost weight . . . you couldn't sleep and you lost interest in going out and were unable to work . . . and that lasted about six months . . . . and then you came into hospital . . . . (*Student summarises the main points of the history so far; by doing this he can check whether he has missed out anything important.*) Have I got things clear? (*Checks the details are correct*)

Patient Yes.
Student Do you think I've missed anything important . . . . . . is there anything else that happened to you during this period? Any other upsets or unusual things? (*Checks for other distressing life events*)
Patient No.
Student Do you know how you came to be admitted to hospital?
Patient My daughter got the doctor round and she got Dr Davies to come and see me. I didn't want to go . . . . but I think they made me in the end . . . . . you know they sectioned me . . . . .
Student Oh . . . . OK. I can check on that. And how are you feeling now?
Patient Oh a lot better. A lot better. After I'd had about four treatments.
Student The electrical treatment?
Patient Yes . . . . I just began to feel a lot better. I've put on a bit of weight. I can enjoy some things now. I'm not back to normal, but I'm getting there. I went out to stay with my daughter at the weekend. That was lovely.

Box 9. After completing the history of the presenting complaint the student (Tom) would go on to take a full history. From the initial part of the history, he has established that Mrs Peters has been suffering from a severe depressive illness (psychotic depression) in the context of a bereavement. As he goes through the history, he should pay particular attention to the points listed in Box 10 as these are particularly important to identify or exclude in patients with depressive disorder.

In the second example (Box 11), a student is asked to take a history from a patient who is agitated and highly aroused. The patient has been brought to the A&E department because he has been shouting at cars and wandering in the road in a dangerous fashion. The psychiatrist has to take over the interview as the patient threatens to leave. He is clearly very ill and has an elevated mood, grandiose ideas, pressure of speech and is experiencing second person auditory hallucinations. The student has been able to elicit these symptoms. She

Box 9
Core skill: communicating with a patient to take a history of the presenting complaint

The setting
Tom has ensured that the history is taken in a private room. He has checked with nursing staff that it is safe for him to interview the patient alone. He and the patient are seated in comfortable chairs, without a desk, slightly at an angle to each other. His chair is closer to the door.

Non-verbal communication
Tom is warm and friendly. He responds with sensitivity to the patient's distress and the tragedy which she has experienced. He is not unsettled by her distress and does not try to ignore it.

Permission
He introduces himself, explains the purpose of the interview and asks permission.

Questioning
Tom uses open questions and only uses closed questions to elicit specific details. He often uses statements to reflect

back the patient's feelings. This encourages further exploration and discussion of her mood.

Verbal and non-verbal cues
He is attentive and picks up cues the patient gives him about her mood state.

Structure
The interview had a clear structure:

- elicits the main problem/symptom
- focuses on the features of the main symptom
- then moves on to other associated symptoms
- summarizes information at the end of the interview.

Tom gives the patient the chance to add information. He applies knowledge whilst taking the history (he knows which symptoms are associated with depression).

Box 10
Important factors to identify or exclude in a patient suffering from a depressive disorder

- A previous history of a depressive disorder
  — any previous bereavements: how did she cope
  — childbirth: any evidence of a puerperal disorder.
- Family history of a depressive disorder or bipolar affective disorder (the severity of Mrs Peters' depression may indicate a genetic predisposition)
- History of parental childhood neglect (predisposes to depression)
- Loss of a parent before the age of 14 (predisposes to depression)
- Premorbid personality (anxious, depressive or obsessional premorbid traits can predispose to depression)
- Any chronic psychosocial stressors (housing problems, financial worries, etc.)

- Social support (lack of social support may make the depression more difficult to recover from)
- Adjustment to the loss of her husband (check for evidence she is coming to terms with this huge loss and is grieving appropriately)
- Prior relationship with husband (very dependent or ambivalent relationships are more likely to cause problems with grieving)
- Alcohol consumption (check she has not been using alcohol to help her to cope with husband's death, and exclude a prior drinking problem)
- Attitude to treatment (compliance with treatment and medication is a good prognostic indicator)
- Insight (good insight and understanding of illness is a good prognostic indicator).

Box 11
History-taking from an agitated patient

Subject: hearing voices
Patient: young adult male
Focus: presenting complaint and history of presenting complaint
Preparation: Duty psychiatrist (Dr Creed) checks whether police or A&E staff have reported that the man has been violent or aggressive. He has not been, but the A&E staff tell the psychiatrist that he's as 'high as a kite'. The psychiatrist can see through the window of the interview room that the man is pacing up and down. He does not appear aggressive. The psychiatrist checks the hospital records for any previous contacts. He is not known to services. The psychiatrist informs staff he is going to interview the patient and asks the police officers, who have brought him to the A&E department, to wait just outside the room in case he needs help. He asks Jane Edwards, a fourth year medical student, whether she would like to accompany him.

Psychiatrist (*Makes eye contact, but does not the shake the patient's hand or touch the patient.*) Hello . . . I'm Dr Creed, I'm one of the doctors who works in this hospital, I'm a psychiatrist. This is Jane Edwards; she's a student doctor. Is it OK if we ask you some questions about how you're feeling and what's been happening to you recently. We'd like to try and help.
Patient Yes. OK.
Psychiatrist Is it OK if Jane asks you some questions?
Patient Yes. She looks OK to me.
The patient is sitting in a chair in the interview room. He looks dishevelled and his pupils are dilated. He has a mild tremor and is sweating. He looks tense but is smiling. Jane and Dr Creed position themselves by the door. Dr Creed has already told Jane to get out of the room if the patient makes any sudden kind of movement. The door opens both ways and there is an alarm button close to where Jane and Dr Creed are standing. Dr Creed suggests they both sit down on chairs near the door.
Student Er. Could I ask you your name?

Patient You can. If that's the name of the game?
(*Laughs and giggles*)
Student OK. What's your name?
Patient Dr Death.
Student Ah . . . . er . . . . . I think the policeman said your name was John Taylor?
Patient It was . . . it was . . . but I'm known to my friends as Dr Death.
Student How old are you?
Patient How old are you?
Student Well er . . . . . I could tell you how old I am . . . . . but what I'm trying to do is to ask you some questions to try to find out what the problem is . . . . . it would help to know how old you are? (*Does not reveal personal information about self but tries to re-direct the interview so the patient is the focus*)
Patient Twenty four
Student What's been happening to you recently?
Patient I'm in love . . . . in love . . . in love . . . . baby, baby . . . . . (*starts singing*)
Student It looks as if you feel pretty good at the moment. (*Picks up verbal and non-verbal cues and tries to establish mood is elevated*)
Patient I'm in love with a wonderful guy (*still singing*).
Student You look really happy (*stays with cue*).
Patient Yes . . . . I feel really good . . . I haven't felt this good for years . . . . . (*turns and looks behind him and then smiles*).
Student How long have you felt this way?
Patient Oh I don't know, a day or so . . . . . I don't know . . . . . ask me something more interesting . . . . umh yes . . she is . . . . . (*turns again to look behind him*).
Student It looks as if you can hear something? (*Student realizes that he is responding to voices and picks up non-verbal cue.*)
Patient It's the angels . . . . . only fools rush in where angels fear to tread . . . . .
Student What are they saying . . . ? (*Tries to establish content*)

Box 11 (contd)

Patient (*laughs hysterically*) I can't tell you . . . . . .
Student It's OK.
Patient You know who you're talking to? (*Said in grandiose manner*)
Student Go on . . . .
Patient You've got a nice arse . . . that's what they're saying . . . and other things . . . . nice . . . nice . . . Bits . . . . . bits and tits . . . . (*Student notes his disinhibited and socially inappropriate comments, tries not to be embarrassed*)
Student They say this to you? (*Using her knowledge of mental illness the student tries to clarify whether hallucinations are second or third person*)
Patient They say such fantastic things
Student Do they talk about you? (*Again trying to clarify the nature of the hallucinations*)
Patient They're my friends, they wouldn't talk about me? (*Establishes that auditory hallucinations are second person*)
Student Do you know how many there are?
Patient Twelve.

Student How do you know.
Patient Mathew, Mark, Luke, Peter, David, John, Joseph, Emanuel, Stephen, Daniel, Jacob, Jeremiah (*says these names very quickly*) (*patient gets up and starts walking back and forth*). I've got to go . . . it's nice talking . . . . but I've got to go . . . . .
Psychiatrist Well, before that . . . I think it may be important for you to stay a little longer . . . . . . The police say you were shouting at cars . . . . . .
Patient I wasn't shouting . . . . . I was blessing cars . . . . I was doing good . . . . .
Psychiatrist I think you nearly got run over . . . . it was quite dangerous . . . .
Patient No . . . . . they can't hurt me . . . . things like that can't hurt me . . . . . I'm invincible . . . . you know . . . I'm made of special things . . . silken threads . . . . beads . . . cheese and beeswaaaaaaaaaaaaax . . . . (*clang association*).

---

has remained calm and focused and taken an excellent history, given the difficult circumstances. She has demonstrated a core skill in being able to communicate with a patient who is elated and disinhibited (Box 12).

It would be impossible to take a full history from this patient as he is aroused and would be unable to cooperate or concentrate for long enough. The provisional diagnosis is hypomania, probably secondary to a drug-induced state, as his pupils are dilated, he is sweating and has a mild tremor. A history from an informant would be essential in this case, and particular points to establish are listed in Box 13. It would also be important to carry out a physical examination and urine drug screen, if the patient would allow this, and to monitor his pulse, blood pressure and fluid intake.

Box 12
Core skill: communicating with a patient who is elated and disinhibited

The setting:
The student has positioned herself close to the door and near an alarm button so she can leave the room quickly or get help if necessary. She is not interviewing him alone. She is with a psychiatrist.

Non-verbal communication
She remains calm, friendly and professional although the patient is making inappropriate remarks about her bodily appearance. She understands that he is ill and is not in control of what he is saying.

Communication style
She uses open-ended questions. She picks up verbal and non-verbal cues to elicit symptomatology.

Box 13
Important factors to identify or exclude in a patient suffering from hypomania

- Previous history of mood swings (either depression or previous episodes of elation)
- Drug history
- Family history of either mood disorders or schizophrenia
- Any history of trauma or physical injury to the brain
- History of epilepsy
- Premorbid personality (evidence of a cyclothymic personality)
- Insight when euthymic
- Compliance with treatment
- Likely abstinence from drugs
- Social support and help from family and friends to stay off drugs.

2.2 Core examination skills

Learning objectives

You should:

- be able to carry out a mental state examination
- be able to carry out a cognitive state examination (CSE).

The mental state examination

The mental state examination (MSE) is a detailed, structured, description of the patient's current mental status.

It is not static and should change according to the patient's degree of illness. In patients who are very ill, it is conducted on a frequent basis to monitor change.

The mental state examination should not include any aspects of the patient's history, as it should only focus on the status of the patient during the most recent assessment by a psychiatrist.

The MSE is divided into the following categories:

- appearance and behaviour
- speech
- mood and affect
- thoughts
- perceptions
- cognitive function.

Appearance and behaviour

Appearance and behaviour refer to how the patient has behaved during the interview. It should include the following:

- dress: appropriate, dishevelled, naked, wearing strange items of clothing, etc.
- facial appearance: normal, decreased facial movement, looked tense or anxious, scars or other abnormal features, etc.
- eye contact: normal, avoids eye contact, makes prolonged eye contact, etc.
- behaviour: normal, socially inappropriate (e.g. invades personal space), agitated (unable to sit in chair, has to keep pacing about), decreased range of bodily movement, etc.

Speech

There are three different aspects of speech that need to be assessed:

- speed: normal rate, slower than normal, faster than normal, so fast the interviewer cannot get a word in (pressure of speech)
- tone: normal modulation, flattened tone
- form: normal grammatical form, circumstantial, loosening of associations, flight of ideas, other forms of thought disorder.

Any abnormality should be recorded and written down verbatim.

Mood and affect

The patient's mood should be described both from an objective and a subjective perspective.

Subjectively, record how the patient describes his/her mood (e.g. 'I can't go on, there's no point, I just want to die, I feel dead inside').

Objectively, record your assessment of the patient's mood (e.g. euthymic, elated, depressed, angry, anxious, fearful, blunted).

Thoughts

The patient's speech obviously reflects their thought processes, but the two are not always the same:

- rate: does the patient describe the speed of his/her thoughts as normal, faster than usual or slower than usual (any evidence of poverty of thought or flight of ideas)
- form: is the flow of thought logical and coherent, or is there evidence of a disruption. Specifically check for circumstanciality, perseveration, loosening of associations, thought blocking, derailment. Are there new words (neologisms)?
- content: main concerns or preoccupations
  — evidence of thought insertion, withdrawal or broadcasting
  — evidence of specific delusional ideas (e.g. passivity experiences)
  — suicidal ideation (strength of intent).

Perceptions

Describe in detail any abnormal perceptual experiences, including the type of abnormality and its content. Specifically check for evidence of illusions, visual or tactile hallucinations, auditory hallucinations (distinguish between second person and first person).

Cognitive state examination

1. Orientation

Describes the patient's level of consciousness (is the patient alert or drowsy?) and orientation for time, place and person.

2. Registration and short-term memory

Registration is tested by the *digit span*. A lengthening series of digits made up by you is read out to the patient who has to repeat them immediately. Healthy individuals can retain 7 or 8 items in this way. Impaired digit span occurs in delirium or advanced dementia.

Also test short-term memory over minutes by asking the patient to remember a *made up address* of 7 items or so. Check first that he has registered it correctly be repeating it back to you. Then get on with other assessments before asking the patient 5 minutes or so later to recall the address. Normal individuals will be able to do this.

3. Long-term memory

Long-term memory can be assessed asking for historical dates or recent current affairs. Avoid asking autobiographical details, such as home address, because there, may be no way to verify this.

4 Visuospatial function

Ask the patient to copy a simple drawn figure such as a circle or square and move to a more complex figure. The person then can be asked to draw a house. Finally, asking to insert the numbers on a pre-drawn clock face will test for deficits of lateralized inattention.

5 Object naming

This test for dysphasias. Ask the person to name objects you point to such as pen, shoe, watch. More subtle dysphasia can be detected by asking names of less common objects such as nib, laces, winder.

6. Attention of concentration

Can be assessed by asking *serial 7s*, subtracting 7s sequentially from 100 or serial 3s from 30.

Insight Record the patient's view of his/her illness, his/her view of treatment and whether he/she will agree to treatment.

Summary

Most of the information that is necessary to be able to carry out a mental state examination can be acquired during history taking. It is helpful, however, as you come to the end of the history, to check mentally whether you have all the details or whether you need to ask the patient some supplementary questions. Box 14 refers back to the example described in Box 8. It shows the supplementary questions that Tom, the medical student, needs to ask Mrs Peters in order to carry out a mental state examination. Box 15 then shows the mental state examination that he recorded.

Box 16 shows the mental state examination that the medical student, Jane Edwards, recorded for Mr John Taylor, following her interview with him in the A&E department

---

Box 14
Mental state examination questions

Subject: depression
Patient: middle-aged female
Setting: Tom is coming to the end of his interview with Mrs Peters. During the interview he has been carefully noting her behaviour and speech. He now goes on to ask specific questions so he can complete his mental state examination
Location: Visitors room; psychiatric inpatient unit

Student   Mrs Peters, we have a few minutes left. I'd like to check I haven't missed anything by asking you a few specific questions. Is that OK?
Patient   Yes that's fine.
Student   You've told me quite graphically how low you've been over the last few months, but I was wondering how you were feeling today?
Patient   Well, I feel fine. Apart from a bit of headache.
Student   Do you feel low?
Patient   No, not at all.
Student   Compared to your usual self, what is your mood like today: normal, a bit lower than normal or a bit higher than normal.?
Patient   I'm not back to normal, but I'm getting there. I've got a little bit further to go.
Student   If normal was 100% and the worst you've ever felt was 0%, where would you put yourself now?
Patient   Oh I'd say 75–80%.
Student   Are you having any problems thinking clearly?
Patient   No.
Student   You're thoughts aren't speeded up or slowed down, or muddled?
Patient   No. I'm quite clear.
Student   Do you have any particular worries or fears?
Patient   No.
Student   You told me that you were worrying that you were to blame for problems on the railways . . . and . .
Patient   Oh that was silly . . . I don't think that now.
Student   And your husband . . . you felt you were to blame somehow . . . ?
Patient   Yes . . . . I still wish I'd kissed him that morning, but I don't feel guilty or to blame the way I did. (*Tom does not ask again about suicidal ideation as he has already*

covered this in the history.)
Student   Have you experienced anything abnormal or strange today?
Patient   What do you mean?
Student   Well anything . . . . . er . . . look strange or hear odd to you? Hear anybody talking about you?
Patient   No.
Student   I know this seems odd, but can I just check you know where you are?
Patient   P6-The Infirmary.
Student   Do you know the date today?
Patient   4th September 2000.
Student   And the time?
Patient   11.30 a.m.
Student   What's the name of the doctor who's in charge of your care?
Patient   Dr Davies.
Student   Now I'd like to ask you some questions to assess your memory and concentration. I'd like to tell you a name and address, and then I'll ask you to repeat it back to me in a few minutes. Is that OK? Its:
   John Moorhouse
   4 Angel Street
   Bingley
   Bradford.
Could you repeat it?
Patient   John Moorhouse, 4 . . . . . er, Bradford.
Student   I'll say it again, it's quite a lot to take in, in one go. Its:
   John Moorhouse
   4 Angel Street
   Bingley
   Bradford.
Patient   John Moorhouse, 4 Angel Street, Bingley, Bradford.
Student   That's fine. I'll ask it you again in a few minutes. Now could you try another test for me. Could you take seven away from 100 and then take seven away from the number you get, and then seven away from that number, and so forth, until you get down to 0.
Patient   Er.
Student   If it was 8 from 100, it would be 100, 92, 84, 76, etc.

Box 14 (contd)

Patient Oh . . . . yes I see, I don't think I'm going to be very good at this (*chuckles*). Er 100, 93 . . . 93 7 from 93 is 86 . . . . 79, 72 7 from 72 is er 65 . . . 58 . . 51 . . . 44 . . . . 37 . . 30, 23 . . . er 7 from 23 is 16 . . . . 9 . . 2 . . .
Student Could I ask you the name and address again?
Patient Er, John Moorhouse, Bingley, Bradford, er, Angel Street, er,
Student The number?
Patient Er 4.
(*Tom repeats this task a three minutes later. Mrs Peters remembers the name and address correctly.*)
Student Could I ask you what sense you make of what's happened to you over the last year?
Patient Well, I didn't at the time, but I think I've been very ill . . . . . very depressed . . . . and I couldn't pull myself out of it . . . . And I got in a bad way with it . . . which is why I needed to come in here.

Box 15
Mental state examination: Mrs Margaret Peters, 4.9.00 Time 11.30 a.m.

Appearance and behaviour
Patient was dressed normally in slacks and a jumper. Her hair was brushed, she was wearing make-up, which had been carefully applied, and her personal hygiene was good. She behaved appropriately throughout the interview and was able to sit in a chair throughout. Her range of body movements was normal (neither increased or decreased). There was no evidence of any socially inappropriate or sexually inappropriate behaviour. She had a wide and varied range of facial expressions, made good eye contact and was warm and cooperative. Her behaviour was congruent with her mood.

Speech
Her speech was normal in rate and form. There were no long gaps before responding to questions and the volume was appropriate. There was appropriate tonal modulation and inflection in her speech.

Mood and affect
Subjectively, she described her mood as, 'Just normal, it's good to feel OK'.
Objectively, her mood was euthymic. There was no evidence of depression.

Thoughts
There was no abnormality in the form and speed of her thoughts.
    She had no specific worries or fears.
    There was no evidence that she still believed any of the abnormal beliefs she held during her illness.
    She did not think she was to blame or responsible for her husband's death or for any problems on the railways.
    There was no evidence of any delusional ideas or obsessional thoughts.
    There were no suicidal ideas.

Perception
There were no abnormalities of perception.

Cognitive function
Mrs Peters was fully orientated for time, place and person. Her level of consciousness was not impaired.
    Her concentration was good. She was able to complete serial 7s in 1 minute 30 seconds without any mistakes.
    Her short-term memory was also good. She required two attempts to register a seven-item name and address, but was able to recall all items at 2 minutes and 5 minutes. At 2 minutes, she had to think very hard to remember one of the items.
    Her long-term memory was well preserved. She was able to give a detailed account of her childhood, which was consistent with historical details at the time she was growing up. For example: The Beatles popularity in 1963 when she was 5 years old: England winning the world cup in 1966 when she was 8 years old, and Concorde's first flight when she was 11.

Insight
She has good insight into her condition. She understands that she has been suffering from a depressive illness, from which she is now recovering. She is able to make an accurate assessment of her mood and level of function. She understands she is receiving ECT (electroconvulsive therapy) and she feels this is helping her. She is compliant with treatment.

Box 16
Mental state examination: Mr John Taylor, 16.11.00 Time 11.30 p.m.

Appearance and behaviour
Patient looked dishevelled. His hair was long, dirty and matted. He was dressed in jeans and a T-shirt, was wearing shoes, but no socks. He had no coat or other kind of warm clothing. It is a cold night and his dress was 'therefore' inadequate for the weather outside. His clothes were stained and crumpled. He appeared tense and was sitting forwards on the edge of his chair. He was constantly fidgeting during the interview and rubbing his hands together. He was sweating and had a mild tremour. He was distractable and kept looking behind him during the interview. He appeared to be responding to voices. His pupils were dilated (both were equal) and he made prolonged and inappropriate eye contact. At times he leaned so far forward in his chair that he invaded my personal space; so I found myself leaning backwards. He was sexually disinhibited and stared inappropriately at parts of the interviewer's body. He had an animated facial expression and laughed and giggled during the interview. His laughter appeared incongruous but was probably related to the content of his auditory hallucinations. He was neither verbally nor physically aggressive or threatening during the interview. Half way through he got up from his chair and began to pace around and said that he wanted to leave. At times he appeared grandiose and inferred that we should

Box 16 (*contd*)

know who he was (the inference being that he was very important). He referred to himself as Dr Death.

Speech
His speech was faster than normal and, at times, he appeared to have pressure of speech (e.g. shouted out the names of 'angels' in a rapid, machinegun-like delivery). The tonal variation of his speech was exaggerated and dramatic. At times he sang. He was difficult to interview and did not respond directly to some questions. The content of his speech was socially inappropriate. The form of his speech was disrupted by clang association (e.g. bits . . . bits . . . and tits . .) inappropriate use of proverbs (it's the angels . . . . . only fools rush in where angels fear to tread). There were no full examples of flight of ideas.

Mood and affect
Subjectively, he described himself as, 'I feel really good . . . I haven't felt this way for years'.
Objectively, his mood was elevated.

Thoughts
He did not describe the speed of his thoughts, although his speech was rapid. The form has already been described in the section on speech.
He did not disclose any specific delusional ideas but implied that he was a very important person. It is possible that he believes he is God or Christ as he said he had been trying to bless cars and he believes angels are talking to him.
His other beliefs were consistent with an elevated mood. He talked (sung) about 'being in love with a wonderful guy'.
There were no suicidal ideas (but he was not asked specifically about this).

Perception
He described second person auditory hallucinations. Angels spoke directly to him, 'You've got a nice arse . . that's what they say'. The voices did not talk about him. He responded to the voices as if he were hearing them in external space and they were real. There were no other abnormalities of perception.

Cognitive function
Orientation was not assessed. The patient was fully conscious.
Concentration was not formally tested, but the patient was distractable and agitated. It is likely his concentration was impaired.
His memory was not formally tested.

Insight
He had poor insight into his condition. He did not understand that he was ill. He believed that his abnormal experiences were real. He is unlikely to accept treatment, but this was not specifically assessed.

(Box 11). Although it was impossible to take a full history, a mental state examination could be performed.

Mini mental state examination

The mini mental state examination (MMSE) is a brief structured assessment of cognitive function. It is widely used and provides the assessment of orientation, registration, short-term memory and language functioning. Some psychiatrists conduct a mental state examination and supplement the assessment of cognitive function with the MMSE. It is a relatively crude measure, and a more detailed assessment of cognitive function should be undertaken if any abnormalities are found. The maximum score is 30. Table 3 shows the scoring system, and Figure 1 shows the figure that patients are asked to draw as part of the test of visual spatial awareness.

It may be helpful to practise carrying out the MMSE on friends, who, hopefully, should have normal cognitive function, before trying to administer it to patients.

2.3 Making sense of psychiatric histories

Learning objectives

You should:

● be able to make a differential diagnosis based on your assessment

● be able to identify predisposing, precipitating and maintaining factors for mental illness in individual patients

● be able to make an informed estimate of prognosis.

A full psychiatric history, and mental state examination, will take between 45 and 90 minutes to complete depending upon the complexity of the patient problem. The information then needs to be organized and placed in a coherent framework (Box 17). You need to state your preferred diagnosis and list the evidence supporting and contradicting your choice. You should then list the differential diagnoses, putting the most obscure possibilities last.

It is important to try to understand why the patient developed mental illness, what factors caused the illness to present at this moment in time and what factors may hinder the patient's recovery (maintaining factors). In order to do this well, you need to have knowledge of the different kinds of mental illness and their causes. This enables you to take particular note of certain parts of the history when you are interviewing the patient, so you can ask about them in detail.

An understanding of the aetiological factors of the patient's illness helps you to develop a treatment plan. The plan should include consideration of whether the

Table 3 The mini mental state examination (MMSE)

Mini mental state examination Name: Date:	Maximum score	Score
Orientation		
What is the year, season, date, month, day (1 point per correct answer)	5	
Where are we: county, city, part of the city, building, ward/floor (1 point per correct answer)	5	
Registration		
Ask permission to test the patient's memory. Name three objects (e.g. penny, orange, chair). Take 1 second to say each one. Ask the patient to repeat the names of all three objects. One point for each correct answer. After this repeat the object names until all three are learned (up to six trials) record the number of times the objects had to be repeated. (*Do not use objects that the patient can actually see, or in some way would prompt the patient to remember*)	3	
Attention and calculation		
Spell world backwards. One point for each letter that is in the right place (e.g. DLROW = 5, DRLOW = 3	5	
Or you can do serial subtractions. Stop after five subtractions. One mark per correct answer		
Recall		
Ask for the three objects repeated above (1 point for each correct answer)	3	
Language		
Point to a pencil and ask the patient to name this object (1 point). Do the same thing with a wrist watch (1 point)	2	
Ask the individual to repeat the following: 'no ifs, ands or buts'	1	
Give the patient a piece of paper and ask him or her to follow a three-stage command. 'Take the paper in your right hand, fold it in half and put it on the floor' (1 point for each correct part) (*Give all parts of the command together, not in stages, as this is a test of comprehension, praxis and memory*)	3	
Show the individual a large message in capitals which says, 'CLOSE YOUR EYES'. Ask the patient to read the message and do what it says (1 point if the individual closes his/her eyes) (*This tests comprehension and reading ability*)	1	
Ask the individual to write a sentence on a blank piece of paper. The sentence must contain a subject and a verb and must be sensible. (1 point) (*This tests expression*)	1	
Show (or draw) the individual two interlocking pentagons (Fig. 1); Ask the patient to copy the design. All 10 angles need to be present and the two shapes must intersect to score 1 point (*This tests for constructional apraxis*)	1	
Total score	30	

patient needs immediate treatment (i.e. admission to hospital or one-to-one nursing supervision). Short-term treatment refers to the days or weeks following presentation and usually involves the treatment of the acute illness. It should include details of drug treatment, nursing care and other acute psychological treatments. Long-term treatment refers to the period of time after the acute illness has resolved. It should include details of drug treatment, supervision, rehabilitation programmes and interventions designed to address factors which may impede or prevent recovery (i.e. maintaining factors) or precipitate another episode of illness.

It is helpful to make an informed estimate of the patient's prognosis, based upon the previous history, the strength and nature of predisposing factors, and the likelihood that treatment interventions will ameliorate maintaining and precipitating factors. Box 18 describes the features of a patient's presenting characteristics. The preliminary diagnosis and formulation of his case is shown in Box 19.

2.4 The assessment of risk

Learning objectives

You should:

- be able to carry out a risk assessment

- be able to maximize your personal safety when working in a hospital or community setting.

All psychiatric assessments should include an assessment of risk of the patient causing harm to another person or to himself/herself. The assessment of risk of suicide is important and is described in Chapter 6. Risk can never be eliminated, and it is extremely difficult to anticipate accurately as risk fluctuates depending upon a variety of different circumstances. A risk assessment can rarely be done by

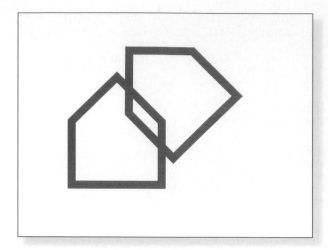

CLOSE YOUR EYES

Fig. 1 Useful cards for the mini mental state examination.

Box 17
Making sense of a psychiatric history

Diagnosis
Preferred diagnosis:
Evidence supporting diagnosis:
Evidence contradicting diagnosis:
Differential diagnosis:

Precipitating factors
What factors caused the development of the illness at this specific moment?

Predisposing factors
What factors made this patient vulnerable to developing the illness?

Maintaining factors
What factors may prevent or hinder recovery?

Treatment
Immediate: e.g. admission to hospital or one-to-one nursing
Short term: acute illness in days/weeks after presentation
Long term: after acute phase

Prognosis
Short tem:
Long term:

Box 18
Mental state examination: Mr Jason Roberts

Background
A 25-year-old man called Jason Roberts was admitted to an orthopaedic ward after suffering multiple injuries as a result of jumping off a motorway bridge. He had been behaving strangely for about 10 days before this incident. His sister described that he became very moody and spent a lot of time by himself. He didn't sleep or eat very much. He began to talk to himself and told her that she shouldn't believe what she read about him in the papers. He told her that the television was telling 'a whole lot of lies about him' and 'he was not a paedophile'. He told her that he'd heard people at college talking about him and people on the bus were also involved. He believed it was only a matter of time before he was going to be attacked and killed. She tried to persuade him to go to hospital but he refused. He began to feel that he was mutating into a demon and that his legs and arms were getting longer. He heard the neighbours whispering about building a gallows to hang him. That night, he ran away from home. He was missing for 4 days before being found by motorway police.

According to his sister, he had not suffered from psychiatric illness before this recent episode. He did not abuse alcohol or drugs. He lived with his parents, sister and younger brother. His father's brother had a history of schizophrenia and committed suicide when he was 35 years of age.

In his personal history, Jason was born after his mother endured a 36 hour labour. Forceps were used to deliver him. His sister did not have any further details. He was a sickly child and developed meningitis when he was 4. He made a good recovery. The rest of his childhood was uneventful. He did well at school and was popular with his school friends. He played football and enjoyed many other sporting interests. He went to university to read physics but dropped out after the second year (when he was 20 years old). He never explained to his parents or family why he did this. He stayed at home and lost contact with most of his friends. He became rather solitary and spent a lot of time on his computer. His sister said the 'spark just seemed to go out'. His parents became more and more dissatisfied with him and his father described him as lazy. Six weeks prior to this illness, his father became very angry and told him that, unless he found a job, he would have to leave home.

When Jason was assessed on the ward his mental state examination was as follows.

Appearance and behaviour
Young male. Lying in bed. Both legs and right arm in plaster. Multiple lacerations and contusions to face and chest. He was physically unable to get out of bed. He looked nervous and frightened. Hypervigilant. Made intense and prolonged eye contact. Kept looking down the ward to the entrance. Quite guarded throughout the interview and suspicious. Kept saying, 'why do you want to know that'. No aggressive or threatening behaviour.

Box 18 (*contd*)

Speech
His speech was normal in rate but he spoke in a whisper. The form was normal.

Mood and affect
Subjectively he described himself as being, 'better off dead . . . . it's just a matter of time . . . .'.
  Objectively: he appeared to be very frightened.

Thoughts
He said his thoughts were normal in rate.
  He described persecutory delusions. He believed that his neighbours, people on the street and people on television thought he was a paedophile and were going to kill him. He did not think hospital staff were involved but was becoming increasingly suspicious of the ward clerk and visitors to the ward.
  He believed he was changing shape and was turning into a monster. He could feel his arms and legs getting longer. He described somatic hallucinations and talked about electricity flowing through his body, which he thought must be coming from the hospital generator.
  He denied any active suicidal ideas but he confirmed that he had jumped off the bridge to kill himself. The fact that he had survived confirmed that he was supernatural. He wished he had died. He believed he was going to suffer a terrible fate. Did not appear to have any thoughts about harming others.

Perception
He did not appear to be experiencing auditory hallucinations during the interview.

Cognitive function
He was fully orientated for time, place and person. The patient was fully conscious.
  Concentration was not formally tested, but the patient was tense and very anxious. It is likely his concentration was impaired.
  His memory was not formally tested. He was suspicious and would not cooperate with the tests.

Insight
He had poor insight into his condition. He did not understand that he was ill. He believed that his abnormal experiences were real. He did not accept he needed treatment.

Box 19
Diagnosis, aetiological formulation and treatment plan

Name: Jason Roberts (assessment described in Box 18).

Diagnosis
Preferred diagnosis: schizophrenia
Evidence supporting diagnosis: third person auditory hallucinations, persecutory delusions, ideas of reference, perplexity, tactile hallucinations (electricity through his body), insidious onset with change in personality over previous 5 years.
Differential diagnoses: symptomatic schizophrenia (drug-induced state, organic conditions), hypomania.

Precipitating factors
No obvious biological factors.
  Threat of eviction from family home by father 6 weeks before illness.

Predisposing factors
Genetic predisposition: family history of schizophrenia.
  Birth trauma: may have resulted in minor damage injury.
  Meningitis as a child may have resulted in minor brain damage.
  No evidence of a schizoid personality (sociable active child and teenager).

Maintaining factors
No insight into condition but this may change with treatment.

Father has been hostile and critical of him recently. If this continues, it may make relapse more likely.

Treatment plan
Immediate: Ward 1 is on the first floor. He needs to be nursed in a ground floor ward or in a room with reinforced glass in the window, so he cannot jump out. May need one-to-one nursing observation. The risk of further suicide attempts is high.
  Short term: treatment with a sedating neuroleptic drug (e.g. chlorpromazine).
  Long term: requires a care plan that includes a detailed assessment of his needs, future treatment plan and social support.

Prognosis
Poor prognostic factors include insidious onset of illness, strong family history of schizophrenia. Good prognostic features include absence of drug and alcohol abuse.
  Further time is required to assess other prognostic factors, which include:
- degree of insight and compliance with treatment and care plan
- Degree to which his family is supportive or critical of him.

---

one person alone and requires access to detailed information from several different sources. Nevertheless, doctors (particularly those working in A&E) are often called upon to make judgements about a patient's risk, without access to detailed information about that person.

The key elements of a risk assessment have been summarized in a report by a Special Working Party on the Assessment and Management of Risk, convened by the Royal College of Psychiatrists (Box 20) (see Further reading).

Box 20
The assessment of risk

History
- Previous violence and or suicidal/behaviour
- Evidence of rootlessness or social restlessness (e.g. frequent changes of address or employment)
- Poor compliance with treatment
- Substance misuse
- Social background that encourages violence
- Identification of precipitants, changes in mental state, that occurred prior to violence or relapse
- Recent severe stress
- Recent discontinuation of medication
- Recent change to any risk factors.

Environment
Does the person have access to potential victims, particularly individuals identified in mental state abnormalities?

Mental state
- Firmly held beliefs of persecution by others
- Firmly held beliefs of jealousy involving a partner
- Intention or thoughts of acting on beliefs
- Beliefs about being controlled by external forces
- Command hallucinations (voices telling the person to be violent)
- Emotions related to violence (e.g. anger, hostility, suspiciousness)
- Specific threats made by the patient.

Conclusions
- How serious is the risk?
- Is the risk specific (i.e. related to a specific person) or general?
- How immediate is the risk?
- How volatile is the risk?
- If an individual is at risk, does that person need to be informed?
- What specific treatment, and which management plan, can best reduce the risk?

Box 21
Maximizing personal safety

Preparation
- Always discuss the patient with a member of staff before seeing him/her
- Check with staff that it is safe to do so
- Check whether the patient has a previous history of violence
- Inform staff where you will be seeing the patient
- Never carry out a community visit by yourself
- Prepare the interview room before seeing the patient
- Position the chairs so that your chair will be closest to the door
- Be aware which way the door opens; never place yourself behind the door, as you can be trapped in the room.
- Check if there is an alarm in the room.

Managing the interview
If a patient becomes aroused or agitated during the interview:
- try to make calming statements
- do not pursue a line of enquiry that is upsetting the patient
- do not disagree with the patient
- avoid becoming a focus for criticism ('Well I can take up your complaint with the ward managers')
- try to bring the interview to a close ('Well, perhaps we could leave things there for today')
- leave the room if you are worried you will be assaulted, run out of the room if necessary
- if you become trapped, shout for help, press the alarm (if there is one)
- if the patient brings a weapon into the room, calmly tell the patient that you will have to terminate the interview; get up and leave
- if the patient demands a prescription for drugs (and does not realize you are a student) and is threatening you with a knife, write the prescription. The pharmacy can be contacted later.

Aftermath
If you are the subject of an assault or serious threat of violence:
- get appropriate physical help
- report the incident to managers and to your consultant and tutor
- review with them whether anything can be learned from the incident (either relating to your own behaviour or hospital procedures)
- discuss whether the perpetrator of the assault should be prosecuted
- talk about your experience with friends and family (even minor assaults or threats can be very frightening); be aware that you may feel upset and aroused after the incident. If you still feel very upset and are suffering from anxiety, panicky feelings and nightmares several weeks after the incident, seek help from your GP or university counselling/hospital occupational health services.

Managing personal safety

There are two different aspects involved in managing safety. Hospitals and other statutory agencies have a duty to provide a safe working environment. This includes the provision of training for staff, adequacy of staff numbers, protocols for dealing with violent incidents and provision of alarm devices and other features to make buildings and other environments more safe. Individuals have a responsibility to attend training courses and follow safety guidelines.

Medical students are very rarely exposed to violent or dangerous incidents. Most psychiatric patients are not violent. However, students must always be aware of the potential for violence and act accordingly. Box 21 provides some helpful guidelines for students to enable them to manage personal safety.

2.5 Investigations

Learning objectives

You should:

- be able to plan appropriate investigations for patients with mental illness

- understand what information can be derived from these investigations and whether this is useful.

Most investigations should only be undertaken to exclude specific physical conditions. It is bad practice to order a battery of tests routinely, without clear thought as to their purpose. Extensive battery testing is often cumbersome and inappropriate for most psychiatric populations; it is also expensive.

Blood tests

A full blood count, urea and electrolytes, and blood sugar are all inexpensive tests. Although anaemia is relatively uncommon in psychiatric patients, a raised MCV (mean cell volume) may indicate excessive alcohol consumption. It is useful to confirm normal renal function and exclude diabetes if pharmacological treatment is to be considered.

Thyroid function tests (TFTs) should be carried out, regardless of symptoms, on women over 50 years, as the prevalence of hypothyroidism in this group is relatively high. TFTs in young women or men are unlikely to be of value unless there is a specific indication, as the prevalence of hypothyroidism is so low (<0.1%).

Liver function tests should be ordered if there is a suspicion of alcohol abuse. In dementia, B_{12} and folate and syphilis serology are indicated.

X-rays examination

Chest or skull radiographs are of little value as routine screening instruments. They may be ordered if indicated by the patient's history and presentation.

Electrocardiogram

An electrocardiogram (ECG) is not carried out routinely on most psychiatric patients but may be required to exclude underlying cardiac disease or to confirm normality before implementing specific treatments such as electroconvulsive therapy (ECT) or lithium.

Electroencephalography (EEG)

Electroencephalography (EEG) is an inexpensive test that is readily available in most hospitals. In patients with reversible diffuse brain dysfunction caused by a toxic metabolic process, the EEG may be diagnostic, while a CT scan is normal. It has three main indications: diagnosis of epilepsy, the detection of mild delirium that presents with psychiatric symptoms, and cognitive dysfunction secondary to degenerative brain disease. Most psychotropic drugs can produce slowing of the EEG. When accompanied by an increase in anterior beta activity, an overdose with a barbiturate, benzodiazepine or tricyclic antidepressant should be considered (Table 4).

Neuroimaging

The main reason for carrying out a brain scan on a patient with psychiatric problems is to exclude an intracerebral lesion as a cause for the symptoms. The main indications are when patients have cognitive impairment or a history suggestive of a prior brain injury or epilepsy.

The two most common types of neuroimaging that are used in psychiatry are computed tomography (CT) and magnetic resonance imaging (MRI). Other methods of imaging the brain such as SPECT (single photon emission CT) are not widely available, although they are utilized for research purposes. The main advantages of CT

Table 4 Type of wave activity seen on electroencephalography (EEG) traces

Activity	Causes
Beta activity (faster than 13 Hz)	Barbiturates, benzodiazepines, tricyclic antidepressant
Alpha activity (8–13 Hz)	Found posteriorly during relaxation, attenuating when eyes are open
Theta activity (4–7 Hz)	Found anteriorly (particularly in children); Stimulant drugs such as LSD (lysergic acid diethylamide) or hallucinogens
Delta (< 4 Hz)	Always abnormal in the awake adult; if localized suggests a structural lesion; many psychotropic drugs produce slow wave activity
Spikes (sharp wave forms of high voltage)	If persistent at one site it indicates a focal electrical charge
Spike and wave activity	Describes runs of spikes and large delta waves: suggest epileptic focus

and MRI scanning in relation to psychiatry have been described by O'Brien and Barber (2000; see Further reading) and are summarized in Boxes 22 and 23.

Box 22
Computed tomography

The advantages of CT in psychiatry are:

- widely available
- inexpensive
- can be performed quickly (so tolerated by patients who are disturbed or agitated).
- good for excluding space-occupying lesions (tumours or subdural haematomas).

The disadvantages are:

- soft tissue lesions are not always well visualized
- images are limited to axial views
- patients are exposed to radiation.

Box 23
Magnetic resonance imaging

The advantages of MRI in psychiatry are:

- can examine the structure of the whole brain in any plane and generate three-dimensional images
- good visualization of white matter lesions and smaller infarcts
- improved resolution and superior soft tissue contrast
- does not use ionizing radiation
- can be used for serial monitoring.

The disadvantages are:

- not widely available
- expensive
- the noise and confinement of the scanner makes some patients feel sick or panicky
- contraindicated in patients with cardiac pacemakers and intracranial aneurysm clips.

2.6 Organization of services and professional attitudes

Services for mentally ill people in the United Kingdom have undergone a dramatic change in the last 20 years. Many psychiatric inpatient facilities have closed, and most patients with mental illness are managed in the community. Although there are very good models of community care across the country, many inner city services face severe pressures, as individuals with severe mental illness are more common amongst inner city populations than in rural or semi-urban areas. This

---

Learning objectives

You should:

- know how services for the mentally ill are organized
- know the main features of the Care Programme Approach
- be aware of the different professional groups that comprise community mental health teams
- adopt a professional attitude towards all people with mental illness
- be aware of stigma and prejudice in relation to mental illness.

---

is partly because people with severe mental illness tend to drift into the inner cities, and most hostels for the mentally ill are located in the inner cities.

Most services for the mentally ill are provided by community mental health teams, who cover a specific, small geographical area. The teams are multidisciplinary and are drawn from both health and social services. They usually consist of a psychiatrist, community psychiatric nurses, social workers, support staff and a variety of other staff, including art therapists, occupational therapists, etc. Specific teams may be developed to provide intensive imput to a small number of individuals with complex needs. Most services have specific teams who provide rehabilitation for patients with schizophrenia, and other teams who focus on patients who are difficult to engage or maintain in treatment. These teams are described further in Chapter 5.

Health and social services have recently been reorganized so that a seamless service for the mentally ill can be provided. As many individuals with mental illness have a range of social as well as health needs, it makes sense to try to coordinate health and social services. Most community services have:

- a single point of entry
- a unified health and social care assessment process
- coordination of the respective roles and responsibilities of each agency in the system
- access through a single process to the support and resources of both health and social care.

Most services have a small number of psychiatric inpatient beds for high-risk patients, and day-hospital or outpatient services. Psychiatrists work closely with the community mental health teams and with primary care. Many psychiatrists meet with GPs on a regular basis to review patients or provide advice about treatment and management.

Services for individuals who are over the age 65 years are provided by old age psychiatry. There are also specific psychiatric services for children, patients with addiction problems, patients who are involved with the criminal justice system (forensic psychiatry) and patients in the general hospital (liaison psychiatry).

The Care Programme Approach

All community mental health services implement the Care Programme Approach (CPA), and all patients with mental illness have a care plan. The CPA was introduced in 1991 to provide a framework for effective mental health care. Its five key elements are listed in Box 24.

Standard and enhanced Care Programme Approach

Many services operate different levels of the CPA according to the patient's needs. Patients who are cared for under the enhanced CPA are almost always those individuals with complex needs, who require multiprofessional and/or agency input to meet their needs, and who benefit from formal coordination of their care (Box 25). Most individuals with schizophrenia fall into this category.

Box 24
Key elements of the Care Programme Approach

1. Systematic arrangements for assessing the health and social needs of people accepted into specialist mental health services
2. The formation of a care plan that identifies the health and social care required from a variety of providers
3. The appointment of a care coordinator to keep in close touch with the service user and to monitor and coordinate care
4. The involvement, in all aspects of the care process, of the user, his/her advocate, carers and others who are appropriate
5. Regular review and, where necessary, agreed changes to the care plan.

Box 25
Characteristics of people who are cared for by the enhanced Care Programme Approach

- They have multiple needs requiring interagency coordination
- They are only willing to cooperate with one professional or agency but have multiple needs
- They may be in contact with a number of agencies
- They are likely to require more frequent and intensive interventions
- They are more likely to have mental health problems coexisting with other problems such as substance misuse.

Box 26
Characteristics of people who are cared for by the standard Care Programme Approach

- Require the support of one agency or discipline or require low-key support from more than one agency or discipline
- More able to manage their mental health problem
- Have an active informal support network
- Pose little danger to themselves or others
- More likely to maintain appropriate contact with services.

Patients who receive standard CPA are those individuals with less complex needs, often requiring input from only one professional (Box 26).

Care planning

Each individual on the CPA must have a care plan. Each individual's care plan must be based on a thorough assessment of their health and social care needs. The plan must be agreed between the patient and the care team, and the patient should receive a detailed copy of the care plan. The care plan must:

- identify the interventions and anticipated outcomes
- record all the actions necessary to achieve the agreed goals
- in the event of disagreement, include the reasons
- give an estimated timescale by which the outcomes or goals will be achieved or reviewed
- detail the contributions of all the agencies involved
- include appropriate crisis and contingency plans.

Support for the service user and their wider family

All individuals who provide regular and substantial care for a person on the CPA should have an assessment of their caring, physical and mental health needs, repeated on an annual basis. They should also receive their own written care plan, which is given to them and implemented in discussion with them.

Mental health professionals

A variety of different professionals work together to form a multidisciplinary team to provide community services for the mentally ill.

Consultant Psychiatrist. Has 5–6 years of undergraduate medical training, 1 year pre-registration training and a minimum of 6–7 years of postgraduate training. Takes clinical responsibility for patients regarding risk, determines treatment and approves care plan.

Community psychiatric nurse. Has 3 years of training in psychiatric nursing, plus 1 year extramural course. Usually spends some time postqualification working in an inpatient setting. Provides regular contact and support for patients, gives depot treatment, monitors medication. Implements basic behavioural programmes.

Social worker. The social worker is employed by social services and has had 3 years of training. May have specific training in the Mental Health Act (1983). Provides regular contact and support for patients. Has particular role in relation to patients treated under the Mental Health Act (1983).

Support workers. These may be employed by social services or other agencies and their training is varied. They provide support for patients and help to engage patients in meaningful activities.

Clinical Psychologist. Has a basic degree in psychology, 1–2 years of experience of research (MSc) or clinical work and a 3 year training in clinical psychology. Many clinical psychologists work independently, either in outpatient services or in specific psychological services for primary care. Some clinical psychologists still provide imput into multidisciplinary community teams. They usually offer specific cognitive or behavioural treatment or will supervise other staff who implement the treatment.

Professional attitudes

Many people have a negative attitude towards the mentally ill. Some of the mentally ill suffer vilification, humiliation and physical harm at the hands of the general public. The Royal College of Psychiatrists is currently conducting a nationwide campaign to increase the understanding of six common mental disorders. The aim is to challenge peoples' preconceptions about mental illness, their fears and ignorance, and provide them with accurate information about mental disorders. In this way, the gap between what health professionals and the public regard as helpful treatments may be closed. Detailed information is available on the Royal College of

Psychiatrists' website or by writing to the college directly (see Further reading).

There are four important guiding principles in relation to the ethical practice of medicine. First, doctors must respect the patient's autonomy and the ability of each individual to determine his or her own right to receive or deny treatment. The Mental Health Legislation in England and Wales (and Scotland) gives powers to doctors to restrict the liberty of patients under certain circumstances. Doctors have to ensure that the judgements they make are based upon objective clinical grounds and are not influenced by prejudice or stigma.

Second, doctors should adhere to a principal of beneficence, which means that they have a duty to carry out actions which will be of most benefit to their patients. In certain circumstances, however, this principle may extend to others, if a patient's illness is putting other people at risk. The doctor has to balance his/her duty to the patient against the risk of harm to others.

Third, doctors should not act in a way that harms people. Most treatments have benefits and risks. Doctors must be clear that any potential benefits of a treatment outweigh the possible negative effects, either on the patient or for others.

Finally, doctors should be aware of a principle of justice. This is a complex area but involves issues to do with fairness and treating patients in an equal manner, no matter how they behave or what they have done. It also involves issues relating to equity and a fair distribution of resources.

Doctors have a duty to act in a professional manner with all patients they see, even those who, at times, exhibit challenging behaviour. Some patients, when they are ill, may make inappropriate sexual advances towards staff or may use racist or other kinds of insulting language. While such behaviour should not be condoned in normal individuals, doctors have to be able to control their emotions and respond to such actions in a calm and appropriate manner.

The General Medical Council is particularly keen that professional attitudes are cultivated at an early stage of

Table 5 Areas within psychiatry that may give rise to ethical or attitudinal problems

Areas	Examples
Confidentiality	Sharing information within multidisciplinary teams Sharing information with carers Balance between the patient's rights and the protection of others
Consent	Capacity for consent Using the Mental Health Act (1983)
Involvement of criminal justice system	Prosecution of the mentally ill Giving evidence in court
Problems with colleagues	Inappropriate behaviour Racist or sexist behaviour

medical training and formally assessed in clinical examinations. There are many ethical and attitudinal problems that arise in psychiatry or in relation to the treatment of the mentally ill. Some of these are summarized in Table 5.

It is important to be aware of the medico-legal framework in which doctors work (Chapter 15), and of relevant guidelines that help doctors to shape their practice (*Good Medical Practice*, General Medical Council, 1998). It is also important to be able to think problems through in a calm and logical manner. There is rarely a right or wrong answer and, if in doubt, the doctor should always seek advice from senior colleagues. Legal advice is usually available from Trust solicitors and other organizations such as indemnifying bodies (the Medical Defence Union or the Medical Protection Society), the General Medical Council or the Mental Health Act Commission.

Further reading and sources

Byrne P 2001 Psychiatric stigma. British Journal of Psychiatry, 178: 281–284

Department of Health 1990 The Care Programme Approach Health Circular ((90)23/LASSL(90)11). Department of Health, London

Department of Health 2000 Modernising the Care Programme Approach. A Policy Booklet. Department of Health, London

General Medical Council 1998 Good medical practice. General Medical Council, London

O'Brien J, Barber B 2000 Neuroimaging in dementia and depression. Advances in Psychiatric Treatment 6: 109–119

Assessment and clinical management of risk of harm to other people. Royal College of Psychiatrists Special Working Party on Clinical Assessment and Management of Risk 1996 (*Council Report 53*). Royal College of Psychiatrists, London

Sources

Royal College of Psychiatrists www.rcpsych.ac.uk/campaigns/cminds Campaign: changing minds.

Royal College of Psychiatrists, 17 Belgrave Square, London SW1X 8PG

Self-assessment: questions

Multiple choice questions

1. The mental state examination:
   a. Reflects the past history of the patient's symptoms
   b. Should remain static throughout a patient's illness
   c. Should not include the patient's verbatim description of mood
   d. Begins with insight
   e. Gives an indication of the patient's current mental status

2. In the assessment of cognitive function:
   a. The serial 7s test is used to assess immediate memory
   b. The serial 3s test should be used to assess concentration in individuals with high-intelligence quotients.
   c. A seven-item name and address is used to assess long-term memory
   d. Registration is tested by asking the individual to remember his/her car registration number
   e. Most people of normal intelligence and average educational achievement can perform serial 7s in under 1 minute

3. The mini mental state examination:
   a. Is a detailed, precise measure of cognitive function
   b. Is used widely in psychiatric assessment
   c. Has a total score of 20
   d. Includes a test of visual spatial awareness
   e. Includes an assessment of orientation

4. In making sense of psychiatric case histories:
   a. Precipitating factors refer to factors that convey a vulnerability to developing psychiatric disorder
   b. Important maintaining factors include a lack of insight and good compliance with treatment
   c. A family history of psychiatric disorder is an important predisposing factor in most individuals who present with psychiatric illness
   d. The sudden discontinuation of medication is a common cause of relapse in patients with serious mental illness
   e. Drug abuse is a common precipitant of psychiatric illness

5. The following factors indicate high risk of violence to others in patients with psychiatric disorder
   a. Specific threats made by the patient
   b. Command hallucinations
   c. Expressed intention of acting on beliefs
   d. Poor compliance with treatment in a patient with a prior history of violence when psychotic
   e. Supportive family environment

6. The five key elements of the Care Programme Approach are:
   a. Systematic arrangements for assessing the health and social needs of people accepted into specialist mental health services
   b. The formation of a care plan that identifies the health and social care required from a variety of providers
   c. The appointment of a care coordinator to keep in close touch with the service user and to monitor and coordinate care
   d. The exclusion of the patient from key decision making
   e. No changes to the care plan

7. Most services for the mentally ill are:
   a. Provided by specialist hospital services
   b. Provided by community mental health teams
   c. Are based around a small, specific catchment area
   d. Multidisciplinary
   e. Drawn solely from health services

8. Magnetic resonance imaging:
   a. Is widely available
   b. Is inexpensive
   c. Does not use ionizing radiation
   d. Can be distressing for patients
   e. Can be used for serial monitoring

9. Before seeing a patient you should:
   a. Check whether the patient has a previous history of violence
   b. Prepare the interview room
   c. Be aware which way the door opens
   d. Inform staff where you will be seeing the patient
   e. Note where the alarm is in the room

10. If threatened by a patient during an interview you should:
    a. Hold your ground and argue your case
    b. Refuse any demands the patient makes
    c. Advise the patient to calm down
    d. Try to prolong the interview so you can bring it to a satisfactory resolution
    e. Take the blame for any grievances or complaints the patient has

Case history questions

History 1

> You are a student on a psychiatric firm. You are given a task of interviewing one of the patients on the ward, Mr Ahmed, and presenting an up-to-date mental state examination at the next ward round.

How would you go about this task in relation to maximizing your personal safety?

History 2

> You are a house officer. A patient you have admitted the previous night is ready for discharge. He was admitted following an episode of self-harm. He is assessed by the deliberate self-harm team, who arrange to see him at home the following day and offer to help him to link up with the addictions service as he is an opiate abuser. He asks you to prescribe methadone for him before he is discharged. You explain that you are unable to do this. He follows you into the treatment room, shuts the door and pulls a knife. He tells you to write him a prescription of methadone. He has stolen a prescription form. You try to reason with him, offer to discuss his wishes with him, if he puts down the knife. He becomes more agitated and threatening.

What do you do?

History 3

> A 25-year-old man presents to psychiatric services with an acute episode of schizophrenia. He has been living rough on the streets for the last 2 years. He abuses alcohol and also uses a variety of street drugs. He has suffered from schizophrenia since the age of 18 but has never engaged with services and often drifts from town to town. He had a difficult childhood, was sexually abused by his father and has no contact with his family. He is currently homeless and has no friends.

Describe what kind of care he requires and how this should be organized.

Objective structured clinical examinations (OSCE)

Stations 1 and 2 are based on the following standardized script for a simulated patient. In an examination, a sim-ulated patient would answer your questions based on this script. Ideally get a friend to read the script and then to answer your questions. If this is not available, list your history with notes on the type of question (open/closed) and the sequence.

Standardized script

You are 40 years old (DoB 11.6.1960), female and married with three children. The youngest is 18 years of age and they have all left home. You married young, when you were 17 years old. You and your husband have drifted apart over the last few years and have very little in common. You do not work outside the home. He is a postman.

You feel anxious and tense most of the time. You cannot relax and find it difficult to sit and watch television. Your stomach churns all the time, your bowels are a little loose and you feel on edge. You pick at your fingers. You feel tense across your shoulders and back. You are hyper-alert. You jump in response to sudden noises and cannot stand loud noise or music. Every type of noise seems louder to you than usual and you find it unbear-able. You worry about minor things. Examples of such worries include paying the milkman on time, paying other bills on time and worrying about being late for appointments. You worry that something dreadful will happen to your children and often wake in the night feeling panicky and scared. If your husband is late home from work, you worry he has been killed in a car crash. Your anxiety started about 12 months ago after your youngest child left home. Since then you have felt lone-ly and isolated. You have thought of getting a job but could not consider it, while you feel so anxious.

You also experience panic attacks. These started about 6 months ago. You were shopping in the super-market, queuing to pay for food, when you suddenly became overwhelmed with fear. Your heart raced, you felt light-headed, you thought you were going to die. It lasted about 5 minutes. You had to leave your shopping and get out of the shop. Since then, you experience sim-ilar attacks, two or three times per week. You dread going out alone and have avoided going to supermar-kets. You try to avoid going out as much as possible and have been spending more and more time indoors. The thought of going out now makes you feel sick and pan-icky. Panic attacks are precipitated by crowded places, the thought of having to go out and being in enclosed spaces. You have occasional panics at home but most occur outside the home. In between attacks, you feel tense and worried. Your symptoms are relieved if some-one accompanies you shopping or goes out with you.

You have difficulty getting off to sleep. You stay up until 2.00 a.m. but then get off to sleep. You then sleep through. You feel tired all the time but cannot relax or have a nap during the day. You have lost about 7 lb in weight and cannot settle to eat or enjoy your food. You find it difficult to concentrate sometimes and cannot settle to read the paper or watch TV. If asked about current affairs, report something accurately that you have heard on the news. If asked about the speed of your thoughts, say they seem a little speeded up. You have the sensation of thoughts whizzing round your brain.

You do not

- feel depressed
- have suicidal ideation or thoughts of self-harm
- experience changes in mood during the day
- feel you do not want to see people; you would like to see your friends but are prevented from doing this by the panic attacks, you are pleased when people visit you or take you out shopping
- have compulsions to clean the house or fears about dirt or cleanliness
- have the sense of resisting the worries you experience
- lose your sense of humour; you can still joke about things
- feel anyone is putting thoughts into your mind or trying to control you.

Behaviour during the interview Throughout the interview, try to appear nervous and fidgety. Sit forward in your chair, change position frequently. Look worried. Try not to smile. Speak quickly and try to inject a tone of concern in your voice. If the candidate starts to ask you a lot of very specific closed questions, look ruffled and become unsure of your answers. Try to keep talking as much as possible and speak quickly. Make a lot of intense eye contact with the candidate.

The candidate may ask you to comply with various tasks regarding memory and concentration. Complete these tasks as you would normally. Say, however, while you are doing them, that you feel anxious and you're sure you're not doing them correctly. In other words, appear anxious but carry out the tests without any mistakes.

If the candidate asks you what you make of your problems, tell the candidate that after talking with your GP you realise you are ill and need help. You've not been like this before and you can't pull yourself out of it. Initially you felt silly and stupid but now you realise you are suffering from anxiety and need help.

Station 1

Take a history of the presenting complaint from this 40-year-old woman who is complaining of anxiety and an inability to relax. You have 10 minutes.

Station 2

Please present the history of the presenting complaint and the mental state examination of the patient you have just seen (described above). You have 10 minutes.

Station 3

You are a house officer. Your are on-call with your senior house officer (SHO). He begins to behave strangely. He starts shouting and ranting at one of the nurses on the ward. He is highly aroused and agitated. (He is usually a quiet, kind and thoughtful person.) He starts picking up notes and drawing pictures of fish on them. He picks up the medication chart of one patient and writes him up for double the dose of digoxin. He chuckles as he does this.

Describe what you would do.

Self-assessment: answers

Multiple choice answers

1. a. **False**. It reflects the patient's immediate mental state.
   b. **False**. It alters as the patient's condition changes.
   c. **False**. It should include the patient's own account of mood.
   d. **False**. It begins with appearance and behaviour.
   e. **True**.

2. a. **False**. Serial 7s is a test of concentration.
   b. **False**. Serial 3s are used if individuals have had a limited amount of schooling.
   c. **False**. Name and address is used to measure short-term memory.
   d. **False**. Registration is tested by asking someone to repeat the items of a name and address immediately after they have been told. Registration can also be tested by asking the patient to repeat three objects immediately after he/she has been told them.
   e. **True**. The vast majority of people can complete the task in under 30 seconds with no mistakes.

3. a. **False**. It is a relatively crude measure.
   b. **True**.
   c. **False**. The total score is 30.
   d. **True**. A figure is given for copying.
   e. **True**. It checks whether patients can say where they are.

4. a. **False**. Precipitating factors refer to factors that provoke the onset of illness or a sudden relapse.
   b. **False**. A lack of insight is usually associated with poor compliance with treatment, which would be an important maintaining factor.
   c. **True**.
   d. **True**. Sudden discontinuation of treatment is a common precipitating factor.
   e. **True**.

5. a. **True**. These must always be taken seriously.
   b. **True**.
   c. **True**.
   d. **True**.
   e. **False**. A supportive family environment is not a risk factor for violent behaviour in a patient with mental illness.

6. a. **True**.
   b. **True**.
   c. **True**.

d. **False**. The user/patient should be closely involved with all decisions about his/her treatment.
   e. **False**. The plan should be regularly reviewed and changed with agreement.

7. a. **False**.
   b. **True**.
   c. **True**.
   d. **True**.
   e. **False**. Services are usually made up of health service and social service staff.

8. a. **False**. It is only available in certain centres.
   b. **False**. It is expensive.
   c. **True**.
   d. **True**. It is noisy and can provoke feelings of panic.
   e. **True**.

9. a. **True**. Check with nursing staff and records.
   b. **True**. Create a good environment, with comfortable chairs at an angle, sit closer to the door.
   c. **True**. This avoids the potential problem of being trapped behind the opening door.
   d. **True**. You should summarize information at the end and allow the patient time to add information.
   e. **True**.

10. a. **False**. Do not disagree or argue with the patient.
    b. **False**. Agree to the patient's demands if it means you can leave the room safely.
    c. **False**. Never tell someone to calm down.
    d. **False**. Try to end the interview as quickly as possible.
    e. **False**. Never draw criticism onto yourself in the company of a patient who is angry and threatening you.

Case history answers

History 1

You need to ask the consultant or registrar (or other relevant staff) about safety issues in relation to this patient. Does he have a history of violence? Has he been disturbed or aggressive whilst an inpatient?

You need to establish from nursing staff whether it is safe to interview him alone. Ask what he has been like that morning. Check whether he is sexually or socially disinhibited.

You need to find an interview room. Establish where the alarm button is in the room. Arrange two comfortable chairs, slightly at an angle to each other. Make sure the alarm button is easily accessible from the chair you will sit in. Make sure you are seated nearest the door and would be able to get out of the room quickly.

Inform the nursing staff you are going to see Mr Ahmed and take him to the interview room, if he agrees to be interviewed. Let them know roughly how long you will be.

Approach Mr Ahmed. Introduce yourself, explain the purpose of your request. Get his permission to be interviewed. Accompany him to the interview room. Make sure he sits in the chair furthest away from the door.

History 2

You ask how much methadone he wants and write the prescription. You give it to him. You let him leave. When you are sure he has gone, you inform the hospital pharmacy you have been forced to give a prescription under duress. You inform hospital security and ask them to go to pharmacy. You then inform the police. If possible, charges should be brought against this man. You inform the deliberate self-harm team and his GP, that this man is dangerous and is carrying a knife. You discuss the incident with your consultant and complete a violent incident form. You allow yourself some time and space to talk about it with friends and family. The incident should trigger a meeting between the ward managers and your consultant to review safety issues on the ward.

History 3

This man will access services at a single point and receive an emergency assessment from one member of the local community mental team. He will probably require admission to hospital and neuroleptic drug treatment. He will be placed on the enhanced level of the Care Programme Approach because he has complex needs, has mental health problems coexisting with substance misuse, will require help from a number of agencies and has failed to engage with services in the past. He will be appointed a care coordinator who will be his main contact with services. An agreed care plan will be drawn up, in discussion with him, which will identify his health and social needs. It will include interventions to address: mental illness, substance misuse, homelessness, poverty, lack of educational achievement, lack of daily structured activity, lack of social support, diet and physical welfare. It will be

signed by his care coordinator and himself. His care coordinator will liaise closely with different members of the multidisciplinary team and other agencies to ensure his needs are met.

OSCE answers

Station 1 answer

Your history-taking should cover the main points outlined below and you would be marked on how well you achieved the objectives in each section. If you were able to take a history from a simulated patient, check how many of these objectives you achieved.

Communication skills
- Introduction: introduced self, asked patient her name
- Consent: asked permission to interview in a way that gave the patient a choice
- Listening skills: listened to what the patient was saying. Did not ask any unnecessary questions about information that the patient had already volunteered
- Style of questioning: used open questions, facilitation (either verbal or non-verbal) to elicit information before moving to closed questions
- Picked up patient's verbal and non-verbal cues
- Summarization: used it intermittently and at the end to clarify all the information that had been obtained
- Responded to patient's concerns and anxiety
- Structured interview appropriately: gave patient warning about the ending, invites questions from patient, ends appropriately.

Content
- Focused upon main symptoms of anxiety and panics before moving to other symptoms or factors
- Elicited a clear description of anxiety
- Elicited a clear description of the panic attacks
- Clarified that the patient suffered from continuous anxiety in addition to panic attacks (i.e. generalized anxiety disorder plus panic disorder)
- Elicited the correct timing and frequency of attacks and the onset of the generalized anxiety
- Elicited symptoms of avoidance
- Identified exacerbating and relieving factors
- Specifically asked questions to exclude depression and self-harm
- Elicited the patient's perceptions and concerns

Station 2 answer

You should have structured your answer as follows:

History

- Starts with name, date of birth, marital status and occupation
- Describes main problem as a 12-month history of generalized anxiety
- Accurately describes main features (tense all the time, unable to relax, hypervigilance, startle response, irrational worries, stomach churning, diarrhoea, muscle stiffness across shoulders)
- Describes 6-month history of panic attacks
- Accurately describes frequency
- Accurately describes main features (sudden increase in anxiety, palpitations, light-headedness, fear of dying)
- Identifies the pattern of avoidance that has subsequently developed
- Identifies potential precipitating factor (final child leaving home)
- Correctly identifies associated symptoms (loss of weight, initial insomnia, poor appetite)
- Correctly identifies important negatives (i.e. excludes depression).

Mental state examination (MSE)

- Structure the mental state examination in the correct order, beginning with appearance and behaviour and ending with insight.
- Present mental state in a competent and efficient manner.
- Accurately assesses each part of the MSE as detailed below.

Appearance and behaviour Describes patient as a middle-aged woman, dressed appropriately in slacks and a cardigan, well groomed, good personal hygiene and no make-up.

Comment on:
- facial appearance: tense, furrowed brow, anxious expression
- eye contact: prolonged
- body language: socially and sexually appropriate but restless and fidgety, sitting on the edge of the chair.

Speech

Comment on:
- rate: slightly faster than normal
- intonation: worried inflexion in speech
- form: normal.

Mood and affect

Comment on:
- subjective experience: describe patient's experience in patient's own words
- objective appearance: tense and anxious.

Thoughts

Comment on:
- form: normal

- speed: subjective sense of thoughts speeded up
- content: irrational worries and fears
- important negatives: no suicidal ideation, no delusions, distinguishes worries from obsessional ideas.

Perception

Comment on:
- heightened sense of perceptual experience
- important negatives: no hallucinations or illusions.

Cognitive assessment

Comment on:
- orientation of patient: fully orientated for time, place and person
- conscious and alert
- concentration: tested by serial 7s as normal
- registration and short-term memory: tested by seven-item name and address as normal (candidate describes procedure)

Insight Describes patient as having full insight into her condition.

Station 3 answer

This is a difficult situation. The candidate should demonstrate a thoughtful and logical approach to the problem. There are several different aspects of this situation that need to be considered.

1. The first element concerns the house officer's responsibility for the welfare of patients on the ward. The SHO is behaving in a manner that could endanger patients. The situation needs to be dealt with immediately.
2. The second element concerns the safety and welfare of the SHO. He is unwell. The nature of his illness is unclear but could include a psychiatric problem, a substance misuse problem or a physical problem, although the last is unlikely.
3. The third element concerns a regard for other staff. The SHO has verbally abused one of the nursing staff and may abuse others, if action is not taken.
4. The fourth element concerns the immediate management of the situation. The house officer should first try to talk to the SHO to see if he can be persuaded to leave the ward and go off duty. If possible, he should be persuaded to see the on-call psychiatrist. If the SHO refuses a psychiatric assessment, the house officer will have to make a judgement as to whether his behaviour will put him at risk if he is allowed to leave the hospital. He should seek advice from his consultant and the duty psychiatrist as to whether he needs to arrange for

security to detain the SHO, so that he can receive a psychiatric assessment.

5. The fifth element involves confidentiality. The house officer or ward manager has a responsibility to inform the managers of the hospital and the consultant about the SHO's behaviour as it has potentially endangered patients. There is not a medico-legal issue of confidentiality as the SHO is not the patient of anyone on the ward. However, the house officer may feel conflict as he may perceive his actions as going behind his colleague's back.

3 Mood disorders

Overview

Depression is a common disorder that affects about 15% of the population at some time in their lives. It is characterized by a pervasive and persistent lowering of mood, sleep disturbance, lowering of appetite and weight loss. It is not the same as unhappiness and is not a state people can 'snap out of'. It is twice as common in females than in males. People with severe depression have a high risk of suicide and it is important they receive appropriate treatment. Severe depressive disorders are best treated with antidepressant medication, while moderate-to-mild disorders can be treated with either psychological treatments or antidepressants, or a combination of both.

Bipolar affective disorder has a lifetime prevalence of about 0.5%. It is characterized by discrete episodes of depression and mania, between which the person usually returns to normal. It usually begins in the early twenties and there is evidence of a strong genetic component. Treatment usually consists of prophylactic treatment with lithium carbonate and specific treatment of the manic or depressive phases.

3.1 Depression

Learning objectives

You should:

- know about the epidemiology of depression and its genetic and social causes
- know the monoamine theory of major depression
- be able to ask about and identify symptoms of depression
- be able to identify psychotic depression
- understand the treatment of depression including severe and psychotic depression
- know the normal pattern of bereavement and how to identify depression in the bereaved
- know the key features of seasonal affective disorder.

Depression is common in primary care and the general hospital. It often goes unrecognized. It is not difficult to recognize but can present disguised as physical symptoms or problems with fatigue or memory, as shown in Box 27.

Epidemiology

Clinically significant depression is called depressive illness or major depression. Major depression used to be called 'endogenous' depression and milder (or minor) depression used to be called 'reactive' depression, with the assumption that it was secondary to life stresses. In fact, life events are important in all forms of depression.

The prevalence of major depression in community surveys in the UK is about 4% in men and 8% in women. The lifetime risk, or the proportion of people who will suffer one or more episodes of major depression at some time in their life, is about 15%. Rates increase with age and are higher in urban areas. Suicide rates in major depression are about 10% over the long term.

Causes

Predisposing causes

There is a genetic predisposition to major depression, as shown by increased rates in first-degree relatives and

---

Box 27
Traps for the unwary: how depression can present in disguise in primary care

- Headache: 'tension headache', which is bilateral, frontal, band-like
- Other pain disorders:
  — atypical chest pain
  — low back pain
  —atypical facial pain
- Fatigue
- Weight loss
- Poor memory

higher concordance rates in monozygotic compared with dizygotic twins. No single major gene has yet been shown to be involved. It is likely that there are many genes each of small effect.

Social and environmental predisposing factors include:

- historical factors: early maternal death, parental neglect, a long period of separation from a parent during childhood, childhood sexual abuse
- current factors: unemployment, lack of a confiding relationship.

Precipitating causes

Major depression can arise out of the blue, particularly in people with a genetic predisposition. Usually, however, it follows one or more stressful life events, particularly where there are predisposing factors. So-called 'loss' life events are especially important, such as bereavement, being made redundant or the break up of a relationship. So-called 'threat' life events are more likely to give rise to anxiety disorders. Physical illness and childbirth are also important precipitating factors.

Biochemical factors

The monoamine theory of depression states that reduced availability of the monoamine serotonin (5-hydroxytryptamine; 5HT) and, to a lesser extent, noradrenaline (norepinephrine) is important in the pathogenesis of depression. Evidence for this includes the finding of reduced levels of metabolites of these neurotransmitters in the cerebrospinal fluid and urine of depressed patients and reduced serotonin in the postmortem brains of suicide victims. The mechanism of action of antidepressant drugs is based on their ability to increase synaptic serotonin and noradrenaline (norepinephrine) (Ch. 17 says more about this). Endocrine changes can also be shown in severely depressed patients: increased plasma cortisol and reduced thyroid-releasing hormone.

Symptoms of depression

The symptoms of depression can be remembered as falling into three main groups: mood and motivation, biological and cognitive (Box 28). How to ask about important symptoms at interview is shown in Table 6.

Mood and motivation symptoms

There are feelings of *sadness*, often with increased *tearfulness*. The person often feels they are unable to cheer up and enjoy things they once did, such as being with friends or watching TV; this loss of pleasure is called *anhedonia*. *Loss of interest* in family, friends and hobbies

---

> **Box 28**
> Key symptoms of depressive disorder
>
> **Mood and motivation symptoms**
> Persistently lowered mood (may be worse in the morning)
> Diminished interest or pleasure in almost all activities
> Social withdrawal
> Loss of energy
> Poor concentration
>
> **Biological symptoms**
> Significant weight loss when not dieting
> Sleep disturbance most days (either initial insomnia or early morning waking)
> Retardation or agitation
> Decreased sex drive
>
> **Cognitive changes**
> Depressive ideation: feelings of guilt, worthlessness, self-blame
> Suicidal thoughts
> Hopelessness

occurs, with *social withdrawal*. People often describe increased *irritability* and snappiness at home. The person reports *low energy* and also *poor concentration*, which can result in absent mindedness and forgetfulness for everyday recent events. Anxiety symptoms, worrying and panic attacks can occur in depression.

Cognitive symptoms

Low mood leads to a deterioration in how people come to think about themselves. This involves inappropriately negative thoughts about the past (*guilt, regrets* and *self-blame*), about the present (*low self-esteem, worthlessness*) and about the future (*pessimism, hopelessness, thoughts of dying* and *suicidal ideas*).

Biological symptoms

Biological symptoms (also called vegetative symptoms) are markers of moderately severe depression and are less evident in milder depressive states (Table 7):

- loss of appetite and weight
- loss of sex drive
- early morning waking: this characteristic symptom involves waking in the early hours of the morning, often 4 or 5 a.m. and being unable to get back to sleep.
- diurnal variation of mood, such that mood is worse in the morning and slowly lifts in the evening.
- non-specific physical symptoms such as tension headache, back pain and atypical chest can also occur.

Very severe depression

In very severe depression, the following features can appear:

Table 6 Depression: asking about symptoms

Symptom	Question
Low mood	How are you feeling in your spirits, in your mood?
Tearfulness	Do you find yourself in tears?
Anhedonia	Can you cheer up sometimes? Do you enjoy the things you used to?
Loss of interest	Are you able to keep interests going?
Fatigue	How is your energy level?
Poor concentration	How is your concentration on things? Can you read the paper or watch TV and take it in?
Irritability	Are you more snappy than usual?
Panic attacks	Do you get panicky at all?
Tension headache	Do you get headaches or other pains?
Diurnal variation of mood	Is your mood worse at any particular time of day?
Initial insomnia. Early morning waking	How is your sleep? Are you able to get to sleep? Do you stay asleep?
Loss of appetite and weight	What about your appetite? Has your weight changed?
Loss of libido	How is your sex drive?
Guilt, self blame	Do you find yourself blaming yourself or regretting things?
Worthlessness, low self-esteem	How do you view yourself, in comparison with others?
Pessimism, hopelessness	How do you see the future?
Thoughts of dying	Step 1: are there ever times when you feel you just want to go to sleep and never wake up?
Suicidal ideation	If yes to Step 1, then Step 2: Have you thought of taking your own life?

Table 7 Biological features in depression

	Mild depression	Moderate-to-severe depression
Sleep	Difficulty getting to sleep (initial insomnia)	Early morning waking
Appetite	Unchanged or increased	Decreased
Weight	Unchanged or increased	Loss
Libido	Unchanged or reduced	Reduced
Daily variation in mood	Worse in the evening	Worse in the morning (diurnal mood variation)

- *Psychomotor retardation*: the person is aware of thinking slowly, and at interview their speech and movements are perceptibly slowed up. In the most severe cases, the patient stops speaking (becomes *mute*) and becomes immobile (a *depressive 'stupor'*).
- *Delusions and hallucinations*: so-called *psychotic depression*. These will have a depressive content to them and can be thought of as extreme versions of the negative cognitions. Delusions can be persecutory, hypochondriacal (the person believes they have cancer), nihilistic (the person believes the world is about to end) or of guilt (the person believes they are to blame for dreadful events). Auditory hallucinations can be of voices insulting the person or saying he/she is evil.

Management of depression

History-taking will include alcohol and drug use and psychosocial history with evidence for supportive relationships. Suicidal risk assessment is important. Physical investigations will include eosinophil sedimentation rate (ESR) and thyroid function and, in older patients, chest X ray and computed tomographic (CT) scan. Major depression is usually treated with antidepressant drugs (Ch. 17); these will be effective in 70%. Cognitive behaviour therapy, interpersonal therapy and psychodynamic interpersonal therapy are also used, if available (Ch. 16). Psychosocial interventions will be important to relieve ongoing stresses of relationship difficulties, financial problems or housing difficulties. In severe depression, antidepressants are superior to psychological treatments and should always be considered as the first-line treatment.

If there is no response to first-line treatment with full dosage antidepressant for 6 weeks, the next step is to change to another class of antidepressant drug, after checking compliance. Maintaining factors such as underlying organic illness or continuing psychosocial stresses must be checked. Adding lithium to antidepressant drug treatment will be effective in some patients.

For severe depression or high suicidal risk, inpatient admission may be needed. Psychotic depression will also need antipsychotic drug treatment, with ECT (electroconvulsive therapy) if no improvement is made.

Special types of depression

Bereavement

A normal grief reaction following the death of a close relative or spouse lasts up to 6 months. There are usually three stages.

1. Shock, with a feeling of numbness and unreality, usually lasting a few days
2. Sadness, with tearfulness and loss of sleep and appetite, sometimes along with anger or guilt at not having been able to do more. Illusions or fleeting hallucinations of hearing or seeing the deceased person around the house can occur and are normal.
3. Acceptance.

Bereavement reactions can be abnormal, for instance if they continue for longer than 6 months, are especially severe or have unusual symptoms. Abnormal bereavement reactions are more likely if the death was unexpected, if the relationship with the deceased was itself abnormal or if the normal grieving process is interrupted. Management of abnormal bereavement may involve use of antidepressant drugs or cognitive behaviour therapy.

Seasonal affective disorder

Seasonal affective disorder (SAD) is an uncommon subtype of major depression where episodes occur as daylength shortens. Melatonin appears to be involved. Exposure to bright artificial light (phototherapy) has been shown to be an effective treatment.

3.2 Bipolar affective disorder

Learning objectives

You should:

- know the definition, epidemiology and causes of bipolar disorder
- know the symptoms of mania
- know about the management of acute mania
- know about the long-term management of bipolar disorder

Bipolar affective disorder used to be called *manic depressive psychosis*. It is a disorder characterized by episodes of major depression and, at other times, mania, where mood is abnormally elated. The terms mania and hypomania mean the same. In some cases, there will never be a depressive episode and the disorder will be recurrent episodes of mania; this is still called bipolar disorder. Between episodes, the person returns to their normal self, usually with good insight into the previous episode. After a first manic episode, the risk of recurrence is about 70%.

Epidemiology

Bipolar affective disorder has a lifetime prevalence of about 0.5%, with men and women equally affected. Mean age at first onset is in the twenties, although the first episode is occasionally in late life. In some people, the disorder is preceded by long-standing mild mood swings, called *cyclothymic disorder*.

Causes

Predisposing causes

Bipolar disorder has a strong genetic component. A family history of bipolar disorder and major depression is common. The concordance rate in monozygotic twins is approximately 50% and it rises to 80% if major depression in the co-twin is counted as well as bipolar disorder.

Precipitating causes

Stressful life events are important in triggering both manic and depressive episodes. Childbirth can be a precipitant. Street drug use, including cannabis, is often a precipitant of manic episodes. Sometimes a first manic episode can be triggered by antidepressant drug treatment or the use of drugs such as steroids.

Symptoms

The depressive episodes in bipolar disorder are the same as in major depression. Mania has a characteristic history. The symptoms may come on after a stressful event or street drug use. Usually, there will be history of increasingly elated mood for a few days or weeks, sometimes with irritability. The person will be more and more talkative and energetic, needing less and less sleep. They will often develop grandiose plans and spend increasing amounts of money. They can become sexually disinhibited. Table 8 shows the key features of mania, grouped according to the different categories of the mental state examination.

Management

A detailed history is required, including family history and drug history. It is sometimes impossible to take a full history from someone with mania, and an account by an informant who knows the patient is important. Acute mania often needs inpatient admission because of the behavioural disturbance. The patient may be at risk of harming himself/herself (e.g. may try to jump off a building because of delusions of being able to fly) or of being exploited or harmed by others (may be mugged, or persuaded to engage in sexual activity which, when well, would be abhorrent to the person). Lack of insight may necessitate formal admission under the Mental Health Act. Physical investigations will include thyroid function to exclude hyperthyroidism. Drug treatment initially will usually involve antipsychotic drugs, with a

Table 8 Symptoms of mania grouped according to the categories of the mental state examination

Category	Symptoms
Appearance	May be dishevelled, unshaven; clothes and make-up may be bright and bizarre
Behaviour	Often restless and overactive; socially disinhibited, with overfamiliarity
Speech	*Pressure of speech*: increased rate and difficult to interrupt; may develop *flight of ideas*, with non-stop ideas connected by puns and rhymes ('clangs')
Mood	Elated and grandiose; often irritable
Thoughts	Describes *pressure of thought*, with accelerated thinking
Abnormal experiences	Auditory hallucinations can occur, with grandiose themes
Abnormal beliefs	Delusions can occur, either *persecutory* or *grandiose*, of grandiose identity (e.g. being royalty) or ability (e.g. having supernatural powers)
Cognitive state	Normal, although may show impaired attention span with *distractibility*
Self-appraisal	Insight is usually lost in acute mania

short-acting benzodiazepine for sedation if needed. After remission, management continues using the Care Programme Approach (Ch. 2), with a named care coordinator to organize the care package. Unlike schizophrenia, remission is usually complete and the care package may be fairly simple and short lived. The person can be expected to return to work. Long-term lithium treatment should be considered if the person has had two or more manic episodes (Ch. 17).

Further reading and sources

Blackwood DH, Visscher PM, Muir WJ 2001 Genetic studies of bipolar affective disorder in large families. British Journal of Psychiatry, 178 (Suppl 41): S134–S136

Bonanno GA, Kaltman S 2001 The varieties of grief experience. Clinical and Psychological Review, 21: 705–734

Burgess S, Geddes J, Hawton K, Townsend E, Jamison K, Goodwin G 2001 Lithium for maintenance treatment of mood disorders (Cochrane Review). In: The Cochrane Library, Vol. 3. Update Software, Oxford

Goodnick PJ, Chaudry T, Artadi J, Arcey S 2000 Women's issues in mood disorders. Expert Opinions in Pharmacotherapy, 1: 903–916

Sachs GS, Koslow CL, Ghaemi SN 2000 The treatment of bipolar depression. Bipolar Disorders, 2: 256–260

von Korff M, Katon W, Unutzer J, Wells K, Wagner EH 2001 Improving depression care: barriers, solutions, and research needs [review]. Journal of Family Practice, 50: E1

Sources

American Psychiatric Association. Useful resource site for information about books, journal articles, etc. www.psych.org

Mental Health Net – Depression treatment. Gives details of the treatment of depression. mentalhelp.net

NDMDA (National Depression and Manic Depression Association). Gives an explanation of these conditions and an overview of treatments. www.ndmda.org

Self-assessment: questions

Multiple choice questions

1. In moderately severe major depression:
   a. Mood worsening during the day is usual
   b. Concentration is usually impaired
   c. Tearfulness is uncommon
   d. Psychomotor retardation may be present
   e. Antidepressant drug treatment is unlikely to work

2. In mania:
   a. 'Knights move' thinking can be seen
   b. Recovery is often incomplete
   c. A family history of depression is common
   d. Insight is usually good
   e. Most people will have a further episode after the first

3. Depression:
   a. Is more common in men than women
   b. Occurs in about 15% of all people
   c. Does not have a strong genetic component
   d. Is the same as mania
   e. Has association with increased libido

4. Antidepressant medication:
   a. Is effective in about one quarter of all those with severe depression
   b. Should never be used in conjunction with lithium
   c. Should be tried for several weeks before deciding whether or not it is effective
   d. Never precipitates mania
   e. Is better than psychological treatment for patients with severe depressive disorders

5. The following are aetiological factors of depression:
   a. Schizoid personality
   b. Family history of schizophrenia
   c. Family history of bipolar affective disorder
   d. Parental neglect
   e. Treatment with steroid medication

Case history questions

History 1

Peter is a married 48-year-old teacher. He had an episode of depression when 25 years of age. He presents now to his GP with a 3-month history of low mood and energy, tearfulness, headaches, early morning waking and weight loss of 5 kg.

1. What aspects of the history are particularly important to clarify at this interview, with regard to management?
2. What physical investigations would you do?
3. What is the probable cause of the headaches? What clinical characteristics would you look for?

History 2

A 33-year-old woman is brought to the A&E department of an inner city hospital. She has been mugged. She had drawn all her savings out of her bank account and had brought the money to the hospital to give it to staff, as she thought they were doing such a wonderful job. She was mugged just outside the hospital by two men who snatched her bag. She sustained bruises to her face and back but was otherwise unhurt. While waiting to be seen, she kept pacing backwards and forwards, smiled to herself and occasionally sang. She kept saying that all nurses were angels and commenting how handsome the male doctors were, who worked in the department. In her past history, she had suffered two previous episodes of severe depression, which had been treated with antidepressants and ECT. Her last episode of depression was 4 years ago and she was not taking any medication.

1. What is the likely diagnosis?
2. What is the most appropriate treatment?

History 3

Mary is a 45-year-old married woman who works in a local supermarket. She has two daughters, who are in their twenties and have recently left home. Her husband died suddenly of a heart attack 18 months ago, at the age of 53. She lost her own mother when she was 9 years old, through breast cancer, and her father was killed in a road traffic accident when she was 23. She has felt desperately unhappy since her husband's death and has found it difficult to cope. She has lost 2 stone in weight and has been unable to go into work for the last 2 months because she feels so tired. She does not socialize and has lost touch with many of her friends. She spends her evenings looking at pictures of her dead husband. She feels low all the time, and his death seems as painful to her now as it was when it happened 18 months ago. She does not sleep well and feels anxious most of the time.

1. Is this a normal grief reaction?
2. Are there any important predisposing factors?
3. What kind of help does she need?

Self-assessment: answers

Multiple choice answers

1. a. **False**. Mood is usually worse in the morning.
   b. **True**.
   c. **False**. Tearfulness is very common.
   d. **True**.
   e. **False**. Antidepressants are more likely to have beneficial effects in moderate-to-severe depression than in more milder depressive states.

2. a. **False**. This is more likely to be seen in schizophrenia.
   b. **False**. Recovery is usually complete.
   c. **True**.
   d. **False**.
   e. **True**. Risk of recurrence is 70%.

3. a. **False**. More common in women.
   b. **True**.
   c. **False**.
   d. **False**. Mood is elevated in mania.
   e. **False**. There is decreased libido.

4. a. **False**. It is effective in about 70%.
   b. **False**. This is a powerful combination in treatment of resistant depression.
   c. **True**. Treatment is required for about 6 weeks.
   d. **False**. It can precipitate mania in susceptible individuals.
   e. **True**.

5. a. **False**. It predisposes to schizophrenia.
   b. **False**. It predisposes to schizophrenia.
   c. **True**. It predisposes to depression as well as bipolar affective disorder.
   d. **True**.
   e. **True**.

Case history answers

History 1

1. A history of a stressful life event is important to assess. Alcohol history is important. In the psychiatric history, what treatment worked for the previous episode. Assessment of suicidal ideation is crucial and the existence of a supportive relationship is important to assess.
2. Full blood count, eosinophil sedimentation rate (ESR), electrolytes and urea, thyroid function. If clinically indicated, chest radiograph.
3. It is likely to be a tension headache, with the following features: tight, band-like pain around the head or over the eyes, bilateral, responds poorly to minor analgesics.

History 2

1. The most likely diagnosis is hypomania in the context of bipolar affective disorder. She has had two previous episodes of depression, so her diagnosis, prior to this most recent episode, would have been unipolar depressive disorder. This diagnosis now has to be revised in the light of her manic episode.
2. She is at risk of being exploited by others and has already lost her life savings. She needs to be in a protected environment until the illness is controlled. She would be offered admission to hospital. She would initially be treated with haloperidol and then started on lithium treatment (this is her third affective episode: two depressive and one manic).

History 3

1. This woman has a depressive illness in the context of an abnormal grief reaction. She has biological symptoms of depression. The grief reaction is abnormal because there is no evidence of any adjustment following her husband's death. After 18 months, there should be clear evidence of her beginning to function again. Instead, her level of functioning is deteriorating.
2. The most important predisposing factor is the loss of her mother when she was a child. This makes her more vulnerable to developing depression when an adult.
3. She requires treatment for her depression with antidepressants and may require psychological treatment to help her to adjust to her husband's death.

4 Anxiety disorders

Overview

Normal worry provides an important function in motivating people to solve dilemmas or problems (Ch. 1). Excessive worry or problematic worrying, however, becomes disabling and counter-productive. Problematic worries, in comparison with normal worries, are more intense and uncontrollable. They are more likely to concern ideas about illness, health or injury, and such concerns result in distress and dysfunction. Anxiety disorders are states of mind characterized by excessive or problematic worrying, as a consequence of which, individuals become distressed or dysfunctional. The main disorders include panic disorder, agoraphobia, generalized anxiety disorder, simple phobias, social phobia, obsessional compulsive disorder and post-traumatic stress disorder. The main features of each disorder are summarized in Table 9. There is much overlap between these conditions, and comorbidity for depression is high. The disorders are usually treated using cognitive-behavioural techniques and/or antidepressant treatment. Different techniques are used for different types of disorder. These are described in more detail in Chapter 16.

4.1 Panic disorder and agoraphobia

Learning objectives

You should:

- know the main features of panic disorder
- be able to distinguish panic disorder from organic disease
- know the main features of agoraphobia
- be familiar with the main treatment approaches.

Panic disorder

Panic disorder is characterized by the presence of recurrent and unexpected panic attacks. The features of a panic attack are described in Box 29. In addition, to those symptoms, approximately two thirds of people with panic disorder show evidence of hyperventilation prior to a panic attack. As they become more anxious, their breathing becomes rapid and shallow, and they blow off carbon dioxide, developing hypocapnia. This is associated with feelings of air hunger, sensations of suffocation and audible gasping. The individual develops lightheadedness and paraesthesiae. Not unreasonably, people become concerned and preoccupied with these experiences, and they may misinterpret their symptoms as being caused by physical illness. The most common concern usually involves heart disease. Chest pain in panic disorder however, is usually sharp in nature and lasts only a few minutes, whereas ischaemic cardiac pain is usually dull, crushing-like and lasts for longer. A subgroup of individuals hyperventilate in response to exercise. In this group,

---

Box 29
Features of a panic attack

A panic attack is an episode of intense fear or anxiety in which four or more of the following symptoms develop quickly and reach a peak within 10 minutes:

- palpitations (pounding of the heart, or an awareness the heart is beating fast)
- sweating
- trembling or shaking
- sensations of shortness of breath
- feeling of choking
- chest pain
- nausea
- dizziness
- derealization (a feeling as if everything around one is unreal) or depersonalization (a feeling of being detached from oneself)
- fear of losing control or going mad
- fear of dying
- paraesthesiae
- chills or hot flushes.

Table 9 Main features of the different anxiety disorders

Type of disorder	Main features
Panic disorder	Recurrent and unexpected panic attacks, with or without anxiety in between attacks
Agoraphobia	Fear or anxiety about being in public places or enclosed situations from which escape may be difficult
Generalized anxiety disorder	Excessive anxiety and worry
Specific phobia	Marked and persistent fear of specific objects or situations
Social phobia	Marked and persistent fear of social situations in which embarrassment may occur
Obsessive-compulsive disorder	Persistent, intrusive, unwanted thoughts or images that are difficult to ignore and are recognized by the person as their own. Associated ritualistic behaviour may develop
Post-traumatic stress disorder	Intrusive, recurrent thoughts or images of a traumatic experience, associated with avoidance of stimuli associated with the trauma

the partial pressure of carbon dioxide fails to rise during the first minute of exercise whereas in normal subjects it rises by about 5 mmHg in the first minute of exercise. These 'fail to rise' patients report previous episodes of chest pain that occur significantly more often on exercise, or with emotion, than in those with normal rises.

Many individuals change their behaviour in response to the attacks and give up work, or become fearful of going out alone in case they experience another attack. If this becomes severe, they may develop agoraphobia (see below), in addition to panic disorder. They may become preoccupied with concerns about physical disease and visit their doctor frequently.

Individuals with panic disorder often report constant or intermittent feelings of anxiety in between actual panic attacks. Depressive symptoms are also common, and approximately half of all people with panic disorder also have major depressive disorder.

Panic disorder is two to three times more common in women than men. The lifetime prevalence is 1.5–3.5% and, at any one time, 1–2% of the population will suffer from the condition. Single panic attacks are much more frequent and at least 20% of the population will experience at least one panic attack during their lives. Twin studies indicate that there is a considerable genetic component to the disorder and first-degree relatives of individuals with panic disorder have a four to seven times greater chance of developing the condition.

Panic disorder typically begins in young individuals (18–35 years), and its onset over the age of 45 years is unusual. The course of the disorder is variable, with some individuals experiencing chronic and persistent symptoms over many years, whereas others have short-lived discrete episodes, often precipitated by life stress.

Psychological interventions such as relaxation training, cognitive techniques and exposure are helpful. Antidepressants are also of benefit. If hyperventilation is present, a hyperventilation provocation test can be carried out to confirm that the patient's symptoms are partly caused by overbreathing. Box 30 shows how the hyperventilation provocation test should be carried out. This test should not be performed without close monitoring of

Box 30
Hyperventilation provocation test

1. The patient is asked to breathe at a rate of 30–40 breaths/minute for 3 minutes and then told to 'stop overbreathing'
2. After about 1 minute, the patient is asked how many symptoms were produced during and/or after overbreathing.

In a positive test, the patient experiences symptoms similar to or suggestive of their panic attacks; dizziness and paraesthesiae usually occur before chest pain. The patient may continue to hyperventilate for 5–10 minutes after the test has stopped.

If coexisting ischaemic heart disease is suspected, the test should only be performed in a hospital setting, with electrocardiograph monitoring and access to resuscitation facilities.

the patient's physical condition if there is a possibility that the patient has ischaemic heart disease or other relevant organic disorder, such as phaeochromocytoma.

Agoraphobia

The essential feature of agoraphobia is a fear or anxiety about being in places or situations from which escape may be difficult. The anxiety leads to avoidance of many social situations and the individual becomes increasingly restricted and 'imprisoned' in his/her own home. The condition often develops as a result of panic disorder. Typical fears include being outside the safety of the home, traveling on public transport, being in crowded places, or having to queue.

Exposure and desensitization are the most common treatment approaches. Cognitive therapy has also been used to good effect.

4.2 Generalized anxiety disorder

The main defining features of generalized anxiety disorder (GAD) is excessive anxiety and worry (apprehensive

Learning objectives

You should:

- know the main features of generalized anxiety disorder
- be familiar with the main treatment approaches.

expectation) occurring more days than not for at least 6 months and occurring about a number of events or activities (such as work or school performance). Other features include restlessness or feeling keyed up or on edge, being easily fatigued, difficulty concentrating or the mind going blank, irritability, muscle tension and sleep disturbance. For these symptoms to constitute a disorder, there must be evidence of significant distress or impairment in important areas of functioning. Patients with GAD overestimate the likelihood of unpleasant events happening to them.

The disorder usually begins in mid-teenage years, but patients often only present to services in their late twenties and thirties. Between 60 and 80% of patients will report having been anxious or worried all their lives. This reflects a consistently high level of trait anxiety. Behavioural techniques, such as exposure, are not helpful in GAD. Cognitive therapy, delivered by experienced therapists, shows good evidence of effectiveness. Two thirds to three quarters of patients show clinically significant improvement following treatment. Therapy should aim to identify, and modify, individual maintaining factors. It is usually unhelpful to focus upon a specific concern or worry as these fluctuate and change. Treatment should focus on commonalities such as ways of dealing with uncertainty, or ways of identifying and controlling worry.

4.3 Specific and social phobias

Learning objectives

You should:

- know the main features of specific phobias
- be aware of the main features of social phobia
- be familiar with the main treatment approaches for specific and social phobias.

Specific phobias

The essential feature of specific phobia is marked or persistent fear of specific, circumscribed objects or situations. Exposure to the feared object results in immediate anxiety or a frank panic attack. There is usually marked avoidance. The fear is considered to be excessive or unreasonable. Specific phobias are extremely common, and approximately 8% of the normal population have a diagnosable disorder. In many cases, however, the degree of impairment is insufficient to warrant treatment, and only 1% of the general population seek treatment. For example, an individual may be scared of snakes but live in a country or a region where such creatures are rare or non-existent. In these circumstances, the phobic condition will not result in significant disability. Specific phobias are twice as common in women than in men.

The most common types of phobia are:

- animal type: this usually begins in childhood and common feared objects are snakes, spiders, dogs, birds, various insects, mice and cats
- natural environment type: the fear is precipitated by aspects of the natural environment, e.g. storms, heights or water
- blood–injection–injury: the fear is cued by seeing blood or undergoing a medical procedure (e.g. dental examination)
- situational type: the fear is cued by specific forms of transportation including flying, crossing bridges, elevators, etc.
- other types: a miscellanous category.

Phobias that begin in childhood (commonly animal phobias) usually disappear or diminish with time. Phobias that begin in adult life tend to run a more chronic course. Where fears are specific and circumscribed, fairly brief interventions can be helpful. Most treatments use behavioural techniques, systematic desensitization and exposure techniques.

Social phobia

Social phobia is characterized by a marked and persistent fear of social situations in which embarrassment may occur. Individuals may worry that others will judge them to be foolish or stupid. Public speaking may be a particular problem. Exposure to social situations results in symptoms of anxiety, which may include blushing or diarrhoea. There may be a vicious cycle of anticipatory anxiety resulting in fearful cognitions and anxiety symptoms in the feared situation.

Fears of being embarrassed in public are common, particularly in young people. It is only appropriate to make a diagnosis if the avoidance and fear associated with social encounters, interferes significantly with the individual's daily routine, occupational activity or social life. Common associated features are:

- hypersensitivity to criticism
- negative evaluation

- low self-esteem
- feelings of inferiority
- lack of assertiveness
- poor social skills.

Estimates of the lifetime prevalence of social phobia ranges from 3 to 13%. Social phobia is more common in women than men, but more males than females are seen for treatment. At any one time, approximately 2% of the general population may suffer from the disorder. It occurs more frequently among first-degree biological relatives of those afflicted with the disorder compared with the general population, but little is known about its genetic profile.

Social phobia usually begins relatively early in life, during the teenage years, and tends to run a chronic course if not treated. The most common treatments include in vivo exposure and social skills training. Cognitive techniques can also be used to help with cognitive restructuring and to combat low self-esteem.

4.4 Obsessive-compulsive disorder

Learning objectives

You should:

- know the main features of obsessive-compulsive disorder
- be familiar with the main treatment approaches.

Obsessive-compulsive disorder (OCD) is characterized by persistent, intrusive, unwanted thoughts or images that the individual finds difficult to control or put out of his/her mind. The thoughts are usually unpleasant and are usually concerned with dirt, contamination, harm to others, sex or blasphemy. The individual recognizes that they are his/her own thoughts and usually tries to resist them. Obsessional doubts can also develop (e.g. thoughts that one has not locked the door of one's house, or one has left the gas cooker turned on) and people can experience obsessional images (e.g. unpleasant images of a sexual or violent nature).

As the thoughts persist, the individual may develop behaviours to try to reduce the anxiety and distress that they cause. For example, if the concerns are related to dirt or contamination, the individual may start to wash their hands repeatedly or engage in other repetitive cleaning behaviours. The individual's anxiety is temporarily relieved but soon returns. Sometimes individuals develop overwhelming urges to carry out some form of forbidden behaviour, e.g. shouting out in church 'God is a wanker'. The individual will be tortured by this compulsion but will invariably never act upon it.

The maintenance of the thoughts may be related to the way in which people appraise them. Individuals with an inflated sense of responsibility (i.e. feel that their action can result in harm to others) are at greater risk of the disorder continuing. Such people are likely to attend to the thoughts selectively, carry out neutralizing behaviours and generally feel bad about themselves: all of which serves to maintain the disorder.

In severe OCD, individuals can become completely crippled by the disorder. They may be unable to walk down a street because they have to keep carrying out checking behaviours, or they will spend the whole day cleaning the house because of their concerns with dirt or contamination. In moderate cases, the thoughts can be extremely distressing and the rituals can be time consuming (take more than 1 hour per day).

In addition to the core features of the disorder, individuals may develop avoidance behaviours (e.g. avoid dirty places or visiting other peoples' houses because of their preoccupation with dirt) or increase other kinds of behaviour (e.g. if their thoughts are related to illness, they may make frequent visits to the doctor). Depression and phobic disorders are also commonly associated with OCD and should be treated in their own right, if present. Substance misuse can also develop as a response to the distress of trying to cope with the disorder.

The estimated lifetime prevalence of OCD is approximately 2.5%, with a 1 year prevalence of 1% in males and 1.5% in females. The condition usually begins in adolescence or early adulthood. Onset is gradual. There is some evidence of a genetic component: there is greater concordance of OCD in monozygotic than dizygotic twins.

Psychological treatment for OCD usually involves a cognitive behavioural approach. If there are prominent rituals or compulsions, graded exposure and response prevention are used (Ch. 16). Cognitive strategies are useful for treating obsessional thoughts.

Treatment with SSRIs (selective serotonin reuptake inhibitors) can also be considered, followed by a trial of clomipramine if SSRIs fail. Patients with disabling OCD may require long-term treatment with antidepressant medication.

4.5 Post-traumatic stress disorder

Learning objectives

You should:

- know the main features of post-traumatic stress disorder
- be familiar with the main treatment approaches.

Box 31
Anxiety disorders in primary care

About one fifth of all patients who consult their GP each year are given a psychiatric diagnosis by the GP. The most common symptoms are those of anxiety followed by depression, fatigue and somatic symptoms. Very few of these patients are referred on to hospital services. Specific psychiatric conditions are less clear-cut in primary care and there is much overlap between depression and anxiety.

In the 1960s and 1970s, anxiolytic medication (initially barbiturates and later benzodiazepines) was used in large quantities to treat emotional disorders in primary care. In many cases, this resulted in dependency and a worsening of the underlying condition. Counselling and advice by GPs is as effective in treating anxiety symptoms as treatment with benzodiazepines, and it does not result in an increased demand on GPs' time. A proportion of patients will require specific psychological treatment, but anxiolytic medication should be avoided. Behavioural and cognitive techniques already described in relation to specific disorders in this chapter may be useful but are not always available. Counselling sessions from a practice counsellor may be helpful for specific emotional problems that are causing the anxiety. A relatively new psychological approach to treatment called problem solving may also be helpful (Ch. 16).

The essential feature of post-traumatic stress disorder (PTSD) is the development of a characteristic set of psychological symptoms following exposure to a serious, traumatic event that involved actual or threatened death, or actual or serious injury, to either the self or others. There are three main types of symptom. First, the person re-experiences the events with recurrent and intrusive thoughts, images, dreams or perceptions. Second, there is persistent avoidance of stimuli associated with the trauma, including deliberate efforts to avoid activities or places that provoke recollections of the event. This may also include a sense of detachment or estrangement from others. Third, there are persistent symptoms of increased arousal including sleep disturbance, irritability, poor concentration, hypervigilance and an exaggerated startle response.

The symptoms usually develop within 3 to 6 months of the trauma. The lifetime prevalence is about 1% but there is great variation from country to country. About 30–40% of women have been reported to develop PTSD following sexual assault, and about 20% of American Vietnam war veterans developed the disorder.

Although it has become fashionable to offer 'counselling' or 'debriefing' to victims immediately following a traumatic event, this can be harmful as it may interfere with, or disrupt, the person's normal methods of coping. Most individuals who experience trauma do not develop PTSD. Treatment should, however, be offered to individuals who do develop the syndrome. Cognitive-behavioural treatments for PTSD include anxiety management, exposure and additional cognitive techniques (including stress inoculation training). Antidepressants may also have beneficial effects.

Further reading and sources

Brewin CR 1996 Theoretical foundations of cognitive-behavior therapy for anxiety and depression. Annual Review of Psychology, **47**: 33–57

Foa EB, Meadows EA 1997 Psychosocial treatments for post-traumatic stress disorder: a critical review. Annual Review of Psychology, **48**: 449–480

James I, Blackburn, I-M 1997 Psychological approaches to anxiety disorders. Current Opinion in Psychiatry, **10**: 481–485

Mendlowicz MV, Stein, MB 2000 Quality of life in individuals with anxiety disorders. American Journal of Psychiatry, **157**: 669–682

Mineka S, Watson D, Clark L 1998 Comorbidity of anxiety and unipolar mood disorders. Annual Review of Psychology, **49**: 377–412

Sources

National Phobics Society. www.phobics-society.org.uk Anxiety Disorders Association of America. Good website with brief details and descriptions of specific disorders. Self tests and information about treatment. www.adaa.org

National Institutes of Mental Health Website. Good resource for information about the various disorders. www.nimh.nih.gov/anxiety/index.htm

Self-assessment: questions

Multiple choice questions

1. The following are symptoms of a panic attack:
   a. Palpitations
   b. Sweating
   c. Drowsiness
   d. Constipation
   e. Chest pain

2. Generalized anxiety disorder (GAD):
   a. Usually begins in old age
   b. Usually occurs in people who report they have been anxious or worried all their lives
   c. Responds to exposure techniques
   d. Responds to cognitive techniques that focus on individual patient concerns
   e. Is characterized by excessive worry and anxiety for at least 3 months

3. Obsessive-compulsive disorder (OCD):
   a. Is three time more common in women than men
   b. Is characterized by delusions of persecution
   c. Is maintained by a variety of factors including a deflated sense of responsibility
   d. Is maintained by a variety of factors, including selective attention to obsessional thoughts
   e. Can be treated with clomipramine

4. The following features are characteristic of post-traumatic stress disorder (PTSD):
   a. Hypervigilance
   b. Startle response
   c. Recurrent dreams of the trauma
   d. Confrontation of the trauma or events similar to it
   e. A sense of detachment

5. Specific phobias:
   a. Are common in the normal population
   b. Usually begin in childhood if they involve fears of creatures
   c. Are best treated by cognitive therapy
   d. Are characterized by intense, reasonable fears of objects
   e. Can involve fears of the natural environment

Case history questions

History 1

> A 33-year-old woman was in the middle of a city centre when a terrorist bomb exploded. She was thrown backwards by the blast and suffered moderate-to-severe lacerations from flying glass. In the months after the bombing, she could not stop thinking about it and experienced vivid nightmares. She was unable to relax and jumped if she heard a car back-firing. She was frightened about going into town and did all her shopping locally. She eventually found it an ordeal even to go to the local shops.

1. What condition is this woman suffering from?
2. What are three key symptoms essential for making the diagnosis?

History 2

> A 25-year-old man visited a public toilet. He learnt afterwards that it was often used by gay men for sexual liaisons. He began to worry that he may have contracted AIDs, although nothing unusual happened to him. He visited his doctor and despite reassurance, insisted on an HIV test. This was negative. This failed to reassure him. When he discussed his worries with his GP, he could see that they were unrealistic but could not get them out of his mind. He began to think that he must have picked up the virus from the toilet seat. He began to wash himself repeatedly. He took a towel and soap to work so he could wash his genitals several times a day. His performance at work began to be impaired as he found it difficult to focus upon anything other than his fears.

1. What condition is this man suffering from?
2. What are the key symptoms?
3. What is the treatment?

History 3

A 33-year-old woman was out shopping one day when she suddenly became very faint and light-headed. She noticed her heart was beating fast and she could not get her breath. She felt she was suffocating and fell to the ground. She thought she was going to die. Passers-by came to her aid and an ambulance was called. She was taken to hospital. Her symptoms subsided and medical examination was normal. Over the next few weeks, she developed further similar attacks. She began to worry that something was wrong with her heart and visited her doctor several times. She began to be afraid to go out in case she had another attack. When she was out, she could not stop checking her pulse in case she had another attack. Her anxiety in relation to going out got worse and worse.

1. What condition is this woman suffering from?
2. What are the major features?
3. What would be the appropriate treatment?

Self-assessment: answers

Multiple choice answers

1. a. **True**. A common symptom of a panic attack.
   b. **True**. A common symptom of a panic attack.
   c. **False**. Patients are usually hyperalert during a panic attack.
   d. **False**. Constipation is not associated with anxiety.
   e. **True**. A common symptom of a panic attack.

2. a. **False**. GAD usually begins in young people.
   b. **True**. Individuals usually have premorbid traits of anxiety.
   c. **False**. Cognitive techniques are required to alter morbid thoughts.
   d. **False**. Cognitive techniques need to focus on underlying worries or concerns rather than individual worries, as once one worry has been tackled, the patient will substitute another worry in its place.
   e. **False**. Excessive worry and anxiety is required for at least 6 months before a diagnosis is made.

3. a. **False**. OCD is slightly more common in women than men.
   b. **False**. Delusions are not characteristic of OCD. Patients usually recognize that their thoughts are unrealistic.
   c. **False**. OCD is thought to be maintained, particularly, in individuals who have an inflated sense of responsibility.
   d. **True**. Selective attention (i.e. focusing on the thoughts) helps to maintain thoughts.
   e. **True**. Clomipramine has been used successfully in OCD, but SSRIs (selective serotonin reuptake inhibitors) should probably be tried first.

4. a. **True**. Individuals with PTSD are hypervigilant.
   b. **True**. Individuals with PTSD jump and startle at loud noises or sounds.
   c. **True**. Experience recurrent dreams or images of the trauma.
   d. **False**. Individuals avoid events that remind them of the trauma.
   e. **True**. Individuals can develop a sense of detachment from the world.

5. a. **True**. About 8% of the general population have specific phobias.
   b. **True**. Animal phobias usually begin in childhood.
   c. **False**. Behavioural techniques such as exposure or desensitization are the preferred treatments (Ch. 14).
   d. **False**. Phobias are intense unreasonable fears of objects.
   e. **True**. Phobias of thunderstorms or similar events are common.

Case history answers

History 1

1. The woman has post-traumatic stress disorder.
2. The three key symptoms are that she shows (i) intrusive memories of the trauma; (ii) avoidance (not going into town); and (iii) a heightened arousal (unable to relax – tension and startle response – jumping if a car back-fires).

History 2

1. Obsessive-compulsive disorder.
2. The key symptoms are obsessional thoughts. He has intrusive repetitive concerns that he cannot dismiss yet knows logically are unrealistic. He has also developed cleaning rituals to reduce his anxiety about contamination.
3. The treatment would involve cognitive therapy to address his obsessional thoughts plus relaxation and response prevention techniques to stop the rituals.

History 3

1. She is suffering from panic disorder in association with agoraphobia.
2. She describes classical panic attacks and hyperventilation.
3. Her panic symptoms require treatment with cognitive therapy and her agoraphobic symptoms require relaxation and graded exposure. Antidepressant treatment may also be helpful.

5 Schizophrenia

Overview

Schizophrenia is a serious mental illness characterized by symptoms of delusions and hallucinations, coupled with dysfunctional symptoms such as apathy and lack of volition. It begins usually in late adolescence and early adulthood. Most people recover from the first episode but subsequently experience further episodes characterized by increasing levels of dysfunction. One fifth remain symptom free. The illness has a strong genetic component and the concordance rate in identical twins is 40%. The condition is usually treated with antipsychotic medication. Education of the patient and family about the nature and management of schizophrenia is very important. Most patients require ongoing care from a community multidisciplinary team.

5.1 Definition and epidemiology

Learning objectives

You should:

- know the definition of schizophrenia
- know the epidemiology of schizophrenia.

Schizophrenia was first recognized as a separate mental disorder in the 1890s. Often misunderstood as 'split personality', it is actually a serious mental illness with psychotic symptoms of delusions and hallucinations that comes on in early adult life. In most cases, it then runs a chronic, relapsing course. This is one reason why it is one of the top five most expensive disorders in all of medicine.

Schizophrenia is defined as a psychotic mental illness, meaning it is a severe disorder with delusions and hallucinations (psychotic symptoms). Sufferers usually have episodes of acute psychotic symptoms, often with more persistent social impairment.

The main facts are given in Table 10. An average GP will see about one new case per year, although, because the illness usually needs long-term treatment, he or she will be involved in the ongoing care of 20–30 schizophrenic patients at any one time.

5.2 Symptoms

Learning objectives

You should:

- know the positive and negative symptoms of schizophrenia
- know about first rank symptoms
- have the ability to assess key aspects of mental state in schizophrenia.

The symptoms of schizophrenia can be divided into positive symptoms and negative symptoms. Positive symptoms are:

- delusions: in schizophrenia these are often bizarre
- hallucinations: these are usually auditory; about 20% of patients will have visual, olfactory or tactile hallucinations
- schizophrenic formal thought disorder.

Some positive symptoms are called *first rank symptoms* because they occur in schizophrenia and rarely in other disorders. They are listed in Table 11.

Negative symptoms are:

- poor self-care
- little spontaneous speech
- 'blunted' affect (mood)
- loss of normal willpower.

You should be alert to the following signs and symptoms in the mental state examination of someone who might have schizophrenia.

Table 10 The epidemiology of schizophrenia

Epidemiology	Characteristics
Incidence (rate of new cases)	2 new cases per 10 000 population per year
Prevalence (number of existing cases)	1 in 200 people
Global rates	Similar in all countries studied, with apparently higher rates in some subgroups, e.g. Black Caribbeans in the UK
Social class	Incidence equal in all social classes
Sex	Men and women equal
Peak age at onset	18–25 years; in men; 20–28 years in women
Family history	Present in one third of cases

Table 11 Asking about first rank symptoms

Symptom	The question you ask	Example of responses
Third person auditory hallucinations	Do the voices ever talk to each other, about you?	They say, "She's a very clever person"
Running commentary	Do the voices ever comment on what you're doing?	"She's going up the stairs now"
Echo de la pensee (thought echo)	Do you ever hear the voices echo your thoughts?	
Delusions–thought insertion/withdrawal	Do you ever experience thoughts from somewhere else being put into your head/taken out of your head?	Radio transmitter beaming thoughts into/taking thoughts out of my mind
Delusions–thought broadcasting	Are your thoughts ever broadcast out to other people?	
Delusions–passivity feelings	Do you ever experience your actions of thoughts being physically controlled by an outside force?	Orbiting satellite makes me change the direction I'm walking
Primary delusion: a delusion that arises suddenly, with no other prior symptoms	Have you suddenly felt things around you have changed? Tell me in a little detail	I was given the change on the bus and I knew then that I was the new Messiah

Appearance and behaviour

Appearance and behaviour may be normal, but watch for three areas.

Abnormal movements as a result of illness. The individual may be restless and agitated. They may be doing unusual things. *Mannerisms* are seemingly purposeful movements done for no reason, such as saluting. *Stereotypies* are repetitive non-purposeful movements, such as rocking or grimacing. Rarely there may be *catatonic signs*, where the person is frozen like a statue, allowing their limbs to be moved to new positions like Plasticine.

Abnormal movements as a result of drug treatment. Antipsychotic drugs can themselves cause involuntary movements (Ch. 17).

Negative symptoms. These include *poor personal hygiene* and *self-care*. Is the person dishevelled or unwashed?

Speech

Speech is often normal. However, about half of patients with schizophrenia have a characteristic disorder of language called *schizophrenic formal thought disorder*. This is an abnormality in the way the person is speaking, which when mild is quite subtle, but when marked is striking. The person's speech loses the usual logical flow between one idea and the next, so that segments of speech become partly disjointed from each other. This is known as *loosening of associations* or *'knight's move thinking'*, after the two-squares-forward-one-sideways move in chess (Box 32).

Concrete thinking describes an aspect of thought disorder that involves the impairment of the ability to think

---

Box 32
An example of knight's move thinking or loosening of associations

Interviewer How have you been feeling today?
Patient Well, in myself I have been okay what with the prices in the shops being what they are and my flat is just round the corner. I keep a watch for the arbiters most of the time since it is just round the corner. There is not all that much to do otherwise.

Comment The word 'arbiter' used here is a made-up or inappropriately used word, known as a *neologism*, in schizophrenic thought disorder.

in abstract ways. This is often most obvious if you ask the person to solve an abstract verbal puzzle or explain a proverb.

Mood

Mood in schizophrenia can be normal. Two particular abnormalities are important to look for on examination.

Blunted affect. This is where mood in conversation can be seen to have lost its usual variability. Instead of the normal play of facial expressions and gestures in a social situation, a person with blunted affect appears to have an unresponsive, unchanging expression. This is one of the negative symptoms of schizophrenia

Incongruous affect. This is where, for no apparent reason, the person will giggle or smile secretively to themselves in a way that is inappropriate to the situation. Incongruous affect is found only in schizophrenia.

Thoughts

The person may be preoccupied with their abnormal beliefs and experiences.

Abnormal beliefs

Table 12 reminds you how to ask about abnormal beliefs. Common in schizophrenia are *ideas of reference*, where the person has the impression that items on the television or radio, or in the newspapers, are referring specifically to them. This can also extend to everyday occurrences in the street, such as the impression that people in the street seem to be looking at the person, or the registration plates of passing cars have a special meaning for the person. These become *delusions of reference* if they become fixed and unshakeable.

Other delusions in schizophrenia can be *persecutory, grandiose, religious* or *hypochondriacal*. They can be extremely bizarre. When a delusion becomes so extensive that it becomes a series of linked, fixed beliefs that govern much of what the person says or does, it is said to be a *systematized delusion*. Delusions in schizophrenia can be *primary*, where they arise out of the blue, often quite suddenly, or *secondary* to pre-existing hallucinations as an attempt to explain them, as the result of a

radio receiver implanted in the brain, for instance. Some delusions are so characteristic of schizophrenia that they are first rank symptoms (Table 11).

Abnormal experiences

Hallucinations are usually auditory, of speech, in schizophrenia. Visual, olfactory or tactile hallucinations can occur in schizophrenia but are unusual and should alert you to the possibility of organic illness. Most sufferers can describe their auditory hallucinations in some detail, as in Table 13.

Cognitive state

This will be essentially normal in schizophrenia, although deficits in concentration and abstract thought may be detected, particularly if the person is acutely psychotic or has chronic negative symptoms.

Self-appraisal

Insight into the illness is usually lost in acute schizophrenia and sometimes is not regained fully after recovery. Insight is not a clear-cut issue. People can retain insight into the fact they have an illness but not agree they need treatment, for example. Assessing self-appraisal is essential in determining what management approaches are possible.

Subtypes based on symptoms

Subtypes of schizophrenia can be based on the balance of symptoms and include *paranoid*, with prominent delusions, and *hebephrenic*, with prominent negative symptoms and poor outcome. *Catatonic* schizophrenia is rare and involves marked mannerisms and posturing.

Psychoses similar to schizophrenia are:

- *schizoaffective disorder*: positive symptoms including first rank symptoms are combined with prominent mood disturbance, either manic or depressed; long-term outcome tends to be better than in schizophrenia

Table 12 Mental state examination: asking about abnormal beliefs

Delusions	Question
Abnormal beliefs in general	Have you had feelings that some things are not quite as they should be? (*Open question*)
Ideas or delusions of reference	Do you sometimes have the impression that things on the TV or radio are about you?
Persecutory delusions	Do you ever feel there might be a plot about you? Or even an experiment?
Hypochondriacal delusions	Has anything strange been happening to your body?
Grandiose delusions	Have you special powers or abilities?

Table 13 Mental state examination: asking about auditory hallucinations

Auditory hallucination	Question
Auditory hallucination in general	Do you ever seem to hear things when no-one is around? (*Open question*) Are they voices?
Hallucinations are heard with the ears, like normal speech	Do you hear them with your ears, like you are hearing my voice now? Or is it in your mind? Where does the voice come from?
Patients can describe the characteristics of the voices: their number, loudness, location, content	How many voices are there? Do they say pleasant or unpleasant things? How loud are they? How often do they happen?
Voices talking to one another about the patient ('He is a clever person') are called third person auditory hallucinations, one of the first rank symptoms	Do the voices ever talk to each other, about you?
A voice doing a running commentary ('She is going up the stairs now') or a voice echoing thoughts, called echo de la pensee, are first rank symptoms	Do the voices ever say a running commentary on what you are doing? Do they ever echo what you are thinking?
Insight or self-appraisal	How do you explain the voices?

- *delusional disorder*: characterized by gradual onset of systematized persecutory delusions, without hallucinations or thought disorder
- *drug-induced psychosis*: has a sudden onset and resolves over a few days after the drug is withdrawn; amphetamine-like drugs, including Ecstasy, are often responsible and the usual difficulty is distinguishing this from drug-induced relapse of schizophrenia
- *organic psychoses*. These can mimic schizophrenia and need to be excluded.

5.3 Causes, onset and course

Learning objectives

You should:

- know the likely age of onset and presenting history
- know the possible causes
- know of the dopamine hypothesis to explain the biological basis of schizophrenia.

Onset

The median age at onset is about 23 years in men and 28 years in women. Onset is very rare under 16, and uncommon over 40. Onset can be relatively acute, over the course of 2 or 3 weeks, or insidious. The typical history is for a period of several months increasingly poor functioning at home, work or school, with noticeable social withdrawal, non-specific anxiety and change in behaviour. Delusions and hallucinations then appear, sometimes after several days in which the person reports his or her surroundings to be changed in some strange way that is difficult to describe: so-called *delusional mood*.

Course

Most people will recover from the first episode, usually within 3 months of taking treatment and 20% will then never have a further episode and return to full functioning. However, 70% will recover but relapse in the future, with increasing levels of negative symptoms between episodes. Even with treatment, 50% of patients will relapse in the first 2 years. Approximately 10% of patients will never recover from their first episode and will need high levels of health and social services input and support for many years. Over the first 5 years of the illness, 5% of patients will die by suicide.

Causes

Predisposing factors

The causes of schizophrenia are still largely unknown. Genetic and environmental factors are important. The risk of schizophrenia is increased 15-fold if a first-degree relative has schizophrenia. The concordance rate in identical twins is 40%, strongly suggesting a genetic effect as well as showing that environmental factors must be operating too. The genetic effect is likely to be several additive genes each of small individual effect: a polygenic model. Linkage studies and genetic association studies have provisionally identified some of these vulnerability genes. Also found in the families of schizophrenic probands are increased rates of a non-psychotic disorder of personality known as *schizotypal disorder*, with social isolation and eccentric thinking; this is genetically related to schizophrenia.

About a third of people who develop schizophrenia have had lifelong abnormalities, with poor social skills and few friends, often with slightly delayed motor and cognitive milestones. These are sometimes called *schizoid* traits.

Environmental risk factors include a range of early neurological insults that slightly increase the risk of schizophrenia many years later: obstetric complications, childhood head injury and childhood encephalitis.

Schizophrenic patients often have minor non-progressive brain changes detectable by computed tomography (CT) or magnetic resonance imaging (MRI) (see below). The most common is minor enlargement of lateral cerebral ventricles, but not to a degree considered definitely abnormal by a radiologist.

Schizophrenia is more common by three- or four-fold in one ethnic subgroup in the UK: second-generation AfroCaribbean individuals. This does not appear to be misdiagnosis nor caused by any increase in a risk factor such as street drug use. It is most likely to be a combination of an increased genetic predisposition and increased social stressors and precipitants, such as racist pressures.

Precipitating factors

Although clear precipitating factors are usually absent, two important classes of factor can trigger the first onset of schizophrenia in predisposed people: stressful *life events* and *street drug use*, particularly of amphetamine-like drugs.

Maintaining factors

Family environment Stressful family environment was once thought to be a cause of schizophrenia. This is now known not to be the case. However, it can cause relapse in someone who has had schizophrenia. Ways of measuring how families interact have been developed. Families who have high levels of criticism, hostility and overinvolvement are said to have high *expressed emotion (EE)* and studies have shown that people in remission from schizophrenia are more likely to have a relapse in such a family environment. Since families are often the principal caregivers for younger people with schizophrenia, techniques to support families and to reduce EE if necessary have been developed and shown to reduce relapse. Family intervention involves education about the illness, then advice about dealing with problem behaviours and how to ask for help when needed. A family support worker may be available, often from the voluntary sector. Families find the negative symptoms the most stressful to deal with.

Other factors Other maintaining factors are *poor compliance* with treatment and continued *street drug use*.

The biological basis: the dopamine hypothesis

The key neurotransmitter involved in schizophrenia is dopamine. The so-called dopamine hypothesis states that the symptoms result from overactivity of dopamine, particularly in the mesocortical pathway projecting from temporal to frontal areas. First put forward in 1963, the hypothesis was based on two clinical observations: (i) amphetamines, which released dopamine, could cause schizophrenia-like positive symptoms if overused; and (ii) antipsychotic drugs caused side effects resembling Parkinson's disease, which was known to be caused by dopamine deficiency. Further evidence was that the clinical potency (number of milligrams to have a clinical effect) of individual drugs could be shown to be closely correlated with their in vitro affinity to dopamine D_2 receptors. Problems with the hypothesis were that it did not account well for negative symptoms and there was no direct evidence showing increased dopamine receptors in the brains of never-treated patients at postmortem or by scanning (positron emission tomography). The hypothesis would not predict the effects of clozapine, the superior efficacy of which is achieved with a relatively low blockade of dopamine D_2 receptors.

Structural brain changes

Structural brain imaging using CT and MRI consistently demonstrate mild non-progressive enlargement of cerebral spaces, such as the lateral cerebral ventricles, in patients with schizophrenia compared with normal individuals. These findings suggest that patients with schizophrenia have slightly less brain tissue, affecting, particularly, cortical grey matter and the limbic system; the latter is involved in the control of emotions and memory. Other structures, such as the thalamus, which is involved in the regulation of the flow of information to the cerebral cortex, have also been implicated.

5.4 Management

Learning objectives

You should:

- be aware of the need for prompt action at initial presentation

- know the management of chronic schizophrenia

- understand the roles of all those involved in community care

- understand the way to communicate the diagnosis to the patient and family.

The first episode

The longer the person has active psychotic symptoms, the worse the eventual outcome, so swift referral from primary to secondary care is important when psychotic symptoms are present. Full history and assessment will lead to the diagnosis in most cases. Physical examination and investigations are essential; these include:

- neurological examination
- full blood count
- erythrocyte sedimentation rate (ESR)
- electrolytes and urea
- thyroid function
- electroencephalograph (EEG)
- CT scan
- urine screen for street drugs.

Care needs to be taken over how the diagnosis is discussed with the patient and family; skills in breaking bad news are important. Management of the first episode will usually involve admission as an inpatient or daypatient, although over a third of patients will be able to be managed at home throughout their first episode, with frequent visits from staff of the community mental health team (CMHT). Most people in their first episode will be young adults. Almost all patients will need antipsychotic drug treatment, although low doses of a conventional drug (e.g. haloperidol 1–2 mg twice daily) or new atypical drug are usually sufficient. Education of the patient and family about the nature and management of schizophrenia are very important. Introduction of the Care Programme Approach (CPA) is needed, with an integrated and documented care plan and a keyworker with responsibility for coordinating the careplan. Continuing involvement of a psychiatrist, community psychiatric nurse and social worker as a minimum are usually needed.

Maintenance after the first episode

Maintenance management after the acute symptoms have resolved will include regular CPA meetings organized by the keyworker. Maintenance antipsychotic drug treatment will be needed. How long this should continue if the person has no symptoms depends partly on how severe the initial episode was. Drug treatment should be continued for a minimum of a year; if the first episode was severe, drugs should continue for at least 2 years. Clear discussion of the 'pros and cons' of continued drug treatment will help compliance.

Acute relapse needs reinstatement, change or increase of antipsychotic drug treatment. Admission to daypatient or inpatient services may be needed. Attempts to clarify reasons for relapse (Box 33) are needed.

Management of chronic schizophrenia

Prognostic factors in schizophrenia are listed in Box 34. Persistent positive symptoms, which fail to respond well to other antipsychotic drugs, will improve with clozapine in about 50% of patients. Recent evidence supports the effectiveness of a modified form of cognitive-behaviour therapy for persistent delusions and hallucinations. Persistent negative symptoms are more difficult to treat. Rehabilitation uses a set of graded techniques in order to reduce partially the negative symptoms that cause most disability. Rehabilitation includes occupational therapy, which starts with assessing the degree of functional disability in terms of doing everyday tasks. People with chronic schizophrenia are often unable to live independently, needing sheltered housing or a residential placement with specialist staffing. Work retraining is an important part of rehabilitation.

Some people with schizophrenia are difficult to engage or maintain in treatment. In the past, such patients were often lost to follow-up as they did not attend for outpatient appointments or treatment. Very intensive forms of community treatment have been recommended by the Department of Health in the UK for such patients.

Intensive community treatments

Assertive outreach involves the delivery of continuous and comprehensive community care and treatment to certain

---

Box 33
Common causes of relapse

The causes are listed from most common to least common.
- non-compliance with drug treatment
- discontinuation, or reduction, of drug treatment
- street drug use
- family stress; high expressed emotion
- life event
- childbirth

Box 34
Prognostic factors in schizophrenia

Good prognosis
- acute onset
- early treatment
- good response to treatment
- female sex
- good occupational and social adjustment previously

Poor prognosis
- early age at onset
- insidious onset
- poor previous adjustment
- negative symptoms
- street drug use

patients. It usually involves a multidisciplinary team, who provide 24 hour support and cover. There is a small patient-to-staff ratio of about 10:1, so that staff can provide close follow-up and contact with patients. Usually each member of the team is familiar with each of the patients, so any member of the team can respond to each patient in an appropriate fashion. It is most suitable for those patients with severe mental illness who are at high risk of self-harm or harm to others, and who will not attend clinic appointments or who are erratic in their pattern of attendance. These people often have multiple social problems and drug abuse in addition to psychosis. Assertive outreach, in the UK, is more effective at keeping patients in contact with services and in treatment than conventional care. It does not, however, result in a better clinical outcome. In the USA, it has been shown to reduce hospital admissions, but there is no evidence that it has such an effect in the UK. This may be because of differences in service delivery in the UK or because assertive outreach is not implemented as intensively in the UK as it has been in the USA.

Case management is another form of intensive community care. It differs from assertive outreach in that one member of staff usually works with a small group of patients to provide intensive follow-up and care. The case manager will be part of a team but, usually, will work exclusively with his/her own patients. Twenty-four hour cover is not usually provided.

Further reading and sources

Larsen TK, Friis S, Haahr U et al. 2001. Early detection and intervention in first-episode schizophrenia: a critical review. Acta Psychiatrica Scandinavica, 103: 323–334

Lewis S, Buchanan RW 1998 Schizophrenia. Fast facts. Health Press, Oxford.

Rector NA, Beck AT 2001 Cognitive behavioral therapy for schizophrenia: an empirical review. Journal of Nervous and Mental Disease, 189: 278–287

Siris SG 2001 Suicide and schizophrenia. Journal of Psychopharmacology, 15: 127–135

Warner R 2001 Combating the stigma of schizophrenia. Epidemiologia Psichiatria Sociale 10: 12–17.

Sources

National Schizophrenia Fellowship. Includes access to varied resources for coping with schizophrenia, covering news, support services, literature, conferences and courses. www.nsf.org.uk

Doctor's Guide to the Internet – Schizophrenia. Access the latest medical news and information on schizophrenia. Includes patient information, discussion groups and clinical studies www.pslgroup.com

Self-assessment: questions

Multiple choice questions

1. Concerning the symptoms of schizophrenia:
   a. Delusions are often of a persecutory type
   b. Tactile hallucinations are common
   c. Ideas of reference are common
   d. Insight is usually impaired
   e. Negative symptoms are strong predictors of outcome

2. Schizophrenia:
   a. Is more common in women
   b. Is mainly a disorder of Western culture
   c. Has a peak age at onset of 23–28 years
   d. Is linked to increased rates of suicide
   e. Is mainly caused by stress

3. Factors that make recovery from schizophrenia more difficult include:
   a. A stable and supportive family background
   b. Continued abuse of illicit drugs
   c. Failure to comply with medication
   d. A strong family history of schizophrenia
   e. Continued abuse of alcohol

4. Good prognostic factors in schizophrenia include:
   a. An insidious onset of symptoms
   b. Being female
   c. An early age at onset (e.g. 14 years of age)
   d. Marked negative symptoms
   e. Early treatment

5. Assertive outreach:
   a. Involves a multidisciplinary team
   b. Monitors patients with the most mild disorders in case they become worse
   c. Provides close supervision and treatment for patients with dual diagnosis and challenging behaviour
   d. Involves a large patient-to-staff ratio
   e. Is of proven efficacy in the UK

Case history questions

History 1

Jane had a normal childhood and did well academically at school. In her second year at university, following the break-up of a relationship, she developed over the course of a week auditory hallucinations of voices talking about her and commenting on what she was doing. She believed firmly that a university lecturer had implanted an electronic device in her head that could control her thoughts. After being seen by her GP, she was referred urgently to mental health services where she was assessed jointly by a nurse and a psychiatrist. She was admitted to the day hospital. After routine investigations were normal, she was treated with haloperidol 5 mg daily. After 3 weeks, her hallucinations had subsided and she recognized that her beliefs had been mistaken. She continued to improve over the next month and was able to return to her studies after a further month.

1. What positive symptoms did Jane have?
2. What is the differential diagnosis?
3. What good prognostic factors are present?

History 2

Jason's childhood was normal. His paternal uncle was treated for schizophrenia. He left school with basic qualifications at age 16. He worked as a forklift truck driver. From age 18 he used cannabis and amphetamines regularly. Following his 21st, birthday, his mother and his friends became concerned that he spent increasing periods of time in his bedroom. His mother found pieces of paper in his room with scribbled messages about the CIA following him. He told a friend that he was being watched because he had invented a machine that converted air to water. He refused to see his GP and began to refuse his food because he believed it was poisoned. He was seen at home by a psychiatrist, social worker and GP. He did not wish to be admitted to hospital. After considering whether involuntary admission was needed, it was decided to monitor and treat him at home. Physical investigations were normal. He took chlorpromazine and improved over the next month but was still concerned that he might be watched. His mother noticed that his self-care was less good than previously. He suffered stiffness and dry mouth from his drug treatment and stopped it secretly. His symptoms returned after 1 month; but he still refused hospital admission. After taking a small overdose of his tablets, he was admitted to a psychiatric unit under a section of the Mental Health Act. After a 6 week admission, he was discharged back home with regular support visits from a community psychiatruc nurse. He was given a monthly depot intramuscular injection of fluphenazine decoanate.

1. What types of delusion did Jason develop?
2. On what grounds was he detained under the Mental Health Act?

History 3

Steven had slightly slower milestones at walking and talking than his elder siblings. At primary school he was a timid child with few friends. At secondary school, he was bullied and for periods refused to attend. At 13, years of age, he was referred to child mental health services because of persistent nightmares. He told the assessment team that he knew his room was haunted and he could hear murmuring from under his bed. He did not reattend the clinic. His schoolteacher noticed that he seemed distracted and was whispering to himself.

At age 15 he was reassessed and admitted to an adolescent mental health unit. He was noticed to be grimacing and smiling incongruously. His computed tomographic scan showed slight enlargement of his lateral ventricles, which was within normal limits. He complained that his movements were being controlled by ghosts. A diagnosis of schizophrenia was made. He commenced low-dose haloperidol, which was changed to risperidone after he suffered a dystonic reaction. His delusions improved but he was still withdrawn and spoke little. He returned to the family home with visiting support but was frightened to return to his bedroom. He left home unannounced the next week. Three months later he was found sleeping rough in a nearby town, dishevelled, emaciated and muttering to himself. He was re-admitted to a psychiatric unit for further treatment.

1. What negative symptoms has Steven developed?
2. What poor prognostic factors have been present?

Objective structured clinical examination (OSCE)

Topic: hearing voices
The following information is given to you on a card by an examiner. You are asked to read it and then to answer a series of questions.

James Kerry is 49 years old. He was brought to hospital by the police on a Section 136 4 weeks ago. He had been found by the police walking along a busy road. He was dishevelled and kept shouting at cars as they passed him. At times he shouted out 'bastards' and 'leave me alone'. In hospital, he appeared to be 'hearing voices'. He told staff that 'the bastards are always taking about me', 'they keep telling each other that I'm rubbish and no good', 'it's driving me mad'. 'I've never touched any children. They keep whispering to each other that I molest children. It's all a pack of lies'.

He believed that he was being followed by Mormons who were planning to kill him. He knew that all people who drove black-and blue-coloured cars were Mormons and were following him wherever he went.

Mr Kerry had a long history of mental illness. He first presented to services when he was 22 years of age and, at that time, suffered from delusions that the IRA were following him. Over the years he had had 10 admissions to psychiatric hospitals following similar presentations. He had no insight into his illness and always defaulted from follow-up and treatment after discharge.

He had worked as a road labourer in his twenties but had not worked for the last 20 years. He often slept on the streets as he had little money and rarely had the social stability or drive to organize benefits for himself.

1. What kinds of phenomenon was the patient experiencing?
2. If your answer is hallucination, define the term and specify what kind of hallucination the patient was suffering from.
3. If your answer is delusion, define the term and specify what kind of delusion the patient was suffering from.
4. What is the clinical relevance of the symptoms?
5. What is the most likely diagnosis?
6. What would be the most appropriate form of community treatment for the patient, after treatment of his initial disorder?

Self-assessment: answers

Multiple choice answers

1. a. **True**. They are often bizarre.
   b. **False**. They occur only in around 20% of patients; auditory hallucinations are common.
   c. **True**. If they become fixed and unshakable, they become delusions.
   d. **True.** Some insight may be retained and this needs to be assessed for management.
   e. **True.** They predict a poor outcome.

2. a. **False**. There is an equal gender distribution.
   b. **False**. It is seen all over the world.
   c. **True**.
   d. **True**. Patients have high rates of suicide.
   e. **False**. Schizophrenia is predominantly a brain disorder.

3. a. **False**. The family is often the principal source of caregivers.
   b. **True**. Street drug use is an important precipitating factor and continued use impairs recovery.
   c. **True**. This is common in those who are erratic in clinic attendance, have no fixed home or refuse regular treatment.
   d. **True**. Risks are increased 15-fold in first-degree relatives.
   e. **True**.

4. a. **False**. This indicates a poor prognosis.
   b. **True**.
   c. **False**. Early onset indicates a poor prognosis.
   d. **False**. These have poor prognosis and are difficult to treat.
   e. **True**. The eventual outcome worsens with the length of time for which active psychotic symptoms are untreated.

5. a. **True**. Usually all members of the team are familiar with the patient.
   b. **False**. It is only for the most severely ill who are difficult to keep engaged in services.
   c. **True**. Dual diagnosis usually implies patients with schizophrenia and illicit drug misuse.
   d. **False**. There is a small number of patients per staff (usually 10:1) as the treatment is intensive.
   e. **False**. Although evidence from the USA has indicated benefit, the results of UK studies are equivocal.

Case history answers

History 1

1. Jane is describing classical passivity experiences in that she has delusional ideas about being controlled by an external agency. She also is experiencing third person auditory hallucinations and a running commentary.
2. The most likely diagnosis is schizophrenia because of the presence of first rank symptoms and the absence of any symptoms indicating a manic episode. In a young person, it is always important to exclude a drug-induced psychosis, which could mimic schizophrenia. Other possible diagnoses include other organic factors that could produce a schizophreniform psychosis.
3. Good prognostic factors include the rapid onset of the condition, precipitated by a life event; the rather florid symptoms; the evidence for a normal childhood without evidence of a schizoid premorbid personality; and the return to normal following the illness without any negative symptoms (e.g. blunting of affect, lack of motivation, etc.).

History 2

1. Jason developed persecutory delusions.
2. He was admitted under the Mental Health Act because he had a mental disorder, he was at risk to himself, he refused to be admitted on a voluntary basis and there was no other reasonable alternative to treatment (Ch. 15).

History 3

1. He showed evidence of lack of self-care, poor motivation and little spontaneous speech.
2. He shows evidence of soft neurological signs during childhood, an insidious onset of the disease, a very early onset of the disease (age 13), negative symptoms, poor compliance with treatment and little insight into his illness.

OSCE answer

The criteria for marking this type of station would involve a global mark based upon the candidate's overall performance. The criteria listed below are features that should have been covered in the answers. An examiner does not necessarily have to award one mark per point made.

1. Hallucinations and delusions. Second person auditory hallucinations (the candidate could also infer the patient may have secondary delusions).
2. Hallucination is an abnormal perception; its quality is that of a real perception; it arises in clear consciousness; it does not arise from material objects (i.e. is not a misperception like an illusion). (A student should be able to provide a clear definition of an hallucination and be able to distinguish an hallucination from an illusion. You should be able to identify that the patient is describing third person auditory hallucinations, possibly also second person auditory hallucinations.)
3. A delusion is a false belief that is held with conviction by the patient and which is out of keeping with his social and familial background. The patient is describing persecutory delusions.
4. The symptoms are suggestive of schizophrenia. Third person auditory hallucinations are first rank symptoms of schizophrenia and persecutory delusions are common in this type of disorder, although they are not specific to it.
5. The most likely diagnosis is schizophrenia.
6. Assertive outreach or case management.

6 Suicide and deliberate self-harm

Overview

Suicide accounts for about 1% of total mortality per year in the UK. The most common methods are hanging, overdose and carbon monoxide poisoning from car exhaust. Men are more likely to commit suicide than women and to use more violent methods. The UK government has made the reduction of suicide a national priority for the health service and has set a target of reduction of suicide by one fifth by the year 2010. The main risk factors associated with suicide are presence of psychiatric illness, family history of suicide, a previous history of deliberate self-harm, older age, severe physical illness, and social isolation. People with severe mental illness have the highest risk of suicide.

Deliberate self-harm is more common in women than men, although the gender difference is progressively narrowing. Most patients are young and are between the ages of 14 and 25 years. Patients who harm themselves are 100 times more likely to kill themselves in the future than members of the general population. Risk assessment should involve the assessment of the lethality of the attempt, current suicidal intent, presence of depressive illness, psychosocial support, the presence of other psychiatric conditions and a history of previous self-harm.

6.1 Suicide

Learning objectives

You should:

- know the epidemiology of suicide
- understand the factors affecting risk
- be aware of the relationship between suicide and mental illness
- know how to carry out a risk assessment for suicide.

Epidemiology

Worldwide, suicide accounts for 300 000–450 000 deaths per year. In Western countries, it is one of the three leading causes of death in young people. For Europe, the rates are higher for northern countries such as the UK, the Netherlands and the Scandinavian countries, whereas suicide is reported less frequently in Spain, and Greece. Many countries have reported an increase in suicide since the 1960s.

In the UK, suicide accounts for about 5 500 deaths per year, 1% of total mortality. The risk for the general population is 1 per 10 000. The most common methods are hanging, overdose and death by carbon monoxide poisoning from car exhaust. Men are more likely than women to use violent methods.

Rates of suicide in most countries are higher in males than in females. China is one important exception, with very high rates in females, especially young women in rural areas. In recent years, several countries have experienced an increase in suicide rates in males, particularly in the younger age groups. In contrast, suicide rates of females have declined, especially in older women, or remained fairly stable, particularly in the young. This pattern is especially marked in the UK with an overall rise in male rates and a decrease in female rates. The reason for this change is unclear, but it suggests that causal factors and, possibly, protective factors have changed in different directions in the two genders.

The UK government has made the reduction of suicide a national priority for the health service and has set a target of a reduction of suicide by one fifth by the year 2010. Consequently all psychiatric services have to address this issue and implement strategies to detect and treat those at most risk of suicide.

Factors affecting risk

The demographic and psychosocial factors affecting risk are shown in Box 34. Unemployment is strongly related to suicide, but this relationship is more enduring and stronger among women. For men, the risk is twice that of those who are employed, and this effect is stronger in the early years of unemployment. In women, unemployment increases the risk of suicide by three times, regardless of the duration of unemployment.

Box 34
Risk factors for suicide

Depressive disorders
Schizophrenia
Substance misuse
Suicidal behaviour in first-degree relatives
Previous history of deliberate self-harm
Unemployment
Male gender
Older age
Emotionally unstable personality disorder
Physical disorder
Living alone

Affective disorder is a very important risk factor for suicide and there is some evidence that the risk varies depending upon the severity of the disorder. The lifetime prevalence of suicide in patients with depression and suicidality treated in an inpatient setting is 8.6%, whereas it is 2.2% for patients treated in an outpatient setting. Elderly patients who present with depression or suicidal ideas should receive a particularly careful assessment.

An increased risk of suicide is associated with chronic physical illness, mostly likely because of the high risk of depression in this group.

Individuals with a forensic history (i.e. have a criminal conviction) are also more likely to kill themselves than the general public.

Suicide and mental illness

People with severe mental illness (who have required inpatient treatment) have the highest risk of suicide above all other groups. The risk is highest in the first 3 months following discharge: 25% of all suicides in this group occurs in the first 3 months following discharge and approximately 50% within the first year. Over 70% of patients use violent methods.

Patients suffering from schizophrenia or depressive disorders are at the greatest risk; schizophrenic patients who commit suicide usually kill themselves within the first few years of the illness. Another high-risk time is in the early stages of relapse, before treatment can be re-instituted. So-called 'command hallucinations' voices, which tell the person to kill himself/herself, should be taken very seriously as patients may act upon these experiences.

For those patients receiving inpatient psychiatric treatment, a recent bereavement, presence of delusions, suicidal ideation, chronic mental illness and a family history of suicide are all associated with a higher risk of suicide while in hospital.

Preventative factors

Changes in natural prescribing habits to reduce the availability of barbiturates dramatically reduced the number of deaths from this cause in the 1960s, but it did not affect the overall suicide rate. A high proportion of patients who commit suicide visit their GP shortly before they carry out the act. Therefore, improved education of GPs to enable them to conduct better-quality risk assessment could potentially have an important preventative effect on the rate of suicide.

The following have been shown to reduce the risk of suicide in patients with mental illness:

- maintenance treatment of the underlying illness in the severely mentally ill helps to ensure fewer relapses.
- general social cohesion in the presence of children protects individuals against suicide.

Risk assessment

It is important to remember that risk is not static. It varies between populations and across age ranges, and within individuals over different periods of time. Clinicians and researchers are not terribly proficient at quantifying and predicting risk. The positive predictive value of most methods of assessment (the proportion of individuals identified as high risk, by risk assessment measures, who are actually high risk) is low. This means it is very difficult in clinical practice actually to predict which patients will take their lives. Despite this, it is good practice to carry out a risk assessment, and failure to do so can have important medico-legal implications.

The doctor should consider the following factors.

1. Always conduct a risk assessment.
2. Be aware of demographic risk factors.
3. Be aware of previous psychiatric and behavioural factors, for example previous illness, previous history of deliberate self-harm, alcoholism, a family history of suicide.
4. Ask about low mood.
5. Ask about suicidal thoughts.
6. Identify the presence of other key symptoms, for example hopelessness and worthlessness.
7. Ask about suicidal actions.
8. Be especially vigilant if the patient is a young male, over 50 years of age, or recently discharged from hospital, or has a serious mental illness that is relapsing.
9. Ask about any protective factors, for examples a supportive partner or family member, supportive accommodation provided by social services.

6.2 Deliberate self-harm

Learning objectives

You should:

- know the prevalence of deliberate self-harm
- understand how the epidemiology of deliberate self-harm is changing
- know how to carry out a risk assessment for suicide in a patient with deliberate self-harm.

Epidemiology

Deliberate self-harm is a common reason for attendance at A&E departments and for acute admissions to general medical beds. It has been estimated that there are over 100 000 admissions per annum in England and Wales for deliberate self-harm. The ratio of women to men with deliberate self-harm used to be 2:1, but in many centres now it is equal. Most patients are young, between the ages of 14 and 45 years, with the highest number of patients falling into the 14–24 year age group. Patients with deliberate self-harm are 100 times more likely than the general population to commit suicide, and 1 in 100 patients who present with deliberate self-harm will commit suicide within 12 months of presentation. The assessment of suicidal risk in these patients is, therefore, extremely important.

Deliberate self-harm is not a psychiatric diagnosis. It is an abnormal behaviour that may or may not signify underlying psychiatric morbidity. It is a culturally determined behaviour that has become very common in the UK, the USA and some northern European countries. It is, however, relatively rare in Southern Europe and less Westernized parts of the world.

Methods

The most common method of deliberate self-harm is self-poisoning (about 90% of all cases) and paracetamol is the drug most commonly ingested. Other methods include self-laceration, hanging and carbon monoxide poisoning.

Precipitating factors

Most episodes of deliberate self-harm are preceded by some kind of negative stressful event that the patient feels unable to cope with. Most of these events involve problems or stresses to do with close relationships in the patient's life, such as a bereavement, the break-up of a marriage or a fierce argument with a spouse. Patients who deliberately self-harm are less able to cope with these problems or find solutions to their stress compared with other individuals who do not harm themselves. Patients who self-harm are often socially disadvantaged and, in addition to adverse acute social stresses, they also experience a high prevalence of chronic social difficulties, such as unemployment, poor housing and poverty. It is often the combination of a sudden change in their lives coupled with chronic background stress that results in the deliberate self-harm episode.

Psychosocial and risk assessment

It is important that all doctors are able to carry out a competent psychosocial assessment on a deliberate self-harm patient, in addition to a physical assessment. The main aim of the psychosocial examination is to carry out a risk assessment for suicide and detect treatable illness.

In order to do this, six aspects of the patient's history and mental state require particular attention:

- the assessment of the lethality of the deliberate self-harm attempt
- the assessment of current suicidal intent
- a history of previous deliberate self-harm
- the assessment of the presence of depressive disorder
- the detection of other psychiatric conditions
- the assessment of the patient's psychosocial support network.

The assessment of the lethality of the deliberate self-harm attempt
A detailed history of the circumstances leading up to the self-harm attempt should be taken. The following features are indicative of a high suicidal intent:

- evidence of planning the attempt
- act unlikely to be discovered
- large number of drugs ingested
- all available drugs ingested
- patient expected act to be fatal and wanted to die
- suicide note
- patient discovered by chance.

The assessment of current suicidal intent
The presence of suicidal ideation, at the time of assessment in hospital, is one of the strongest predictors of suicide and should be taken very seriously. The patient should be asked whether he/she is still thinking of harming him/herself. If the patient answers positively, it is important to find out the strength of the patient's suicidal ideas, and how likely the patient is to act upon them in the near future.

A previous history of deliberate self-harm
Those patients with a previous history of self-harm are more likely than others to harm themselves again in the near future and are more likely to commit suicide.

The assessment of the presence of depressive disorder

The presence of a persistently lowered mood state for several weeks (at least 2) before the self-harm attempt is suggestive of a coexisting depressive illness. Other features may include:

- disturbed sleep with waking in the early morning
- poor appetite
- weight loss
- poor concentration
- loss of interest in usual activities.

In addition, the patient may have very strong feelings of hopelessness and worthlessness and may view the future in a pessimistic way. The presence of such feelings heightens the risk of suicide.

The detection of other psychiatric conditions

Alcohol abuse is especially common in deliberate self-harm and many patients may have taken alcohol in association with tablets or other some method of harming themselves. They may still be intoxicated at the time of the examination; if so, they should be asked to wait until they can answer questions in a clear and coherent fashion. Other common psychiatric conditions associated with deliberate self-harm are:

- anxiety states and panic disorder
- personality disorder.

Schizophrenia is relatively uncommon, but all patients with schizophrenia who self-harm should be taken very seriously. They may wish to harm themselves because they feel depressed or because they are acting upon psychotic symptoms related to the schizophrenia.

The assessment of the patient's psychosocial support network

Those patients who live alone and have few friends or family to support them are more at risk than those who have a strong supportive network who rally round after the deliberate self-harm attempt.

The demographic and psychosocial factors associated with an increased risk of suicide are described in Box 34.

Repetition of deliberate self-harm

Of patients who attend hospital after an episode of self-poisoning, 12–25% will take another overdose within a year. Repetition is more common and occurs more frequently in those patients with a previous history of self-harm. Men and women are equally likely to repeat and most repeat within 12 weeks of the index episode. Early intervention is, therefore, required.

A small group of patients present repeatedly with deliberate self-harm or self-mutilation. The episodes themselves can be quite minor or extremely serious. Patients who repeatedly harm themselves have a relatively high risk of killing themselves eventually, although the immediate short-term risk may be low. These patients can be difficult to manage and cause frustration amongst medical and nursing staff. The most common psychiatric diagnosis is that of personality disorder, as patients often have difficulties in many areas of social functioning. A childhood history of sexual or physical abuse is common, plus alcohol or drug addiction difficulties during early adulthood.

Management

The management of patients with deliberate self-harm varies widely between different hospitals. Some general hospitals have a policy to admit all patients overnight to a general medical bed or short-stay ward. A detailed psychosocial assessment is usually carried out the following day. Other hospitals only admit those patients who are medically unwell and require further treatment. Patients who are medically fit receive a psychosocial assessment in the A&E department prior to discharge.

Patients deemed to be at high risk of suicide should be admitted to a psychiatric bed or equivalent service for further observation and assessment. Those at moderate risk of suicide can be managed in the community provided they have good psychosocial support and access to community psychiatric services. Those patients at low risk of suicide can be discharged home. Patients who have a depressive illness will require treatment for this. If they are at low risk of suicide, treatment can be managed by their GP. Patients with severe symptoms of depression will require treatment from a psychiatrist and referral to specialist services.

Patients who repeatedly self-harm should be assessed for immediate suicidal risk; if this is low, management should be directed towards encouraging the patient to find alternative ways to deal with distress. Staff should be encouraged neither to be punitive towards such individuals nor to encourage unwanted behaviour. Admission to hospital (unless the patient is suicidal) may re-inforce self-injurious behaviour, and if possible, alternative ways of managing the patient should be attempted.

Asking about suicidal ideas

Some medical students find it difficult to ask patients about suicidal ideas. It is best to broach this subject in the context of enquiring about the patient's mood. If the patient reports feeling low, going on to enquire about suicidal ideation seems natural and entirely appropriate (Box 35).

Doctor I'd like to know a little about how you've been feeling recently (*open question*).
Patient What do you mean?
Doctor Er . . . . how you've been feeling in yourself . . . . in your spirits (*open question*).
Patient Not so good . . . .
Doctor Umh . . . (*facilitation*)
Patient Very fed up . . . I can't seem to pull myself out of it . . .
Doctor You've been feeling down (*said in tentative way: reflection and picks up cue*).
Patient Yeah . . . very down . . . .
Doctor I'd like to understand this a bit more, can you describe to me how you've been feeling inside? (*Exploration of mood*)
Patient I feel . . . dead . . . I can't feel anything . . . just a kind of empty feeling.
Doctor Umh . . . like there's nothing inside you?
Patient Yeah . . . .
Doctor Umh . . . does this feeling vary? Come and go? Or is it there all the time? (*Closed questions*)
Patient All the time.
Doctor Is it especially bad at any time?
Patient In the morning, when I wake up . . . I just . . . well it's unbearable.
Doctor When it's unbearable and you feel really empty . . . what goes through you're mind? (*Begins to enquire about suicidal ideas*)
Patient I just don't want to carry on . . . .
Doctor Have you thought about harming yourself? (*More specific enquiry*)
Patient Yes, but it's silly.
Doctor Well . . . I don't think it's silly . . . can you tell more about this
Patient I don't know . . . what do you mean
Doctor Well, I'd like to get an idea of what you have thought of doing (*further exploration*)
Patient Taking my tablets . . . I've been saving some up . . . I take them out of the bottle and look at them.
Doctor So you've got pretty close to taking them (*clarification*).
Patient Yes I suppose so.
Doctor How often has this happened?
Patient Only once or twice.
Doctor What's actually stopped you from taking them? (*Assesses barriers to overdose*)
Patient I've thought of my daughter . . . what she would think . . . how she would cope.
Doctor When did you last have these thoughts?
Patient This morning.
Doctor And sitting here with me now, have you thought about killing yourself? (*Specific question re current suicidal intent*)
Patient No . . . it's just when I wake up.
Doctor Well . . . you and I need to take this very seriously and we need to think through how best to manage this . . . .

In the example in Box 35, the patient is suffering from a depressive disorder, has marked suicidal ideas and is clearly at high risk of acting upon them. The doctor would then complete the assessment and discuss with the patient the most appropriate form of management.

If the patient does not have a low mood, it is still important to ask about suicidal ideas. The best phrase to use is, 'Can I ask whether you had any thoughts of harming yourself at all?' This is less shocking than using the terms such as 'suicidal thoughts' or 'thoughts of killing yourself'. The patient may ask for clarification, in which case you can go on to use such phrases as 'thoughts about ending your life' or 'thoughts of taking tablets or hurting yourself in some other way'. Most patients will not feel insulted if the questions are asked in a sensitive manner.

Specific psychological treatments for deliberate self-harm

Brief psychological treatments have been developed specifically for patients with deliberate self-harm. They

Some patients who attend the A&E department following deliberate self-harm refuse treatment for their medical condition. This is a difficult situation and a complex medico-legal area. If the patient is unconscious or confused, the common law justification of 'necessity' can be used to justify medical intervention (Ch. 15). If the patient is alert and conscious, he/she is presumed competent to refuse treatment, in the absence of any evidence to rebut this. His/her mental capacity to decline investigation and treatment must be assessed as a matter of urgency. The key issue is whether the patient has some impairment or disturbance of mental functioning that prevents him/her from making an informed decision. A psychiatrist is best placed to make this assessment. If the patient is deemed to lack capacity, treatment can be instituted.

In some circumstances detention under the Mental Health Act 1983 may be appropriate. This will involve an application for admission to hospital by an approved social worker or the patient's nearest relative and the involvement of one or two doctors, depending upon which part of the act is used for admission. This should only be done if the patient is deemed to be suffering from a mental disorder, is at risk to him/herself or others, and there is no safe alternative to inpatient treatment. Medical treatment for the patient's mental disorder can be given under Section 63 of the Act, which includes the consequences of a suicide attempt that results from the patient's mental disorder. The law in relation to this difficult area of management is unclear and may change with the introduction of the new Mental Health Act (Ch. 15). At present (2001), the UK government is still considering how patients who make an attempt to end their own life and decline treatment should be managed within a legal framework.

are derived from cognitive behavioural therapy or interpersonal therapies. They all have a problem-solving component. The therapies attempt to help patients to find more socially acceptable ways to deal with difficulties or emotional distress, other than by self-harming. Several randomized controlled trials have demonstrated that psychological treatment results in improved psychological well-being and social adjustment but does not have a significant impact on repetition, for most patients. For patients who repeatedly self-harm, intensive psychological treatment results in a reduction in repetition in addition to improved psychological status. Such treatment is not, however, widely available.

Further reading and sources

Appleby L, Shaw J, Amos T et al. 1999 Safer services. Report of the National Confidential Inquiry into Suicide and Homicide by People with Mental Illness. Department of Health, London

Hawton K, Townsend E, Arensman E, Gunnell D 2001 Psychosocial and pharmacological treatments for deliberate self harm. In: The Cochrane Library, vol. 2. Update Software, Oxford [http://www.cochrane.org /cochrane/revabstr/ ab001764.htm]

Hawton K, van Heeringen K (eds) 2000 The international handbook of suicide and attempted suicide. John Wiley & Sons, Chichester, UK

Sources

American Foundation for Suicide Prevention. Organization funds research, education and treatment programmes. Explores such categories as depression, survivor support and assisted suicide. http://www. afsp.org

The Samaritans. Telephone helpline and counselling service for anyone who is suicidal.
46 Marshall Street
London W1V 1LR
Telephone 08457 90 90 90

Self-assessment: questions

Multiple choice questions

1. The following are true:
   a. Deliberate self-harm is much more common in young women than in young men
   b. Deliberate self-harm is a common reason for attendance at the A&E department
   c. Patients with deliberate self-harm have a low risk of suicide
   d. The most common class of drug used in self-poisoning are antidepressants
   e. Deliberate self-harm is a major health problem in most European countries

2. In a patient with deliberate self-harm, the following are suggestive of a high suicidal risk:
   a. The overdose was impulse
   b. The patient says that he still wants to kill himself
   c. The patient describes feeling completely hopeless about the future
   d. The patient took tablets in front of his wife
   e. The patient drove to a secluded spot without telling anybody and connected a hosepipe from the exhaust of his car to the interior

3. In patients who repeatedly self-harm themselves
   a. The risk of eventual suicide is low
   b. The best management is admission to hospital
   c. The most frequent psychiatric disorder is schizophrenia
   d. The episodes of deliberate self-harm are usually of very low risk
   e. Alcohol abuse is rare

4. The following aspects of history should be particularly noted in patients with deliberate self-harm:
   a. A history of 6–8 weeks of depressed mood prior to the attempt
   b. A previous attempt of deliberate self-harm
   c. Whether the patient lives alone
   d. Whether the patient smokes
   e. Whether the patient drinks alcohol heavily

5. Psychological treatment of deliberate self-harm:
   a. Reduces the degree of psychological distress
   b. Is derived from either cognitive behavioural therapy or interpersonal therapies
   c. Reduces the general rate of repetition of deliberate self-harm
   d. Reduces repetition in patients who frequently harm themselves
   e. Teaches patients the skills to manage stress and solve problems in a socially acceptable manner

6. Risk factors for suicide include:
   a. Suicidal ideation
   b. Previous history of deliberate self-harm
   c. Being an air stewardess
   d. Obsessional personality traits
   e. Good social support

7. Males:
   a. Are more likely to commit suicide than females
   b. Are more likely to self-harm than females
   c. Are more likely to use violent methods to kill themselves than females
   d. Are increasingly at risk of committing suicide at a young age
   e. Never take alcohol before an episode of deliberate self-harm

8. Features of the mental state that increase the likelihood of suicide are:
   a. A history of deliberate self-harm
   b. Feelings of hopelessness
   c. Low mood
   d. Second person auditory hallucinations telling the person to kill himself or herself
   e. Clouding of consciousness

9. The suicide rate:
   a. Is declining in the UK
   b. Is high in southern European countries
   c. Is high in Scandinavia
   d. Is approximately 1 in 10 000 in the UK
   e. Is low in Arabic countries

10. High rates of suicide are found in the following groups:
    a. Doctors
    b. Those with a chronic illness
    c. Teachers
    d. Farmers
    e. Those with alcohol abuse.

Case history questions

GPs, staff in A&E and general physicians and surgeons need to be able to assess suicidal risk. In particular, the immediate, and short-term risk need to be assessed, and doctors need to know when to refer on for specialist psychiatric assessment. For Histories 1–5, answer the following questions.

1. What is the risk of suicide immediately and in the short and long term?
2. What should the patient's management be in the light of the assessment of the suicide risk?

History 1

A 56-year-old man visits his GP. He says that he has been feeling very tired and miserable and cannot sleep. His wife died from breast cancer 3 months previously and since then he has not coped very well. He lives alone with few other social contacts, and says that he has not been eating or looking after himself very well. He burst into tears during the interview. The GP asks about suicidal ideas and the man says that he desperately wants to join his wife, he has nothing to live for, his life has been destroyed and he cannot go on. That morning he awoke at 4 a.m. and thought about driving to the cemetery and then gassing himself in his car.

History 2

A 44-year-old woman is assessed at home by her GP. The health visitor has asked the GP to visit because she is concerned about the welfare of the woman's 2-year-old daughter.

The woman took an overdose the previous week, 30 aspirin and paracetamol, and has a long-standing problem of alcohol abuse. The GP called at 11.30 a.m., after morning surgery, to find that the woman is already intoxicated. Her speech is slurred and she is irritable. She is alone in the house with her 2-year-old daughter. The child is crying and has a nappy on that is soiled and old.

The woman tells the GP that she is fed up, the child keeps crying and she is getting on her nerves. The woman says that she is depressed and wants treatment for this. She says she is frightened the child will be taken away from her by social services. Two of her previous children are in care. The woman has no plans to kill herself and does not appear depressed. Her sleep is disturbed but her appetite is good. She has a long history of alcohol abuse but no previous history of depression.

History 3

A 26-year-old woman is brought to the A&E department having taken six aspirin, three diazepam tablets (5 mg each) plus alcohol. She is a mature student and has just started at university. She tells the A&E officer that she made a silly mistake. She is now regretful. She has no suicidal ideas but has been feeling low for 4 months. She has lost weight and cannot sleep or concentrate.

She has had two previous episodes of depression both of which required treatment.

History 4

A 29-year-old man is visited at home by his GP at his parents' request. He has schizophrenia but has been well for the last 2 years. He stopped all treatment 3 months previous and disengaged from psychiatric services. He is very quiet and looks preoccupied. He is muttering to himself. His mother reports that she found him sitting on the window ledge of his bedroom with his legs over the side of the window. He has told her that 'they are coming to get him'. The previous time he was acutely psychotic, he tried to jump off a bridge.

History 5

A 64-year-old man is brought to the A&E department having taken 70 paracetamol tablets. He was found by chance by a neighbour. He has vomited in the ambulance and is now saying that he is feeling better. He says that it was all a dreadful mistake and he doesn't want to bother anyone. He wants to go home. The A&E officer asks him whether he has been feeling low and he says not. He denies any other symptoms of depression. The doctor notices, however, that he is unkempt and there is no change in his facial expression, which is flattened. The A&E officer asks him to stay to have his paracetamol levels checked, but the man says that he is now alright and wants to go home.

History 6

A 23-year-old man presents to the A&E department. He has taken 30 paracetamol tablets. He took the tablets the day after his wife left him. Their marital relationship has been poor for several months. He did not plan the overdose and telephoned his brother shortly after taking the tablets to tell him what he had done.

1. What other areas of history do you need to ask about?
2. What aspects of his mental state do you need to assess?
3. If these are negative, what is the risk of suicide in this case?

History 7

A 56-year-old man was brought to the A&E department by his daughter. She had called to see him unexpectedly. She had found him in bed with an empty bottle of tricyclic antidepressant tablets beside the bed. He was drowsy and difficult to wake up. He became more alert in the A&E department and said that he wanted to go home.

1. What is the suicidal risk in this case?
2. What would you do?

History 8

A 23-year-old woman came to the A&E department having lacerated both her arms. The lacerations were superficial and from a medical perspective required no treatment. This was her third attendance for deliberate self-harm at the department in the last month. She told the A&E officer that she felt depressed and suicidal and would kill herself if she was sent home. She smelt of alcohol and said that she had been thrown out of her accommodation that evening because the landlord 'didn't like her'. Although she described feeling depressed, she did not feel down continuously, and she had been able, at times, during the last few weeks to enjoy herself. She had no other symptoms of depression.

1. What is the suicidal risk in this case?
2. What would you do?
3. What should the psychiatrist do now?

The duty psychiatrist assesses her 1 hour later. In the interim she has been noticed by staff to be sitting happily in the waiting room, chatting and laughing with other patients. The duty psychiatrist telephones her landlord to find out why she was asked to leave her lodgings. The landlord tells the psychiatrist that she has been drunk and abusive most nights and has made it difficult for the other residents to sleep. The psychiatrist reviews her psychiatric notes and sees that she has been diagnosed as having borderline personality disorder. She is under the care of one of the consultants in the department and is being supported on a weekly basis by a community psychiatric nurse. The psychiatrist re-assess her. She has no evidence of a depressive illness, and although she states she will kill herself if asked to leave, she has no specific plans and also talks about things she hopes to do in the following week. She finally admits that she is frightened about being thrown out of her accommodation and wants somewhere to stay.

Objective structured clinical examination (OSCE)

Topic: assessment of deliberate self-harm

At this station, you are presented with the following case card.

A 29-year-old man is brought to the A&E Department having taken an overdose. He has taken 50 paracetamol tablets plus four cans of beer and a bottle of vodka.

List the questions you would ask in order to assess this patient from a psychiatric perspective. Do not concentrate on the physical aspects of management.

Self-assessment: answers

Multiple choice answers

1. a. **False.** Deliberate self-harm is now virtually equally common in males and females.
   b. **True.** Deliberate self-harm accounts for approximately 2% of all A&E attendances.
   c. **False.** Patients who present with deliberate self-harm are 100 times more likely to kill themselves than the general population.
   d. **False.** Paracetamol is the most common drug used for self-poisoning.
   e. **False.** Deliberate self-harm is relatively uncommon in Spain, Portugal and Italy, whereas it is very common in the Northern European countries such as Germany and the Netherlands.

2. a. **False.** An impulsive overdose implies a lack of careful planning or forethought.
   b. **True.** Current suicidal ideation is high predictor of suicide.
   c. **True.** Feelings of hopelessness are high predictors of suicide.
   d. **False.** This suggests that the patient knew that he would be discovered and action to help him would be taken.
   e. **True.** The patient took steps not to be found and the attempt was serious.

3. a. **False.** Patients who deliberately self-harm have a high long-term risk of suicide.
   b. **False.** Unless the patient is actively suicidal, hospital admission is best avoided, as it may lead to an escalation of the self-harm behaviour.
   c. **False.** The most common psychiatric diagnosis is personality disorder.
   d. **False.** The episodes of deliberate self-harm can be of high or low risk.
   e. **False.** Alcohol and drug abuse are common.

4. a. **True.** This is both an indicator of future suicide or further episodes of deliberate self-harm.
   b. **True.** Low mood for 6–8 weeks is suggestive of a depressive illness.
   c. **True.** If the patient still has suicidal thoughts, the risk of suicide may be greater if he/she lives alone and has no social support.
   d. **False.** Smoking does not increase the risk of suicide.
   e. **True.** Alcohol abuse is common in patients who deliberately self-harm and may require treatment in its own right.

5. a. **True.** Psychological treatment results in decreased levels of depression and anxiety
   b. **True.** Most psychological treatments for deliberate self-harm are derived from cognitive behavioural therapy or interpersonal therapy.
   c. **False.** Psychological intervention has not been demonstrated to reduce the rate of repetition significantly in most patients.
   d. **True.** Intensive psychological treatment can reduce the repetition rate in patients who repeatedly self-harm.
   e. **True.** Psychological treatment tries to help patients to develop alternative, more socially acceptable, ways of dealing with distress or stressful life events.

6. a. **True.** One of the most important risk factors.
   b. **True.** Patients who have self-harmed are at high risk of suicide.
   c. **False.** There is no increased risk with this particular job.
   d. **False.** Obsessional traits may be protective. No evidence that they increase risk.
   e. **False.** Good social support is not a risk factor for suicide.

7. a. **True.**
   b. **False.** Females are more likely to self-harm than males, although the gender difference is narrowing.
   c. **True.**
   d. **True.** There has been an increase in young male suicides in the 1990s.
   e. **False.** Alcohol is commonly ingested.

8. a. **False.** A history of deliberate self-harm does increase the risk of suicide but it is not part of the mental state.
   b. **True.**
   c. **True.**
   d. **True.**
   e. **False.** Patients who are acutely confused are very unlikely to kill themselves as they are too disorganized. They may be at risk of coming to harm but this is not the same as deliberate self-harm.

9. a. **False.** It is increasing particularly in young men.
   b. **False.** It is lower in southern European countries than northern countries.
   c. **True.**

d. **True.**
e. **True.**

10. a. **True**.
    b. **True**. Probably linked to the high risk of depression.
    c. **False**.
    d. **True**.
    e. **True**.

Case history answers

History 1

1. Immediate risk: this man has a high risk of killing himself. His GP recognized the risk and specifically enquired about suicidal ideas. This man has biological symptoms of depression in the context of a severe bereavement and he is socially isolated.
2. He needs to be assessed by a psychiatrist with a view to either inpatient treatment or 24 hour intensive community treatment. If he declines, he would require assessment for compulsory admission to hospital under the Mental Health Act. His GP would have to contact the local psychiatrist and mental health worker.

History 2

1. The immediate risk of suicide is low as she does not have active suicidal ideation or evidence of a depressive illness. The short-term risk is moderate as she has a recent episode of deliberate self-harm, is socially isolated and is suffering from alcohol abuse.
2. The GP should not agree to her request for antidepressants but should try to persuade her to have treatment for her alcohol problems. Her mood will only improve if she stops drinking. She is under considerable social pressure and social work involvement is required despite her fears that the child will be taken into care. The GP has a duty to contact social services so that a clear risk assessment in relation to the safety of the child can be conducted.

History 3

1. The immediate and short-term risk in this patient is low. However, she is at long-term risk of suicide if her depression is not treated.
2. The A&E officer should ask the on-call psychiatrist to assess her and provide follow-up.

History 4

1. There is an immediate risk of suicide with this young man. He is acutely psychotic, and it is difficult to assess his thoughts.

2. He acquires immediate hospital admission. The GP calls an ambulance.

History 5

1. The immediate risk of suicide in this case is high. Although the man says he is alright, he took a serious overdose and the A&E officer suspects that he is depressed, although the man denies it.
2. The A&E officer should try to persuade the man to stay in casualty until he can be assessed by the duty psychiatrist. If the man insists on leaving, the A&E officer would have grounds to detain him, under common law, until he could be assessed by a psychiatrist. He is also medically at risk from the amount of paracetamol ingested.

History 6

1. Although ingestion of 30 paracetamol tablets is potentially lethal, the circumstances of the overdose imply that the suicidal intent was low. It is important to enquire about a previous history of deliberate self-harm, depressed mood over the previous few weeks or months and alcohol intake over the last few weeks and months. The two latter points are important as the patient's marriage might have broken up either because he has been depressed or because he has been drinking heavily.
2. It is important to assess his current suicidal intent and to check whether there is evidence of any depressive ideation, including feelings of hopelessness and worthlessness.
3. The risk of suicide is low.

History 7

1. Although you have very little information about this man, the deliberate self-harm episode is very serious. He was found by chance, had taken all his tablets and the tablets that he had taken are potentially lethal. He is also older than most patients who harm themselves and this is an additional risk factor.
2. This man needs to stay in hospital so that his physical status can be assessed. He also requires a full psychosocial assessment. The doctor should gently explain the situation to him and should try to find out more about his mental state and recent psychological health. It is likely that he is suffering from a depressive illness, and that he is currently under treatment for this (otherwise he would not have had access to tricyclic medication). The assessing doctor should ask him to be reviewed by the duty psychiatrist. Independently of his medical

condition, he may require admission to hospital for further assessment of his mental state under the Mental Health Act (1983). It may be appropriate to admit him to a medical ward in the first instance, if his medical condition needs to be monitored. His agreement to this would have to be clarified, and if he refuses, his capacity to decline further investigation and treatment (cardiac monitoring) would need to be assessed.

History 8

1. It is difficult to assess this woman's suicidal risk as she has some features suggestive of high risk, and others suggestive of a low risk. The deliberate self-harm attempt was not serious, and she does not appear to have a depressive illness. She does, however, say that she is suicidal and she has a previous history of deliberate self-harm. The assessment rests upon how seriously the assessing doctor believes that she will actually act upon her beliefs.
2. This is a difficult judgement to make, and the assessing doctor should always ask for a specialist opinion in these circumstances.

3. The psychiatrist discusses her case with a duty social worker and arrangements are made for her to spend the night at a women's hostel for the homeless. The psychiatrist says that she will speak with the patient's community pychiatric nurse in the morning.

OSCE answer

An examiner would expect the student to ask questions that elucidated the following:

1. The patient's suicidal intent in relation to the overdose
2. The patient's suicidal intent now
3. Any feelings of hopelessness
4. The lethality of the overdose (planned/impulsive; note/made efforts not to be discovered, etc.)
5. The presence of depressive illness.
6. Any previous psychiatric history and any previous self-harm episodes.

A mark would be given for each point covered plus marks for any other questions that were relevant and for overall performance.

7 Eating disorders

Overview

This chapter describes the main types of eating disorder: anorexia nervosa and bulimia nervosa. Eating disorders are 10 times more common in women than men and usually begin in late adolescence. Both disorders are characterized by an abnormal fear of fatness and a distorted body image. The other main features of anorexia nervosa are severe weight loss and amenorrhoea (in women), with or without bingeing. Bulimia nervosa is characterized by repeated episodes of bingeing in the absence of significant weight loss. Psychological treatment is the treatment of choice for all of the disorders, although antidepressants and other psychotropic drugs are helpful in treating comorbid disorders. The prognosis for bulimia nervosa is good, with the majority of individuals making a full recovery in the short term. However, about half of all patients with anorexia nervosa remain symptomatic many years after the onset of the disorder.

7.1 Types of eating disorder

Learning objectives

You should:

- know the definitions of the main types of eating disorder
- know the prevalence of the disorders.

Preoccupation with dieting and body image is common amongst young women. The majority of female university students have a distorted body image and regard themselves as being fatter than they are in reality. The ideal feminine figure according to fashion magazines is an emaciated, waif-like creature, whereas young males are portrayed as muscular, active and well-nourished beings. For each individual, the development of an eating disorder will depend upon a variety of factors, and biological, hormonal, psychosocial and familial factors have all been implicated in the aetiology of eating disorders. It is unlikely, however, that there will be a reduction in the prevalence of eating disorders until the social pressures on young women to diet are reduced.

Both the disorders discussed in this chapter involve attempts by the individual to control or reduce their body weight. It is important to remember, however, that obesity, particularly severe obesity, is also a disorder of eating, and one that may have serious long-term health implications. Obesity, however, is so common in developed countries, it has not until recently been considered a disorder. It is not discussed further in this chapter, but individuals with severe obesity may require psychological help, in addition to other methods, to help them to control their calorific intake.

The characteristic features of anorexia nervosa are given in Box 37 and those of bulimia nervosa in Box 38.

Box 37
Criteria for the diagnosis of anorexia nervosa

Body mass index (weight (kg)/height (metres) less than 17.5 (18.5 is suggestive of low weight)
Body weight less than 85% of that expected for height
Morbid fear of fatness and weight gain
Absence of at least three consecutive menstrual cycles in postmenarchal woman
Overconcern with body weight or shape and a distorted body image

---

Box 38
Criteria for the diagnosis of bulimia nervosa

Recurrent episodes of binge eating
A lack of control over eating
Minimum average of two binges per week for 3 months
Recurrent behaviour to limit effects of binge eating on weight (e.g. purgatives, self-induced vomiting, diuretics, fasting, etc.)
Overconcern with body weight and shape
Does not have anorexia nervosa

Prevalence

Both disorders are about ten times more common in women than men. Eating problems are usually manifested in early to late adolescence. They can, however, present later, but this usually implies a poorer prognosis. The exact prevalence in the general population is unclear. In the USA, studies suggest 4.5% of female college students have a history of eating problems. In the UK, one study found 1.9% of women attending a family planning clinic had a formal bulimic disorder. The lifetime prevalence of anorexia nervosa is 0.5–3.7%. The lifetime prevalence of bulimia nervosa is 1.1–4.2%.

First-degree female relatives of patients with anorexia nervosa have higher rates of eating disorders than would be expected, as do twin siblings of patients with either anorexia or bulimia nervosa. The concordance rates are higher in monozygotic than dizygotic twins. Families of patients with bulimia nervosa also have higher rates of substance misuse disorders than expected. The genetics of eating disorders are unclear, but there is probably a genetic and familial component.

7.2 Anorexia nervosa

Learning objectives

You should:

- know the clinical features and prognosis of anorexia
- know the management of anorexia.

Anorexia nervosa can be of two types:

- restricting type (i.e. weight controlled by restriction of food intake and exercise)
- binge-eating type (characterized by episodes of self-induced vomiting, binge eating or purging).

The main features of anorexia nervosa are described in Box 37. There are however, many subsidiary symptoms, some of which are secondary to the effects of starvation. The condition may start with the young woman becoming preoccupied with her weight and regarding herself as too fat. This is not unusual in itself as most young women tend to regard themselves as being larger than they are in reality. The young woman may start to diet and gradually becomes more and more preoccupied with the process. Her diet becomes more and more restricted; at the same time she becomes more and more preoccupied with food. She may start to cook more for the family yet eat very little of what she has made herself. She may begin to hoard food or have vivid dreams about it. She may start to eat very slowly so that the rest of the family become irritated and annoyed with her. Despite the small amount of food that she eats, if questioned, she will profess to have eaten large amounts.

Some young women with anorexia nervosa begin to binge and vomit at some stage of the condition, while others continue with a purely restrictive pattern of eating. The bingers and vomiters have a poorer prognosis than those who solely restrict their food. The bingeing usually begins in response to overwhelming feelings of hunger as the body is essentially subject to extreme conditions of starvation. The young woman is usually mortified after she has binged and makes herself vomit so as to avoid putting on weight.

Throughout the condition, the young woman's perception of her own body remains distorted. Some patients with severe forms of the disorder, despite only weighing 4 stone (25 kg), will consider themselves as being overweight.

Other features of the disorder can be grouped into categories.

- behaviour targeted at weight reduction
  — excessive exercise (running, cycling, swimming)
  — overactivity to ward off feelings of hunger
  — use of slimming pills
- physiological changes
  — decreased body temperature
  — compensatory lanugo body hair
  — decreased heart rate
  — decreased respiration rate
  — decreased metabolic rate
  — hypocalcaemia: decreased bone density, decreased calcium from teeth
  — decreased libido or failure to develop libido if condition begins around puberty
  — poor tolerance of the cold
  — poor peripheral circulation resulting in chilblains
  — sleep disturbance
  — oedema
  — gastrointestinal discomfort
  — coarse and dry skin, hair loss
- additional physiological complications of purgative use
  — hypokalaemia
  — cardiac arrest
  — melanosis coli
- additional physiological complications of self-induced vomiting
  — electrolyte imbalance
  — cardiac arrhythmias
  — dehydration
  — loss of tooth enamel
  — callous formation on dorsum of phalanges
- emotional changes
  — depression

— low self esteem

— irritability

— passive, withdrawn manner, punctuated by outbursts of anger

- cognitive changes

  — poor concentration

  — poor memory

  — increasingly distorted body image

- social changes

  — social withdrawal and isolation

- abnormal eating behaviours

  — extremely slow eating

  — playing with food, without eating it

  — eating alone

  — pretending to eat but disposing of food later

  — hoarding food

  — interest in preparing food for others

  — leaving the table during meals or immediately after to vomit.

Investigations

All patients require a thorough physical examination and routine blood tests with appropriate further investigations depending upon physical findings. Table 14 lists key investigations that may be necessary in some patients with anorexia nervosa.

About 50% of patients with anorexia nervosa have a good long-term outcome; 25% have an intermediate outcome, and 25% remain chronically underweight and socially disabled. Poor prognosis is indicated by:

- an older age at onset
- a previous history of mental health and personality difficulties
- a long duration of illness
- lack of social support or disturbed family relationships

- severe low weight
- an inability to engage in treatment or show motivation to change.

Management

The majority of patients are treated in the community, but those who are severely underweight require inpatient treatment. For patients who are seriously underweight, the goals are to restore weight, normalize eating patterns, achieve normal perceptions of hunger and satiety, and correct biological and psychological sequelae of malnutrition. Most inpatient programmes can achieve a weight gain of 2–3 lb (1–1.5 kg) per week without compromising the patient's safety. As the patient's weight and nutritional status increases, other eating disorder symptoms and distorted cognitions about body size tend to diminish. Mood improves and patients may become more socially interactive.

As weight increases, psychological treatments, including individual psychotherapy and family therapy, may be introduced. There are very few systematic trials of psychological therapies for anorexia nervosa, although results of a recent study provide support for family therapy and individual psychodynamic therapy. However, most of the evidence comes from case reports or case series. Treatments may be targeted at the symptoms themselves or at underlying psychosocial problems, such as relationship difficulties and family dysfunction.

Antidepressants may be used as an adjunct to treatment if there is evidence of significant depression. Mood state and suicidality should be regularly monitored. Anti-psychotic drugs may be used in low doses to reduce anxiety.

On rare occasions, the Mental Health Act (1983) may have to be used if the patient is dangerously below weight. Refeeding has been classified as a treatment for

Table 14 Investigations in anorexia nervosa

Symptoms or signs	Investigation
Pallor	Full blood count (FBC) with white cell differential Serum iron; total iron-binding capacity; ferritin, vitamin B$_{12}$ and folate levels may be indicated if FBC indicates patient is anaemic
Palpitations, weakness, dizziness, peripheral vasoconstriction	Electrocardiograph to exclude bradycardia, arrhythmias, Q-T elongation
Bone pain on exercise, short stature	X-ray or bone scan for pathological stress fractures; assessment of bone density to exclude osteoporosis
Arrested psychosexual development, which does not recover after re-instatement of normal body weight	Secretion of luteinizing hormone and follicle-stimulating hormone
Cold intolerance, diuresis, low body temperature	Cortisol, thyroid function tests
Bruising	FBC to exclude anaemia, neutropenia, thrombocytopenia
Gastrointestinal symptoms	Gamma scintigraphy to assess delayed gastric emptying
Apathy, poor concentration, severe cognitive impairment	Computed tomography may show ventricular enlargement; magnetic resonance imaging may show decreased grey and white matter

anorexia nervosa for the purposes of the Act and can be given under Section 63 (Ch. 15).

7.3 Bulimia nervosa

Learning objectives

You should:

- know the clinical features, course and prognosis of bulimia nervosa
- understand its management.

Binge eating is characterized by eating large amounts of food over a very short period of time. Typically, the individual carries out binges when alone and has the sense of being out of control, and being unable to stop eating. The binge usually stops because the individual is unable to eat any more food.

In addition to episodes of bingeing, the individual may develop a variety of other symptoms. These include repeated vomiting and purgative abuse, which have already been described. Other symptoms include acute dilatation of the stomach as a result of overeating; electrolyte imbalances, leading to brain seizures; abnormal electroencephalograph features; muscle cramps and stiffness; liver disease and kidney failure; and sleep disturbance and fatigue.

Little is known about the long-term outcome of bulimia nervosa. The short-term outcome is relatively good with about two thirds of individuals reporting an improvement in symptoms. Poor prognosis is indicated by:

- poor motivation to change
- previous history of personality difficulties
- other associated symptoms such as self-laceration
- continuing dissatisfaction with body image.

Assessment and treatment

As most eating disorders begin in adolescence, when the young person is still at home, a detailed personal and family assessment is important. The young person should be asked to keep a diary of her dieting behaviour over a period of 2 weeks. Any emotional difficulties within the family should be identified and the family should be discouraged from re-inforcing any of the young person's abnormal eating behaviour. Attempts should be made to restore a normal pattern of eating and to help the young person to feel more comfortable and accepting about being a normal weight, or about increasing her weight.

About 40% of patients with bulimia nervosa have significant medical complications; the most serious metabolic changes occur as a result of purging. As potentially fatal complications can arise in both anorexia and bulimia nervosa, patients with moderate-to-severe problems should receive a full physical examination (in the presence of a chaperon) and basic laboratory investigations (Table 14).

Psychological treatment, either cognitive-behavioural therapy or interpersonal therapy, is effective provided it is instituted at a relatively early stage of the disorder. Patients usually require treatment on a one-to-one basis for up to 16 weeks. Antidepressant treatment may also be helpful, if the patient is very depressed. There are a variety of self-help agencies, help lines and support groups that offer advice and help (see Further reading and sources).

Hospital admission is rarely indicated and should only be considered if the young person:

- is severely underweight
- has suicidal ideation
- has physical complications of dieting behaviour that puts her life at risk.

Further reading and sources

Agras WS, Walsh BT, Fairborn CG, Wilson GT, Kraemer HC 2000 A multicenter comparison of cognitive-behavioral therapy and interpersonal psychotherapy for bulimia nervosa. Archives of General Psychiatry, 57: 459–466

Andersen AE 2001 Progress in eating disorders research. American Journal of Psychiatry. 158: 515–517

Dare C, Eisler I, Russell G, Treasure J, Dodge, L 2001 Psychological therapies for adults with anorexia nervosa: randomised controlled trial of out-patient treatments. British Journal of Psychiatry, 178: 216–221

Various authors 2000 Practice guideline for the treatment of patients with eating disorders. American Journal of Psychiatry 157 (Suppl): 1–39.

Sources

American Anorexia Bulimia Association. National non-profit organization dedicated to the prevention and treatment of eating disorders. http://www.aabainc.org

The Eating Disorders Association. Offers help, advice and support to those suffering from anorexia, bulimia, binge eating as well as other eating-related illnesses. http://www.edauk.com

King's College London Institute of Psychiatry: Eating Disorders Research Unit. One of the few inpatient centres for the treatment of patients with severe anorexia nervosa. http://www.iop.kcl.ac.uk/IoP/Departments/PsychMed/EDU/index.stm

Self-assessment: questions

Multiple choice questions

1. The main features of anorexia nervosa are:
   a. Weight gain of greater than 15%
   b. Amenorrhoea of at least 3 months
   c. An abnormal fear of fatness
   d. A distorted body image
   e. A desire to put on weight

2. Anorexia nervosa:
   a. Is more common in males than females
   b. Has a better prognosis if the condition starts later in life
   c. Never requires hospital inpatient treatment
   d. Has a poorer prognosis if there is a previous history of personality difficulties
   e. Is best treated with pharmacotherapy

3. The main features of bulimia nervosa are:
   a. Severe weight loss
   b. Repeated episodes of bingeing
   c. Amenorrhoea
   d. Distorted body image
   e. Fear of fatness

4. The following are recognized abnormal patterns of eating that occur in anorexia nervosa:
   a. Eating small amounts of food
   b. Cutting food up into very small pieces
   c. Eating alone
   d. A hatred of cooking for others
   e. Hoarding food

5. Complications of self-induced vomiting include:
   a. Electrolyte imbalance
   b. Cardiac arrhythmias
   c. Water intoxication
   d. Loss of tooth enamel
   e. Callous formation on palmar side of phalanges

6. Body mass index is calculated by:
   a. Weight in lb/height in inches
   b. Weight in grams squared (g^2)/ height in metres
   c. Weight in grams/height in metres
   d. Weight in kg/height (in metres)^2
   e. Weight in kg × height in metres

Case history questions

History 1

A 31-year-old woman who is 5 feet 7 inches tall (1.67 m) weighs 4 stone 8 lb (29 kg) when she is admitted to hospital. She is severely emaciated and her body is covered in lanugo hair. She has been underweight for the last 15 years and has been amenorrhoeic since she was 20 years of age. She is preoccupied by her weight and feels that her stomach is too fat. She severely restricts her diet and usually only eats oranges, other fruit and slimming rye breads. She lives at home with her mother and has an extremely restricted social life. She has never had a sexual partner. She resents being admitted to hospital and does not accept she has a problem with weight gain.

1. What is her diagnosis?
2. What is the prognosis?

History 2

A 23-year-old geography student presents to her GP with a 2 year history of bingeing and vomiting. She is slightly overweight. Her symptoms began following the break-up of a serious relationship with a man she had been going out with for 3 years. She had been persuaded by her friends, with whom she lived, to seek help. She described starving herself all day so as not to put on weight, but then bingeing at night time when she would lose control and eat a whole box of cornflakes, plus a loaf of bread, plus biscuits and chocolate. She would then feel dreadful about herself and make herself sick. She did not use any other methods to limit her weight. She regarded herself as being grossly overweight and felt she was ugly and unattractive.

1. What is her diagnosis?
2. What treatment would be appropriate?

History 3

A 28-year-old nursery nurse has suffered from type I diabetes since she was 14 years of age. Her diabetes has always been poorly controlled and she has begun to develop renal complications. On her most recent admission to hospital (for ketoacidosis) the nursing staff suspect she is making herself sick in the ward toilets after meals. She rarely eats hospital food but is seen eating chocolate and sandwiches, which are brought in by her family.

When asked about her eating habits, she denies that there is a problem. She says she eats all the hospital food given her, despite clear evidence from nursing staff that this is not the case. Her body mass index is within normal limits. She denies trying to lose weight, and she denies any misuse of her insulin regime.

How would you manage the situation?

Self-assessment: answers

Multiple choice answers

1. a. **False**. Weight loss of at least 15%.
   b. **True**. In those postmenarche.
   c. **True**. There is often a distorted sense of body size.
   d. **True**.
   e. **False**.

2. a. **False**. It is 10 times more common in females than males.
   b. **False**. The prognosis is worse if anorexia nervosa begins in older age groups.
   c. **False**. Hospital admission is required if the young person is suicidal, has a dangerously low body weight or other serious risk factors.
   d. **True**.
   e. **False**. Psychological treatment approaches are preferred.

3. a. **False**. Body weight is usually normal or slightly higher than normal.
   b. **True**.
   c. **False**. Menstruation is normal or irregular.
   d. **True**.
   e. **True**.

4. a. **True**.
   b. **True**.
   c. **True**.
   d. **False**. There is often a desire to cook and make food for others, although the individual will not eat it herself.
   e. **True**. Individuals with anorexia nervosa may collect or hoard tins of food.

5. a. **True**.
   b. **True**.
   c. **False**. Dehydration is more likely.
   d. **True**. This is caused by the acidic stomach contents.
   e. **False**. Callous formation on dorsum of phalanges.

6. a. **False**. Body mass index is given by weight (kg)/height (metres)^2.
   b. **False**.
   c. **False**.
   d. **True**.
   e. **False**.

Case history answers

History 1

1. This woman is suffering from a severe form of anorexia nervosa Her current weight is well below 15% of what should be her normal weight; she has been amenorrhoeic for at least 3 months, she has a distorted body image and an abnormal fear of fatness.
2. Her prognosis is poor as she has had the condition for over 10 years and is poorly motivated to change.

History 2

1. This young woman has bulimia nervosa. She describes recurrent episodes of binge eating and a lack of control over eating. She shows recurrent compensatory behaviour to prevent weight by vomiting after she has overeaten. The behaviour happens at least twice a week and has been present for more than 3 months. She has a distorted body image.
2. She would be best helped by brief psychological treatment, either cognitive-behavioural therapy or psychodynamic interpersonal therapy.

History 3

This young woman may have an eating disorder that is contributing to her poor diabetic control and frequent hospital admissions. She has denied any problems with eating when asked about this by staff. It will be important to establish if one member of staff, either a ward nurse or diabetic nurse, can build up a relationship with her so she feels she can talk about her symptoms. The team could also consider referral to a liaison psychiatrist, with her permission, to see if the liaison psychiatrist could help her to confide more openly about her problems. Until she can be helped to do this, treatment is unlikely to be of help.

8 Alcohol and drug abuse

Overview

Alcohol and illicit drug problems are a major cause of mortality and morbidity in the Western world. Problems with alcohol should be viewed on a continuum. The recommended safe drinking limits are <14 units alcohol per week for women and <28 units for men. Drinking above these levels on a persistent basis places individuals at risk of physical complications from alcohol abuse such as cardiovascular disease, hypertension and stroke. Large amounts of alcohol consumption on a regular basis result in severe physical and psychosocial sequelae, including neurological damage, liver cirrhosis, depression and brain damage. Alcohol dependence syndrome refers to individuals who become physically addicted to alcohol and suffer physical withdrawal symptoms from the drug if it is stopped. This condition is potentially fatal and should be treated in a hospital setting. Controlled withdrawal regimens, however, can be carried out in the community. There are now effective treatments for alcohol abuse, and a range of statutory and voluntary help is available.

Illicit drugs vary in their effects and withdrawal syndromes. Opiates, cocaine and amphetamines have clear withdrawal syndromes, whereas hallucinogens, cannabis and inhalants do not. The treatment approaches for illicit drug abuse are similar to those for alcohol-related disorders. For some patients with opiate addiction, methadone maintenance treatment may be appropriate. Drugs which decrease craving for opiates may play a greater role in treatment in the future.

8.1 Prevalence of alcohol-related problems

Learning objectives

You should:

- know the prevalence of alcohol problems in different settings (e.g. community and general hospital)
- know the recommended safe limits of alcohol consumption
- be familiar with the different terminology used to describe alcohol-related problems
- be aware of the costs to society of alcohol-related problems.

The degree of alcohol consumption in the community has risen since the 1980s. In a recent survey in the USA, 52% of the population regularly drank alcohol and 9% met criteria for either alcohol abuse or dependence. Alcohol problems were more common in whites than non-whites. The overall consumption was higher in males than females, but drinking was particularly increasing in young women. The highest rates were seen in young males (late teenage years to early twenties). The general level of alcohol consumption within the community is important as the higher the average consumption, the greater the number of people who will be drinking excessively. Age of onset is also important. Individuals who begin drinking alcohol before the age of 14 have four times the risk of lifetime dependence in comparison with those who begin after the age of 20 years.

In the hospital setting, 10–30% of inpatients have alcohol-related problems, and approximately 40% of ambulatory attenders at A&E departments have alcohol-related disorders. Detection is important, as the general hospital or A&E department may be the patient's first contact with treatment services.

Differences between men and women

Women begin using alcohol later than men and are strongly influenced by partners or spouses. They report different reasons for maintaining the use of alcohol, are more likely to drink in secret, but enter treatment earlier in the course of their illnesses than do men. Women have a higher prevalence of comorbid psychiatric disorders, such as depression and anxiety, than do men, and these disorders typically predate the development of alcohol use problems. Women, however, are more likely to engage in treatment than men and are more responsive to treatment than men.

Genetics

Children of alcoholics are more likely than the general population to be either teetotal or develop alcohol problems themselves. The role of familial, environmental and genetic factors, however, are difficult to disentangle. It is possible that individuals may inherit either a vulnerability to alcoholism or a vulnerability to organ damage by alcohol. Genes might play a role by influencing temperament or personality in such a way as to predispose individuals to alcoholism. Studies have shown there is greater concordance of alcohol dependence in male, monozygotic twins than male, dizygotic twins. The same is not true for female twins. Adoption studies have also confirmed that the adopted children of alcoholics preferentially develop alcoholism as adults.

A potential marker (the dopamine D_2 receptor) is currently being studied as it is found more often in alcoholics than in non-alcoholics. In animal studies, this marker has been associated with brain functions relating to reward, reinforcement and motivation.

Two basic experimental techniques are being used to search the human genome for specific genes related to alcoholism. The first, the candidate gene approach, involves hypothesizing that particular genes are related to the physiology of alcoholism based on our knowledge of biology and physiology and then individually testing these genes for linkage. The second approach, scanning the human genome, involves characterizing piece by piece the entire length of DNA and finding genes that related to alcoholism without proposing candidate genes.

Additionally, researchers can use animal models to study the genetics and biology of alcoholism. A new animal model of alcoholism has been recently developed. Rats derived from this model show certain characteristics. They have an incentive demand to consume alcohol and exhibit relapse-like drinking even after a very long time of abstinence. They show tolerance to alcohol and have mild signs of physical withdrawal during the onset of abstinence. During abstinence, they also exhibit a psychological withdrawal syndrome consisting of enhanced anxiety-related behaviour and hyperactivity to stressful situations. Anti-craving drugs such as naltrexone (see below) suppress the alcohol deprivation effect.

Costs

The costs incurred in the treatment of alcohol-related problems, or the adverse effects of alcohol morbidity and mortality on productivity, are enormous. Treatment and prevention of alcohol problems and related health conditions are estimated to have cost $18.8 billion in 1992 in the USA. Alcohol and drug abuse caused more than 1107 360 deaths in 1992, and the estimated loss of productivity resulting from deaths attributable to alcohol was $31.3 billion. The estimation of lost productivity caused by alcohol was $66.7 billion in 1992. These figures do not include costs related to other consequences of alcoholism such as crime and social morbidity.

Safe levels of alcohol consumption

Since the early 1980s, there has been a change in the way alcohol misuse is viewed. Instead of a previous dichotomy between 'alcoholism' and 'normal drinking', alcohol consumption is now viewed as a spectrum of disorders. *Hazardous drinking* refers to a pattern of drinking that confers risk of harmful consequences, and *harmful alcohol use* (alcohol abuse) refers to actual physical harm or social problems caused by drinking.

The consumption of alcohol is measured in terms of units. A unit of alcohol or standard drink is equivalent to the consumption of:

- half a pint of beer
- a standard measure of spirits
- a glass of wine.

The safe limits of alcohol consumption are 14 units per week for women and 21 units per week for men (including at least two alcohol-free days). Hazardous consumption is equivalent to 21–42 drinks per week for men and 14–28 drinks per week for women. At this level of drinking, there is an increasing risk of problems such as raised blood pressure, stroke or liver cirrhosis. Sustained drinking of above 42 units per week for men or 28 units for women is likely to cause physical, mental or social problems. *Alcohol dependence* refers to the state of being physically addicted to alcohol.

8.2 Alcohol history and physical examination

Learning objectives

You should:

- be able to take an alcohol history from any patient

- be familiar with brief screening questions for problem drinking and alcohol abuse

- be able to conduct a relevant physical examination to detect physical sequelae of alcohol abuse

- be able to conduct a mental state examination to detect psychological and cognitive sequelae of alcohol abuse.

Taking an alcohol history

An alcohol history consists of the following elements:

- age first began drinking
- amount consumed in teenage years, and each subsequent decade
- amount consumed in the past week, itemized on a day-by-day basis
- time points when average alcohol consumption either increased or decreased (reasons for change)
- pattern of drinking (binge or regular consumption)
- evidence of physical dependence upon alcohol and age this first occurred
- signs and symptoms of alcohol-dependence syndrome (see below)
- blackouts or memory losses
- attempts to reduce consumption or become abstinent
- longest period of abstinence and what factors contributed to this
- contact with services and compliance with treatment
- motivation to stop drinking (stages of awareness: does the patient accept there is a problem; does the patient recognize change has to occur; how willing is the patient to make changes and accept treatment; see below)
- any psychological sequelae of alcohol (e.g. depression, excessive anxiety, jealousy, persecutory ideation)
- any physical sequelae of alcohol consumption (e.g. convulsions, accidental injuries, head injuries, peptic ulcer, gastritis, pancreatitis, liver disease, peripheral neuropathy, proximal myopathy, etc.)
- any cognitive sequelae (short-term memory impairment, dementia, frontal lobe damage)
- any social sequelae of excessive alcohol consumption (e.g. drink driving offences, assaults, problems at work, domestic difficulties and violence).

The details will need to be checked by taking a history from an informant, as people often underestimate their own alcohol consumption and the degree to which their lives have been affected by drinking.

Screening for alcohol problems

It is not feasible to conduct a detailed alcohol history on every patient, but all medical and surgical patients should be asked routinely about their levels of alcohol consumption and whether they have ever experienced any symptoms of withdrawal. Unfortunately, alcohol problems often remain undetected in the medical setting, which can result in patients suddenly going into acute withdrawal on a medical ward. This should never happen and is easily avoided by taking a brief alcohol history where a high consumption of alcohol is suspected.

Several brief screening questionnaires have been developed to detect problem drinking. A relatively new screening questionnaire, the Alcohol Use Disorders Identification Test (AUDIT), is able to detect over 90% of hazardous drinkers in a range of clinical and non-clinical settings. The questionnaire was developed from a series of World Health Organization (WHO) collaborative studies on brief interventions for hazardous alcohol use. Once hazardous drinking has been detected, 5 minutes of structured advice from an alcohol counsellor or health worker (GP) results in a reduction in hazardous drinking by 30%. These findings suggest that all doctors should be familiar with this questionnaire and the screening questions it contains (Box 39).

Physical examination and investigations

A careful physical examination should be undertaken, looking for the following signs of the physical effects of alcohol abuse.

1. Check whether the patient smells of alcohol, has slurred speech or other signs of intoxication.
2. Observe whether the patient is sweating and has signs of a coarse tremor.
3. Check for palmar erythema, spider nevae and other signs of liver disease.
4. Check for scars or signs of old injuries.
5. Cardiovascular system: check for rapid pulse and low blood pressure.
6. Neurological system: check for tone and power and reflexes in upper and lower limbs. Check for proximal muscle weakness or tenderness, decreased sensation in lower limbs, up-going plantars. Check eye movements for nystagmus. Check for

Box 39
Alcohol Use Disorders Identification Test (AUDIT)

Please circle the answer that is correct for you

1. How often do you have a drink containing alcohol?

   | never | monthly or less | 2–4 times a month | 2–3 times a week | 4 or more a week |

2. How many standard drinks containing alcohol do you have on a typical day when drinking?

   | 1 or 2 | 3 or 4 | 5 or 6 | 7 to 9 | 10 or more |

3. How often do you have six or more drinks on one occasion?

   | never | less than monthly | monthly | weekly | daily or almost daily |

4. How often during the last year have you found that you were not able to stop drinking once you had started?

   | never | less than monthly | monthly | weekly | daily or almost daily |

5. How often during the last year have you failed to do what was normally expected from you because of your drinking?

   | never | less than monthly | monthly | weekly | daily or almost daily |

6. How often during the last year have you needed a drink in the morning to get yourself going after a heavy drinking session?

   | never | less than monthly | monthly | weekly | daily or almost daily |

7. How often during the last year have you had a feeling of guilt or remorse after drinking?

   | never | less than monthly | monthly | weekly | daily or almost daily |

8. How often during the last year have you been unable to remember what happened the night before because you had been drinking?

   | never | less than monthly | monthly | weekly | daily or almost daily |

9. Have you or someone else been injured as a result of your drinking?

   | no | yes, but not in the last year | yes, during the last year |

10. Has a relative or friend or a doctor or other health worker been concerned about your drinking or suggested you cut down?

   | no | yes, but not in the last year | yes during the last year |

Scoring: Questions 1–8 are scored 0, 1, 2, 3, 4 (left to right); questions 9 and 10 are scored 0, 2 and 4 (left to right). A total of ≥8 = hazardous drinking; >13 in women and >15 in men is likely to indicate alcohol dependence. From Saunders et al. (1993).

visual–spatial awareness and hand eye coordination. Observe the patient's gait.

7. Perform the following investigations:
   a. Full blood count. Check for evidence of anaemia, either iron deficiency or vitamin B$_{12}$ and folate. Mean Cell Volume (MCV) is raised in about 60% of problem drinkers.
   b. Blood alcohol. Detects recent alcohol consumption.
   c. Liver function tests. Gamma-glutamyltranspeptidase (GGT) is raised in about 80% of problem drinkers.

More detailed investigations may be required, which will be dependent upon the signs and symptoms elicited at interview.

Mental state examination

In the mental state examination, the following areas require particular attention:

- check that the patient is fully oriented
- check the level of arousal (in the early stages of acute withdrawal, patients are easily startled and hyper-aroused)
- note whether the patient is sweating and has a tremor
- note whether the patient smells of alcohol
- note whether the patient is aggressive or argumentative (take precautions for safety if this is detected)
- check whether the patient's speech is slurred
- can the patient understand what you are saying and respond appropriately?
- check the patient's mood with special reference to depression and suicidal ideation
- does the patient have any abnormal ideas, in particular ideas of reference or persecutory ideas
- check for evidence of visual hallucinations or illusions, tactile hallucinations, and second person auditory hallucinations
- does the patient have any specific ideas of jealousy in relation to his/her partner
- if the patient is fully conscious, test the following in detail: concentration, and short-and long-term memory.

8.3 Psychological and physical sequelae of alcohol abuse

Learning objectives

You should:

- know the major psychological and social sequelae of alcohol abuse
- know the major neuropsychiatric sequelae of alcohol abuse
- know the key features of alcohol-dependence syndrome
- know and be able to detect the major physical sequelae of alcohol abuse.

The psychological effects of excessive alcohol consumption

In small quantities, alcohol has an anxiolytic effect, and it is often used by people to reduce anxiety or stress. However, excessive consumption results in a depressive effect upon mood, with increased anxiety in-between drinking. Unfortunately, these effects encourage further drinking, with the possibility of dependence or other adverse consequences.

Psychological changes as a result of excessive alcohol consumption can be grouped into three categories:

- psychiatric syndromes that develop without overt evidence of brain damage
- alcohol-dependence syndrome
- psychiatric syndromes that result from organic damage because of either the direct toxic effects of alcohol or the indirect effects of malnutrition.

Psychiatric syndromes

The most common psychiatric syndromes that develop without overt evidence of brain damage are shown in Table 15. As alcohol has a toxic effect on the brain, the development of all these conditions is probably related to some degree of subtle brain damage, although overt cognitive function may not be impaired. Excessive alcohol consumption can also result in changes of personality, with increased self-centredness and a lack of concern for others.

Alcohol-dependence syndrome

Physical dependence upon alcohol is associated with a characteristic constellation of symptoms (Box 40). All individuals who are dependent upon alcohol will show these characteristic features.

Neuropsychiatric effects of alcohol excess

Chronic alcoholism results in brain damage and dysfunction, leading to a constellation of neuropsychiatric symptoms including cognitive dysfunction, the Wernicke–Korsakoff syndrome, alcoholic cerebellar degeneration and alcoholic dementia. It is likely that these conditions are caused by a synergistic combination of the direct, toxic effect of alcohol upon brain cells and indirect effects via malnutrition, metabolic disturbances and damage following accidental or violent trauma. Alcohol and its metabolite acetaldehyde are directly neurotoxic. Alcoholics are thiamine deficient as a result of poor diet, gastrointestinal disorders and liver disease. In addition, both alcohol and acetaldehyde have direct toxic effects on thiamine-related enzymes in the liver and brain.

Table 15 The psychological effects of excessive alcohol consumption

Psychological sequelae	Symptoms
Depressive illness	Continuous low mood, poor sleep
Anxiety symptoms	Tension, heightened arousal, nervousness, restlessness, autonomic symptoms
Suicidal behaviour and deliberate self-harm	Alcohol abuse is associated with high rates of suicide. Between 5 and 20% of patients with alcohol abuse commit suicide. Alcohol abuse, or a family history of alcoholism, is particularly associated with an increased risk of suicidal ideation in men
Sexual dysfunction	This can be a direct effect of intoxication, a consequence of a deterioration in the relationship with the sexual partner or an indirect effect of the physical sequelae of alcohol abuse
Alcoholic hallucinosis	In this rare condition, the individual experiences second or third person auditory hallucinations of a derogatory nature in the absence of delirium. They often develop secondary persecutory ideas but usually settle within a few weeks. If the symptoms do not settle, it is indicative of schizophrenia
Pathological jealousy	Irrational suspiciousness of partner's sexual fidelity. Delusional syndrome is rare, but mild-to-moderate jealousy is common, probably compounded by poor sexual performance and deteriorating relationship

---

Box 40
Features of the alcohol-dependence syndrome

- A compulsion to drink
- Primacy of alcohol above all other social activities (e.g. eating)
- Altered tolerance (ability to drink greater amounts of alcohol before experiencing a feeling of intoxication: in the late stages of drinking tolerance falls)
- Withdrawal symptoms (including tremor, agitation, sweating, wretching, hallucinations or illusions); begin within 6 to 8 hours after last drink
- Relief drinking (drinking to counteract the withdrawal symptoms): most commonly detected by asking the patient whether he has a drink first thing in the morning (so-called 'hair of the dog')
- Salience of the drinking repertoire (the patient loses the ability to vary his alcohol intake in relation to social cues, as he has to drink regular and consistent amounts to control withdrawal symptoms; most people's alcohol intake varies according to different circumstances)
- Reinstatement after abstinence (the patient's withdrawal symptoms and physical dependence upon alcohol quickly return if the patient starts to drink again)

In the past, it was thought that alcoholics developed discrete brain syndromes through the differing effects of alcohol on the brain. It is likely, however, that chronic alcoholism is characterized by a continuum of brain dysmorphology, and that clinical signs only develop after substantial brain damage has already occurred. Alcoholic dementia may be a more severe form of alcoholic Korsakoff syndrome. The main clinical syndromes are described below, although there is much overlap between them, and they probably share the same aetiological pathway.

The Wernicke–Korsakoff syndrome (the amnesic syndrome)

The Wernicke–Korsakoff syndrome is characterized by a prominent disorder of recent memory in the absence of generalized cognitive impairment. The amnesic syndrome may follow from an acute neurological syndrome originally described by Wernicke. This is an encephalopathy, and the main features include clouding of consciousness, memory defect, disorientation, ataxia and ophthalmoplegia. Once the acute illness has subsided, the patient can register events as they occur but is unable to remember them a few minutes later. The patient's ability to perform everyday tasks is grossly impaired, as he/she easily becomes disorientated. The patient may have little insight into the condition and may often confabulate (make up unlikely stories) in order to cover up gaps in memory. Classically, memory for remote events is more com-

plete, although many patients have disturbances in long-term memory as well. The affect of the patient can appear rather blunted or fatuous, and motivation may also be impaired.

The most common cause of the syndrome is thiamine deficiency secondary to prolonged alcohol abuse. The pathology is characterized by neuronal loss, gliosis and vascular damage in regions surrounding the third and fourth ventricles and the cerebral aqueduct. Other non-alcohol-related causes include carbon monoxide poisoning, vascular lesions, encephalitis, malnutrition caused by gastrointestinal surgery, and tumours of the third ventricle. Recent evidence suggests that the circuit involving the mammillary bodies, the mammillo-thalamic tract and the anterior thalamus, rather than the medial dorsal nucleus of the thalamus, is particularly critical in the formation of new memories. The relationship of these deficits to thiamine depletion remains a topic of current investigation, as does the purported role of neurotransmitter depletions in the cholinergic, glutamate/gamma-aminobutyric acid (GABA) and catecholamine and serotonergic systems. Neuroimaging studies have confirmed postmortem findings of more widespread structural and metabolic abnormalities, particularly involving the frontal lobes.

Alcoholic dementia

Detoxified chronic alcoholics often display mild-to-moderate cognitive deficits. Memory for visuospatial stimuli is often worse than for verbal material, which parallels findings that these patients tend to show greater dysfunction in visuospatial skills relative to verbal abilities. Relatively young alcoholics (in their thirties) may show little neuropsychological impairment, and older alcoholics may show improvement in cognitive functioning after at least 5 years of sobriety.

Box 41 Ethical issues in alcohol abusers

The Mental Health Act may have to be used with patients with Korsakoff's syndrome in the early stages of the illness when they are acutely confused. This will depend upon how cooperative they are with treatment, and the length of time that restraint or treatment may need to be given against their will. At a later stage, guardianship provision might need to be considered (this gives powers to ensure the patient resides at a particular place and attends treatment, although he/she may refuse any treatment offered). Additional legal measures may be required to manage the patients' financial affairs. Patients with Korsakoff's syndrome are often relatively young, and the balance between their rights and liberties and the risk of further harm by continued alcohol consumption, or the risk to themselves because of disorientation, needs to be carefully considered.

Some chronic alcoholics, however, develop a global dementia that persists despite abstinence from alcohol. Widespread cerebral atrophy can result from prolonged alcohol abuse and computed tomography (CT) shows enlarged ventricles and widened cerebral sulci. Most patients will also have diencephalic pathology; therefore, rigorous attention should be paid to their nutritional status. Alcoholic dementia is typically characterized by severe impairment of memory, conceptualization, problem-solving and visuospatial abilities. The memory disturbance is characterized by rapid forgetting of information over time, rather than retrieval or encoding difficulties. Sustained abstinence can result in moderate improvement of cognitive performance with associated improvements on CT scan.

Acute withdrawal

Withdrawal symptoms usually begin within a few hours of the patient's last drink, as blood alcohol levels begin to fall. Withdrawal symptoms follow a characteristic pattern in most patients unless they are stopped, by either treatment or further drinking. The main features are described in Box 42. They begin within a few hours (6–24 hours) of the person's last drink. *Delirium tremens* may develop 24–48 hours after the last drink. In very heavy drinkers, withdrawal symptoms can be triggered by a reduction in the amount of alcohol drunk rather than complete cessation.

Alcohol withdrawal syndrome is a potentially fatal condition that requires immediate medical management and hospital admission if delirium has developed. Patients can die because of fluid loss followed by cardiovascular collapse. Patients can undergo supervised withdrawal regimens in the community. These are planned and managed by members of community alcohol teams. The patient is prescribed an appropriate

---

Box 43
Management of acute alcohol withdrawal

1. Appropriate nursing care: manage patient in well-lit room, close observation, reassurance and continual orientation of patient (i.e. tell patient the time, place and who you are)
2. Parenteral vitamins B and C (Pabrinex)
3. Monitor blood glucose levels
4. Adequate fluid balance: intravenous fluids may be required
5. Benzodiazepines every 4–6 hours (dose proportional to patient's symptoms) (patient may require 100 mg chlordiazepoxide or 40 mg diazepam every 4–6 hours). Dosage should be reduced after 2–4 days, and the patient placed on a reduction regimen. Medication should not be required after 7–10 days.

---

amount of medication to control any physical symptoms of withdrawal and is monitored on a daily basis.

Box 43 describes the basic principles of the medical management of a serious alcohol withdrawal state.

Physical effects of excess alcohol consumption.

The main, adverse physical effects of excess alcohol consumption are listed in Box 44.

Box 44
The physical effects of chronic excess alcohol consumption

- **Hepatic effects**
  — fatty inflammation
  — alcoholic hepatitis: acute illness with deep jaundice, right upper quadrant pain, tender hepatomegaly, fever, raised white cell count, elevated prothrombin time
  — cirrhosis: palmar erythema, gynaecomastia, testicular atrophy, more than five spider naevi on the face or upper trunk, evidence of portal hypertension (splenomegaly, ascites, oesophageal varices, haemorrhoids), evidence of deranged synthetic function, cerebral dysfunction (dementia)
- **Pancreatitis**: central abdominal pain that radiates through to the back, with tenderness, rigidity and guarding, pallor, sweating, shock (hypotension, poor peripheral perfusion and tachypnoea)
- **Gastritis**: dyspepsia, bleeding
- **Peripheral neuropathy**: symmetrical glove and stocking loss of sensation, paraesthesiae
- **Cardiomyopathy**: heart failure
- **Effects on the fetus**: low weight, low intelligence, facial abnormality
- **Other effects**: oesophageal carcinoma, peptic ulcer, cerebellar degeneration, epilepsy, anaemia, episodic hypoglycaemia, myopathy, obesity, decreased fertility in women

---

Box 42
Alcohol withdrawal syndrome

Nausea, retching and vomiting
Tremor (usually course)
Paroxysmal sweats (in full syndrome, patient will be drenched)
Anxiety
Increased arousal, agitation, restlessness
Headache and fullness
Sensitivity to light
Withdrawal fit
Visual hallucinations (mild, ill-formed to severe, terrifying, vivid hallucinations in full-blown syndrome)
Tactile disturbances (itching in mild form to severe hallucinations of bugs crawling on skin)
Auditory disturbances (sensitivity to noise in mild form to severe, continuous hallucinations)
Clouding of conscious with disorientation and confusion

8.4 Services and treatment for alcoholic disorders

There are a range of services available to help people with alcohol misuse problems. There are several well-recognized and respected organizations that operate completely independently of the NHS. These include Alcoholics Anonymous (AA), Alcohol Concern and Turning Point. All offer a variety of different kinds of education, support and counselling. Alcohol services in the NHS are mainly community based. Community alcohol teams consist of experienced health workers (community alcohol nurses or social workers), who arrange to assess patients, counsel them about their drinking, organize withdrawal regimens if necessary, and link people up with other alcohol services in the voluntary sector. There are relatively few inpatient beds for the treatment of alcohol problems in the UK. Most regions in the UK have specialized treatment centres for patients with the most severe problems, which have a small number of beds. Several of the alcohol charities run hostels or dry houses for recovering alcoholics. These are places where individuals can live for several months after they have stopped drinking to help them to adjust to a new lifestyle and protect them from the temptation to drink. Dry houses have a complete ban on alcohol, and individuals are immediately discharged if they drink alcohol while resident.

Proposals for a national alcohol strategy

The UK Government has declared its intention to introduce a national strategic approach to alcohol (Department of Health, 1999a). Targets that were set in 1992 (Department of Health, 1992) to reduce the numbers of people drinking above safe limits have not been met, and there has been an increase in the numbers of young women and young adult men drinking above safe limits. Potential preventative as well as treatment strategies have been proposed by the charity Alcohol Concern and include:

- maintaining or increasing taxation
- reducing alcohol-related crime and nuisance in and around drinking venues and city centres
- reducing drink driving offences
- controlling the promotion of alcohol
- promoting responsible drinking
- screening for alcohol problems in primary care and hospital settings
- brief treatments within primary care, hospital and alcohol service settings
- longer-term specialist remedial treatment, including detoxification and counselling services in supported and day-care settings, or residential units
- self-help support groups
- support for children and partners of individuals with alcohol abuse.

Many of these are likely to be incorporated into the Government's final strategic document, and they have implications for not only psychiatric services but also for primary care and general hospital services.

Treatment

The response to treatment in substance misuse may depend upon how readily the individual is able to accept that he/she has a problem and is willing to do something about it. Different treatment strategies are required for individuals who have different views of their drinking. If someone does not accept that they have a drinking problem, strategies aimed at treatment will not be successful. Instead, strategies are required to help the individual to gain insight and desire for change (so-called *motivational strategies*). The stages of change through which individuals pass in relation to finally obtaining mastery over their drinking have been described by Prochaska and Velicer (1997). They are summarized in Box 45.

Box 45
Stages of change in mastering a drink problem

Precontemplative stage
No recognition of problem. Motivational interviewing techniques required.

Contemplative stage
Awareness of problem but wants to continue drinking. Motivational interviewing techniques required.

Preparation stage
Willingness to change behaviour. May seek treatment. Treatment required.

Action stage
Engages in treatment. Follows a treatment plan.

Maintenance stage
Maintains abstinence or reduction in drinking

Brief interventions

Brief interventions are appropriate for people with hazardous drinking or harmful drinking that has caused relatively few medical problems. Such strategies have been shown to be effective in primary care and the general hospital setting. The interventions are primarily educational and consist of either one or two sessions of counselling. The interventions work because individuals with drinking problems are detected at a relatively early stage and can alter their behaviour before either psychological or physical dependency develops.

For most individuals with hazardous drinking, abstinence is not a necessary goal. The aim should be to help the individual to drink within safe limits. Abstinence is required, however, if the individual has already developed physical or organic mental illness as a result of his/her drinking or is physically dependent upon alcohol.

Specific treatments

Intensive treatments are required for individuals who have developed physical dependency upon alcohol or have other serious sequelae of alcohol abuse. There are a variety of different treatment approaches; most, however, use a combination of individual and group treatments. The maintenance of long-term abstinence usually requires individuals to alter their lifestyles completely including work and social life (which may revolve around drinking). They will require specific strategies to help them to not drink, and also psychological treatments to solve some of the difficulties (e.g. low self-esteem) that may have led them to drink in the first place. Cognitive-behavioural coping skills therapy (CBT), motivational enhancement therapy (MET) (based upon motivational interviewing techniques) and 12-step facilitation therapy (TSF) (based around the principles to treatment developed by AA: see below) appear to be equally effective for the long-term treatment of patients with alcohol dependence. Significant and sustained improvements in drinking outcomes are achieved by all therapies. CBT and TSF appear to produce effects more quickly than MET, and patients with a history of severe psychiatric problems do better with MET than CBT. Three years after treatment, 30% of subjects (in all groups) are totally abstinent, and those who do report drinking remain abstinent two thirds of the time.

Long-term support is available from many of the voluntary sector alcohol agencies. Individuals who obtain help for a drinking problem and participate in treatment (either formal treatment or participation in AA) have a better outcome, both in the short and long term, than those who do not engage in treatment.

Alcoholics Anonymous: Twelve Step Programme of Recovery AA meetings take several different forms but all involve alcoholics (term used by the society) talking about what drink did to their lives and family, what actions they took to deal with this and how they are living their lives today. The meetings are run by alcoholics who have recovered from drinking. AA does not believe in a cure and maintains that individuals should continue to attend meetings and put into practice what they learn at meetings (from each other) to keep sober. Some meetings are open (i.e. friends or other interested parties such as medical students, can attend), while others are closed. All respect a strict code of anonymity and confidentiality. There are regular meetings most days of the week in most areas of the UK.

AA recommends individuals follow a 12-step programme of recovery. The organization was founded in 1934 and the programme reflects the experience of the earliest members of the society. They are summarized in Box 46. Although emphasis is placed upon the role of God, the organization itself is not a religious organization, and 'God' can be used in either a literal or a metaphorical way by members. We have listed the 12 steps in this book as most doctors should be aware of AA and the kind of approach it offers.

Pharmacological treatments

Disulfiram (Antabuse) or citrated calcium carbimide (Abstem) have been used to good effect in some patients to deter the impulse to drink. Both substances react with

---

Box 46
The Twelve Step Programme of Alcoholics Anonymous

1. Admitted we were powerless over alcohol and that our lives had become unmanageable.
2. Came to believe that a Power greater than ourselves could restore us to sanity.
3. Made a decision to turn our will and our lives over to the care of God as we understood him.
4. Made a searching and fearless moral inventory of ourselves.
5. Admitted to God, to ourselves and to another human being the exact nature of our wrongs.
6. Were entirely ready to have God remove all these defects of character.
7. Humbly asked Him to remove our shortcomings.
8. Made a list of all persons we had harmed and became willing to make amends to them all.
9. Made direct amends to such people wherever possible, except when to do so would injure them or others.
10. Continued to take personal inventory and when we were wrong promptly admitted it.
11. Sought through prayer and meditation to improve our conscious contact with God as we understood Him.
12. Having had a spiritual awakening as the result of these steps, we tried to carry this message to alcoholics and to practise these principles in all our affairs.

Box 47 Alcohol misuse in the primary care setting

Alcohol misuse is common in the primary care setting. A recent WHO study involving countries in Europe, the USA and Australia showed that 18% of subjects in primary care had a hazardous level of alcohol intake, and 23% had experienced at least one alcohol-related problem in the previous year. GPs should be key players in the detection and treatment of alcohol problems. The first three questions from AUDIT (Box 39) can be used as a brief screening tool in primary care. These three questions about alcohol consumption are a practical, valid primary care screening test for the detection of heavy drinking and/or active alcohol abuse or dependence.

Brief interventions, such as alcohol counselling, motivational interviewing techniques, and various problem solving and cognitive-behavioural techniques can be easily adapted for use in primary care. Brief interventions have been shown to be effective in reducing the alcohol consumption of hazardous drinkers treated in primary care.

Box 48
Factors that predispose to the development of illicit drug abuse

Genetic predisposition (possibly mediated via anxiety traits)
Risk-taking personality
Cigarette smoking at a young age (below 12 years of age)
Drug use by peers and/or family
Depression or anxiety
Social stressors
Personality disorder
Schizophrenia
Childhood adversity (either neglect or abuse, or parental separation or divorce)
Underachievement at school
Truancy and delinquency
Unemployment

alcohol to form acetaldehyde, which results in highly unpleasant consequences: sickness, severe headache and palpitations. Some ability to abstain from alcohol must be demonstrated prior to either drug being prescribed. Patients with severe liver or cardiovascular problems should not be given these drugs as the resulting effects, if they drink, could be fatal.

Recent interest has focused on the use of opioid antagonists in the treatment of alcoholism. There is preliminary evidence that naltrexone may attenuate or prevent the recommencement of alcohol consumption in patients with alcohol dependence. However, further evidence of its efficacy will be required before it could be recommended routinely.

8.5 Illicit drugs

Learning objectives

You should:

- know the prevalence of illicit drug disorders
- the costs to society of drug disorders.

In English-speaking countries, approximately 3% of adult males and 1% of females meet the criteria for an illicit drug disorder, although approximately one third of adults aged 16 to 59 years in England and Wales will have used illicit drugs at some point in their lives. The prevalence of drug disorders decreases with age,

with the highest rates seen in the 18–34 year age band. The risk factors for illicit drug abuse are listed in Box 48.

Approximately 25 000 deaths occurred in 1992 in the USA because of drug abuse. The estimated costs related to mortality and morbidity from drug abuse was $28.8 billion for the same year. The medical and psychological treatment of drug abuse cost $9.9 billion.

The following points apply in general to illicit drug misuse. The route of absorption is an important factor in determining its effects. Routes of administration which produce more rapid and efficient absorption into the bloodstream result in a more intense intoxication and an increased likelihood of an escalating pattern of substance use, leading to dependence. Relatively short-acting substances tend to have a higher potential for the development of dependence. The half-life of the substance parallels aspects of withdrawal. The longer the half-life, the longer the time between cessation and the onset of withdrawal symptoms, and the longer withdrawal is likely to last.

Drug use can be classified as:

- experimental: initial use of a drug prompted by curiosity or peer pressure
- recreational: continued use of a drug on either a regular or an occasional basis that does not constitute dependency
- dependent: compulsion to take the drug either to experience it's pleasurable effects or to prevent the discomfort of abstinence
- problem drug use: social, psychological or physical problems associated with the use of illicit drugs.

8.6 Opioids

Learning objectives

You should:

- be familiar with the signs and symptoms of opiate withdrawal
- know the basic principles for managing withdrawal
- be aware of methadone maintenance treatment
- be aware of pharmacological methods to reduce craving.

Heroin is the most common opioid that is used on an illicit basis. It induces a state of euphoria and calm. When taken intravenously, the person experiences an exquisite sensation of well-being somewhat analogous to sexual orgasm. This has been called a 'rush'. Physical dependence is common, especially if the drug is injected intravenously. However, the most common form of ingestion is burning followed by inhalation (so-called chasing the dragon). Risks from the actual drug are relatively rare but include respiratory depression and accidental overdosage. Most of the physical problems occur as a result of intravenous administration and include infections (e.g. human immunodeficiency virus (HIV), septicaemia, abscesses, etc.) and embolic episodes, causing strokes and leading to limb amputation or death.

Iatrogenic dependence can also occur through the regular prescription of morphine or codeine for chronic, painful conditions.

The signs and symptoms of withdrawal from opioids are shown in Box 49. The withdrawal condition in itself is not life-threatening, unlike withdrawal from alcohol. It is, however, extremely unpleasant. Benzodiazepines can be prescribed to ameliorate the symptoms of withdrawal, but caution is required as the person may also

Box 49
Opioid withdrawal syndrome

Misery, distress
Intense craving for the drug
Yawning
Sweating
Pilooerection, shivering
Abdominal cramps, vomiting and diarrhhoea
Insomnia
Dilated pupils
Restlessness and agitation
Hyperaethesia
Paraesthesia
Muscular cramps
Depression

be addicted to benzodiazepines. A variety of detoxification methods have been utilized for the treatment of heroin withdrawal. *Methadone* in gradually reducing doses is still the preferred procedure, and a withdrawal regimen will take approximately 10 days to complete. Most withdrawal regimens are conducted on an outpatient basis, although inpatient withdrawals have a much higher success rate. The initial doses of any methadone withdrawal regimen needs to be titrated according to the patient's symptoms. Enough drug should be given for the patient to feel safe and comfortable. Methadone should be prescribed in a liquid form, as tablets can be crushed and injected. Methadone only needs to be taken twice a day and should be dispensed to patients on a daily basis, if the withdrawal is being conducted in the community. Treatment should be reviewed regularly by a nurse or doctor.

Rapid and ultrarapid withdrawal protocols using clonidine (a centrally acting α–adrenergic agonist), lofexidine (a clonidine analogue that has fewer side effects) and opiate receptor antagonists have been proposed.

Management

Treatment and management of drug addiction is provided by a combination of statutory and voluntary services. Most district services have a community drug team who offer assessment and treatment on a community basis. A small number of inpatient units exist that provide intensive treatment programmes for a small minority of patients.

Most treatment interventions emphasize the importance of psychosocial change in addition to stopping the drug. As with alcohol, most individuals who attain abstinence do so by completely changing their social environment and support networks. Psychiatric services work closely with social services and the probation service, as many addicts have numerous drug-related offences. Treatment can be made a condition of probation for those individuals convicted of drug-related offences.

Re-inforcement based intensive outpatient treatment programmes that link abstinence to the provision of housing, food, and access to recreational activities have produced promising results in the short term but require further long-term evaluation before widespread implementation.

One of the important consequences of treatment for opiate addiction is the reduction in crime. A recent large national UK study of over 750 patients found that the number of crimes committed by patients in the year following treatment was reduced to one third of the number committed in the year prior to treatment. This reduction in crime provides immediate benefit to society through the reduced economic costs of crime and a reduction in psychological crime-related trauma suffered by victims.

Complete abstinence may be difficult for some patients, and methadone maintenance treatment has been shown to be effective for selected patients with opioid dependence. With this form of treatment, patients are legally prescribed methadone on a regular basis, together with psychosocial support. Some patients can be maintained in this fashion and helped to live relatively normal lives for several years. Heroin usage is decreased as are HIV risk behaviours. Recent evidence has been published suggesting methadone maintenance treatment may be cost effective, although it remains a somewhat controversial therapy.

Maintaining abstinence from opiates

Naltrexone is a long-acting competitive antagonist at opioid receptors. It blocks the effects of opiates as well as the development of physical dependence. It can be used as an adjunct to the management of opioid dependence for patients who intend to remain abstinent. It is well tolerated by most patients but some develop nausea or severe headache. It should never be given as a sole treatment for opiate addiction and should be combined with individual or group support and counselling.

8.7 Cocaine

Learning objectives

You should:

- be familiar with the effects of cocaine intoxication
- be familiar with the symptoms of withdrawal from cocaine
- be aware of the physical and psychiatric sequelae of cocaine abuse.

Cocaine is a naturally occurring substance produced by the coca plant. It is grown in Central and South America. Native populations chew the leaves of the plant, which results in a euphoric effect. Cocaine hydrochloride is a white powder that is snorted through the nostrils or dissolved in water and injected intravenously.

Crack cocaine is a cocaine alkaloid that is extracted from cocaine hydrochloride by mixing it with sodium bicarbonate and allowing it to dry into small rocks. Crack cocaine is easily vapourized and inhaled, so its effects have an extremely rapid onset.

Cocaine intoxication

Cocaine produces a feeling of euphoria with enhanced vigour, hyperactivity, alertness, hypervigilance, interpersonal sensitivity, talkativeness, anxiety, tension, alertness, grandiosity, anger, and impaired judgement. Physiological changes include: tachycardia or bradycardia, pupillary dilation, elevated or lowered blood pressure, perspiration or chills, nausea or vomiting, weight loss, psychomotor agitation or retardation, muscular weakness, respiratory depression, chest pain, or cardiac arrhythmias, and confusion, seizures, dyskinesias, dystonias, or coma.

Cocaine is highly addictive, and use of crack cocaine often results in individuals having to use the drug on a very frequent basis to maintain their sense of euphoria. All other aspects of the individual's life will become secondary to the maintenance of the addiction. Important responsibilities will be grossly neglected and the individual may become involved in crime in order to fund his/her habit.

Withdrawal symptoms

Cocaine withdrawal produces a lowered mood that comes on within a few hours of stopping the drug, plus fatigue, vivid unpleasant dreams and insomnia or hypersomnia. A proportion of individuals may have no discernable symptoms on stopping the drug.

Psychiatric and physical sequelae

Cocaine can cause a syndrome of acute emotional and behavioural disturbance that mimics schizophrenia. Individuals can develop paranoid ideation, auditory hallucinations and an altered affective state. Tactile hallucinations can also occur. The symptoms usually resolve within a few hours after the drug has left the patient's system, although in certain individuals, who may be predisposed to developing schizophrenia, the drug can precipitate schizophrenia. Cocaine abuse is also associated with a variety of other psychiatric disorders including eating disorders, anxiety states and sleep disorders. Myocardial infarction, stroke and sudden death from respiratory or cardiac arrest have been associated with cocaine use in otherwise healthy young people. These complications may arise because of its local anaesthetic properties and effects on membrane ion channel activity. Traumatic injuries are not uncommon and result from fights or disputes when the individual is highly aroused or very angry. Violence is also associated with the illicit drug trade. For those individuals who inject the drug, the potential complications are similar to those already described in relation to intravenous opiate abuse. Polydrug abuse is common and cocaine use by patients on methadone maintenance treatment is a widespread problem.

Treatment

The psychosocial treatment for cocaine follows the principles outlined previously for alcohol and opiate addiction. Success is dependent upon the individual's readiness and desire to change.

Promising results in the treatment of cocaine addiction have been achieved using disulfiram, even in patients who do not have comorbid alcohol problems. Disulfiram inhibits dopamine beta-hydroxylase, resulting in an excess of dopamine and decreased synthesis of noradrenaline (norepinephrine). Since cocaine is a potent catecholamine re-uptake inhibitor, it is possible disulfiram may blunt cocaine craving or alter the 'high', resulting in a decreased desire to use cocaine. Pharmacological treatment should always be prescribed in the context of a formalized treatment programme.

8.8 Amphetamines

Learning objectives

You should:

- be familiar with the effects of amphetamine intoxication
- be familiar with the symptoms of withdrawal from amphetamine
- be aware of the physical and psychiatric sequelae of amphetamine abuse.

'Amphetamines' is used to include all substances with a substituted phenylethylamine structure, such as amphetamine, dextroamphetamine and methamphetamine (speed). It also includes substances that are structurally different but also have amphetamine-like action, such as methylphenidate and other agents used as appetite suppressants. Amphetamines are usually taken orally or intravenously, although 'speed' can also be snorted. A very pure form of methamphetamine, called 'ice', can be smoked to produce an immediate and powerful stimulant effect.

Most of the effects of amphetamines are similar to those of cocaine, except that they do not have local anaesthetic activity and so are less likely to cause cardiac arrhythmias. The psychoactive effects of amphetamines last longer than those of cocaine; consequently, the drugs are usually taken on a less frequent basis. Usage may be chronic or episodic, with binges (speed runs) interspersed with periods of abstinence.

Psychological and physiological effects

Psychological effects include:

- euphoria or affective blunting
- changes in sociability
- hypervigilance
- interpersonal sensitivity
- severe anxiety, tension or anger
- impaired judgement.

Physiological changes can occur with amphetamines, including:

- tachycardia or bradycardia
- dilated pupils
- elevated or lowered blood pressure
- perspiration or chills
- nausea and vomiting
- weight loss
- agitation or retardation
- muscular weakness, respiratory depression
- confusion, seizures, dystonias or coma.

Withdrawal syndrome

Withdrawal symptoms develop within a few hours to several days after stopping the drug. They include fatigue, vivid and unpleasant dreams, insomnia, increased appetite, psychomotor retardation or agitation.

Psychiatric sequelae

The most concern regarding the abuse of amphetamines is in relation to their propensity for causing a schizophrenic-like psychosis. Whilst intoxicated with the drug, individuals can develop paranoid ideation, auditory hallucinations and tactile hallucinations. The symptoms usually disappear once the drug is out of the individual's system. These drugs, however, can precipitate the onset of psychosis or schizophrenia in individuals with underlying vulnerability for the disorder, and they can seriously jeopardize recovery if patients continue to abuse such substances. Amphetamines can also produce sleep disorders and cause severe sexual dysfunction.

8.9 Cannabis

Learning objectives

You should:

- be familiar with the effects of cannabis intoxication
- be aware of the psychiatric sequelae of cannabis abuse.

Cannabinoids are substances that are derived from the cannabis plant. Marijuana refers to the upper leaves of the plant, which are dried and rolled into cigarettes. Hashish is the dried resinous exudate that seeps from the tops and undersides of the cannabis leaves. Cannabis is usually smoked but can be taken orally. The psychoactive part of the plant is the cannabinoid delta-9-tetrahydrocannabiol (THC). The THC content of cannabis, and, therefore, the psychoactive power of the drug, varies enormously from as little as 1% to 15%.

Although illegal, cannabis is widely available and used by a large number of young people. It produces a sense of euphoria and calmness. If large amounts are inhaled, it can cause grandiosity, inappropriate laughter, impaired judgement, impaired motor performance and lethargy. Occasionally, severe anxiety can occur with paranoia. Physiological changes include conjuctival infection, increased appetite, dry mouth and tachycardia.

Chronic use is associated with lethargy, blunted affect and a lack of drive or volition. Cannabis takes a very long time to be excreted from the body, and individuals can test positive for the drug up to 2 weeks after last taking it. This may account for the relative lack of withdrawal symptoms when stopping the drug.

Psychiatric and physical sequelae

Many individuals use the drug on an intermittent basis without obvious adverse effects. Heavy use, however, can cause severe anxiety states, panic attacks and acute paranoid states. In patients with schizophrenia, cannabis exacerbates the symptoms of the condition and interferes with treatment.

There are relatively few adverse physical effects of the drug. The main problems arise from smoking and include persistent cough, bronchitis, emphysema and lung cancer. Marijuana smoke contains larger amounts of known carcinogens than tobacco.

8.10 Hallucinogens

Learning objectives

You should:

- be familiar with the effects of hallucinogens
- be aware of the psychiatric sequelae of their abuse.

There are a wide variety of different hallucinogens. They include lysergic diethylamide (LSD), phenylalkylamines (such as mescaline), and MDM (3,4-methylenedioxymethamphetamine) better known as Ecstasy.

The drugs produce a sense of euphoria, wakefulness and alertness. Perceptual changes include a subjective intensification of perceptions, depersonalization and derealization, illusions and hallucinations. Physiological changes include pupillary dilatation, tachycardia, sweating, palpitations, blurring of vision, tremors and incoordination.

Some drugs such as Ecstasy primarily produce euphoric changes with associated increased energy and hyperarousal. Other drugs such as LSD cause visual illusions and frank hallucinations.

Dependence

Physical dependence or a withdrawal syndrome as such does not occur. The drugs have very long half-lives and individuals can spend days recovering from the effects of the drug. Individuals find the euphoric and psychedelic effects of the drug diminish with increased use, and there is cross-tolerance between LSD and other hallucinogens. Individuals who use Ecstasy describe a hangover the day after use characterized by tiredness, insomnia, drowsiness, headaches and sore jaw muscles from teeth clenching.

Psychiatric and physical sequelae

Whilst under the influence of the drug, some individuals may act on their experiences and place themselves in danger (e.g. if they believe they can fly). A syndrome called persisting perception disorder has been described in which individuals experience transient perceptual disturbances that are reminiscent of those experienced whilst taking an hallucinogen but which occur spontaneously without ingestion of a psychoactive substance. These episodes usually diminish in frequency over time but can persist for many years in some individuals. Other psychiatric states include anxiety and panic disorders, and psychotic states. Sudden death from respiratory or cardiac arrest has been recorded in healthy young adults who take Ecstasy.

8.11 Inhalants

Learning objectives

You should:

- be familiar with the effects of inhalants
- be aware of the psychiatric sequelae of inhalant abuse.

Glue sniffing is the inhalation of the aliphatic and aromatic carbons that are found in substances such as glue, paint thinners and spray paints. Several methods are used to inhale intoxicating vapours. Substances can be inhaled directly from containers or from aerosols sprayed in the mouth or nose. A rag soaked in the substance can be applied to the mouth or nose. The substance can be placed in a paper or plastic bag and the gases in the bag inhaled.

Intoxication results in a sense of wellbeing, apathy, impaired judgement and sometimes belligerent or aggressive behaviour. Physiological changes include dizziness, nystagmus, incoordination, slurred speech, unsteady gait, lethargy, tremor, muscle weakness, depressed muscle weakness, blurred vision, stupor and coma.

A possible withdrawal syndrome beginning 1–2 days after cessation of use has been described and consists of symptoms of sleep disturbance, tremor, irritability, nausea and fleeting illusions.

Psychiatric and physical sequelae

Inhalant intoxication can cause changes in perceptual awareness including visual, auditory and tactile hallucinations. Frank paranoid states can develop and abuse is also associated with anxiety states and panic disorder. Most abuse of inhalants occurs in young adolescents and may be part of a wider picture of disturbance. Inhalants are widely available and very cheap, so crime is rarely a secondary effect of this form of substance abuse. Physical effects include coughing, sinus problems, dyspnoea, sinus discharge, abdominal pain and vomiting.

Further reading and sources

Department of Health 1992 The health of the nation: a strategy for health in England. HMSO, London

Department of Health 1999a Saving lives: our healthier nation. Stationery Office, London

Department of Health 1999b Drug misuse and dependence: guidelines on clinical management. The Stationery Office, London

Prochaska JO, Velicer WF 1997 The transtheoretical model of health behaviour change. American Journal of Health Promotion, 12: 38–48

Project MATCH 1998 Matching alcoholism treatments to client heterogeneity: Project MATCH three-year drinking outcomes. Alcohol and Clinical Experimental Research, 22: 1300–1311

Saunders JB, Lee NK. 2000 Hazardous alcohol use: its delineation as a subthreshold disorder, and approaches to its diagnosis and management. Comprehensive Psychiatry, 41(Suppl 1): 95–103

Saunders JB, Aasland OG, Babor TF, de la Fuente JR, Grant M. Development of the alcohol use disorders identification test (AUDIT): WHO Collaborative Project on Early Detection of Persons with Harmful Alcohol Consumption II. Addiction 88: 791–804

Welch S, Strang J 1999 Pharmacotherapy in the treatment of drug dependence: options to strengthen effectiveness. Advances in Psychiatric Treatment, 5: 427–434

Working Party of the Royal Colleges of Psychiatrists and the Royal College of Physicians 2000 Drugs Dilemmas and Choices, Gaskell Press, London

Sources

Al-anon. An organization for friends and family of alcoholics www.al-anon-alateen.org

Alcohol Concern: National agency on alcohol misuse set up in 1984. It has a key role in promoting and advising on the development of national alcohol policy and in promoting public awareness of alcohol issues www.alcoholconcern.org.uk

Alcoholics Anonymous. www.alcoholics-anonymous.org.uk

DrugScope. www.drugscope.org.uk

Narcotics Anonymous World Services. www.wsoinc:com/index.htm

National Institute on Alcohol Abuse and Alcoholism. National, American government agency. Provides detailed information about a variety of different aspects of drug- and alcohol-related disorders www.niaaa.nih.gov

Self-assessment: questions

Multiple choice questions

1. The prevalence of alcohol problems amongst the general population:
   a. Has fallen in the last 20 years
   b. Is more common in men than women
   c. Is higher in individuals over 45 years of age
   d. Is directly related to the degree of alcohol consumption of the general population
   e. Is particularly increasing in young women.

2. Women:
   a. Are more likely to drink in secret
   b. Begin drinking alcohol at a later age than men
   c. Have lower rates of comorbid psychiatric disorders
   d. Are harder to engage in treatment than men
   e. Are more responsive to treatment than men

3. In the general medical setting:
   a. Alcohol problems are more common in women than men
   b. Problem drinkers are easily identified by medical staff
   c. Problem drinkers are usually confined to wards that specialize in liver problems
   d. Patients are routinely screened for alcohol problems
   e. Alcohol counselling provided by a specialist nurse results in significant reductions in harmful use of alcohol by patients with alcohol problems

4. The following are features of the alcohol dependence syndrome:
   a. Loss of memory
   b. Relief drinking
   c. A compulsion to drink
   d. Moderation of drinking behaviour in relation to social cues
   e. Altered tolerance

5. In alcoholic hallucinosis:
   a. Visual hallucinations are common
   b. The patient usually experiences auditory hallucinations of a derogatory nature
   c. The patient is delirious
   d. Primary delusions are a cardinal feature of the condition
   e. The condition usually settles within few days or weeks of abstinence

6. The following are withdrawal symptoms associated with opiate dependence:
   a. Elation
   b. Constipation
   c. Fatigue
   d. Hypersomnia
   e. Shivering

7. In relation to withdrawal regimens for opiate dependence:
   a. Methadone should be prescribed in tablet form
   b. Methadone only needs to be prescribed twice per day
   c. Methadone should be dispensed on a weekly basis if the withdrawal is being managed in the community
   d. No medication should be prescribed to cover withdrawal symptoms
   e. The withdrawal regimen should take about 4–5 days

8. Naltrexone:
   a. Is a long-acting competitive agonist at opioid receptors
   b. Has no effect on the development of physical dependence to opiates
   c. Is poorly tolerated by most patients
   d. Should not be used to treat alcohol-related disorders
   e. Should not be given as a sole treatment for drug addiction

9. Cocaine:
   a. Is highly addictive
   b. Has local anaesthestic properties
   c. Produces a feeling of depression
   d. Withdrawal is characterized by difficulty in sleeping
   e. Can result in a syndrome that mimics schizophrenia

10. Cannabis:
    a. Has a marked and clearly delineated withdrawal syndrome
    b. Does not cause psychiatric sequelae
    c. Is associated with lethargy and a lack of drive or volition if used on a regular basis
    d. Is rapidly excreted from the body
    e. Has serious physical consequences

Case history questions

History 1

Mr Thompson, a 41-year-old man, attends the A&E department at 2.00 a.m. one Saturday morning. He smells of ketones and is dirty and unkempt. His clothes are ragged and shabby. His speech is slightly slurred and he is unsteady on his feet. He has a wide gait. He says that he is fed up and miserable. He feels tense and nervous and cannot sleep. He has nowhere to stay, he has no friends, his family have disowned him, and he has no money. He is desperate and says that he has thought of killing himself. He would rather be dead than go on. He is very edgy and jumps when he is touched. He is sweating profusely and has a coarse tremor.

He has not had a drink for 24 hours as he was robbed the previous day, of what little money he had.

He tells the doctors that, although he had been living on the streets for several months, 5 years previously he had been married, employed as an electrician and financially secure. As his drinking became excessive, his wife had been unable to cope with his possessiveness, jealousy and violence, and she had left him. The more he drank, the more unreliable he became at work, until eventually he was sacked. His social, psychological and physical status then gradually declined over the next few years until, eventually, he ended up living on the streets.

1. What possible alcohol-related problems may this man be suffering from?
2. What immediate management is required?
3. What long-term treatments may he benefit from?

History 2

A 27-year-old man called Simon is admitted to hospital following a grand mal fit. He has no prior history of epilepsy or blackouts and there is no family history. He makes a quick recovery. As part of a routine history and examination, the house officer asks him whether he drinks much alcohol; he says he just drinks an average amount. Later that day, the alcohol counsellor visits the ward and discusses the patients who have been admitted overnight with the ward sister. She decides to speak with Simon and takes a detailed alcohol history from him. He also tells her that he only drinks an average amount.

She asks him how often he drinks and he tells her most days. On a typical day, he has a couple of pints at lunchtime with his workmates and then 2–4 pints in the evening. At weekends (i.e. Friday and Saturday night), he usually drinks 6–8 pints plus 2 or 3 shorts. The night prior to his fit, he had drunk 10 pints and

had 6 shorts. The counsellor worked out that on average he was drinking 86 standard units of alcohol per week. He did not think he had a problem with drinking as most of his mates drank similar amounts.

1. Why did the house officer fail to detect that Simon was a harmful drinker?
2. What will the alcohol counsellor do?

History 3

A 47-year-old woman attends her GP feeling run down and tired. She has felt low for the last 6 months, lacks energy and has had trouble sleeping. The GP thinks that she is suffering from depression but also performs a routine physical check. Physical examination is normal. The GP takes a full blood count (FBC) and urea and electrolytes, and he arranges to see her again the following week. Before leaving, he checks that she does not have any suicidal ideas.

When he reviews her the following week, she is still feeling low. She tells the GP that she has no particular worries and does not understand why she feels so fed up. The GP is about to prescribe a course of antidepressant treatment, when he realizes that her mean cell volume (MCV) (on the FBC) is raised. She is not anaemic. He then takes a drinking history and finds out that she has been drinking a bottle of wine per night for the last 5 years. She lives by herself, has few friends and drinks the wine watching television. He works out she is drinking approximately 49 standard units of alcohol per week.

1. Should the GP prescribe antidepressants?
2. What is the safe amount of alcohol this woman can drink?
3. Why is she depressed?

Objective structured clinical examination (OSCE)

Station: alcohol history

At this station, you are asked to take an alcohol history from a patient. Ideally get someone else to read the history below and then answer your questions. You have 10 minutes in which to take the history. If you cannot do this, read the history and list the questions you would ask. An examiner would assess whether the history was taken in a coherent and structured way and whether all important areas were covered.

A patient aged over 30 years.

You drink 1 bottle of vodka per day plus 6–8 cans of special lager (be vague about how much you drink initially, try to underestimate what you drink, the student should ask you very specific questions).

You began drinking when you were 15 years of age

You used to drink beer and wine socially but for the last 5 years have drunk the same roughly each day

You drink at home alone

You start drinking in the morning when you wake up

You are sweaty and shaky in the mornings and you feel sick

A drink helps you 'get going' and relieves these symptoms

You find that drink doesn't touch you now, you rarely feel or look drunk

You get very shaky and tremulous if for some reason you can't have a drink

You have never stopped drinking for longer than a few days

You think you do have a problem

You sometimes can't remember what you did the night before, but you don't appear drunk

You get down most of the time, but drinking helps you to forget your worries

Your memory for recent events is poor (you forget where you have put your keys etc.)

You sometimes black out and have been to casualty following falls

You have lost your job because you were always late and missed a lot of time (you used to work in a shop)

Your wife/husband left you because of drink

You have a lot of debt but you don't really care

You have never been aggressive or violent or been involved with the police

No one in your family has a history of alcohol problems

No one has a psychiatry history

You have never had any previous treatment for alcoholism

Apart from feeling sick in the morning, you do not have any other physical symptoms

Self-assessment: answers

Multiple choice answers

1. a. **False**. The prevalence of alcohol problems has increased.
    b. **True**. Alcohol problems are much more common in men than women.
    c. **False**. Alcohol problems are more common in young people.
    d. **True**. The pattern of alcohol consumption by the general population is represented by a normal distribution. Hence the higher the average amount drunk by the general population, the larger the number of hazardous or harmful drinkers, as the distribution curve is shifted to the right.
    e. **True**. Although there are fewer alcohol problems in women than men, the number of alcohol problems in young women is showing a sharp increase.

2. a. **True**. Men rarely drink alone. Women, however, are often secret drinkers.
    b. **True**. Women begin drinking alcohol at an older age than men.
    c. **False**. Women have higher comorbid psychiatric disorders than men.
    d. **False**. Women are more likely to engage in treatment than men.
    e. **True**. Women are more likely to respond to treatment than men.

3. a. **False**. Alcohol problems are much more common in males than females.
    b. **False**. Medical staff are poor at detecting hazardous or harmful drinkers.
    c. **False**. Patients with alcohol problems can present with a variety of different physical complaints.
    d. **False**. Patients are rarely screened properly for alcohol problems.
    e. **True**. Even brief interventions by a specialist nurse result in significant reductions in alcohol use after discharge.

4. a. **False**. Loss of memory may well coexist with alcohol dependence syndrome but it is not a feature of the condition.
    b. **True**. Relief drinking (i.e. using alcohol to control symptoms of withdrawal) is a feature of alcohol dependence syndrome.
    c. **True**. A compulsion to drink is key feature of the syndrome.

    d. **False**. Individuals become unable to moderate their drinking behaviour in relation to social cues.
    e. **True**. Individuals find that they can drink more alcohol without appearing drunk or feeling intoxicated.

5. a. **False**. Auditory hallucinations are typical.
    b. **True**. This is the key feature of the disorder.
    c. **False**. The symptom must occur in clear consciousness for the diagnosis to be made.
    d. **False**. Primary delusions are a feature of schizophrenia. Delusions can occur in this disorder but are usually secondary to the auditory hallucinations.
    e. **True**. If the condition continues for more than 6 months, it is considered to be schizophrenia, i.e. not related to alcohol abuse.

6. a. **False**. Opiate withdrawal is associated with misery and depression.
    b. **False**. Individuals experience diarrhoea.
    c. **False**. Fatigue is not a prominent symptom.
    d. **False**. Individuals find it difficult to sleep.
    e. **True**. Shivering is a symptom of opiate withdrawal.

7. a. **False**. Methadone should be prescribed as a liquid.
    b. **True**. It should be given twice per day.
    c. **False**. It should be dispensed on a daily basis to prevent abuse.
    d. **False**. Although opiate withdrawal is not life-threatening, it is extremely unpleasant and patients should be prescribed medication to help them to tolerate the withdrawal.
    e. **False**. The regimen usually takes about 10 days.

8. a. **False**. It is a competitive antagonist at opioid receptors.
    b. **False**. It helps to prevent the development of physical tolerance.
    c. **False**. It is well tolerated by most patients.
    d. **False**. It has been used with caution in alcohol-related disorders.
    e. **True**. It should not be regarded as a stand-alone treatment and should always be given in conjunction with psychosocial treatment.

9. a. **True**. It is highly addictive.
    b. **True**. It is a local anaesthetic.
    c. **False**. It produces euphoria.

d. **False**. Cocaine withdrawal is characterized by hypersomnia.

e. **True**. It can cause auditory hallucinations and persecutory delusions, which can be identical to those of schizophrenia.

10. a. **False**. There is no clear withdrawal syndrome.
    b. **False**. It can cause persecutory states.
    c. **True**. This is a well-recognized problem associated with prolonged and regular use.
    d. **False**. It remains in the body for many hours. It has a half-life of about 20 hours.
    e. **False**. If smoked, serious physical consequences do occur but the main problems arise from smoking rather than from the drug itself.

History 1

1. The most obvious problem is that Mr Thompson is in an acute alcohol withdrawal state. He has not drunk for 24 hours and he is sweating, hyperaroused and has a coarse tremor. He is at risk of fitting and will become confused and develop delirium tremens if he is not urgently treated. The description also states that he has a wide stepping gait. This may suggest he has developed neurological problems as a result of his drinking and is ataxic. He will require a full neurological assessment after he has been treated for alcohol withdrawal. His mental state will also need careful assessment, as he may have cognitive deficits associated with drinking excessively with poor nutrition (he has been living on the streets); a risk assessment regarding his suicide risk needs to be carried out. He may have developed a depressive disorder, although as alcohol depresses mood, his mood may spontaneously improve after a few days.

2. This man requires urgent admission to hospital for the management of acute withdrawal. If a bed cannot be arranged quickly, he requires sedation in the A&E department to control his withdrawal symptoms and to reduce the risk of fitting. Diazepam or chlordiazepoxide should be prescribed. He also requires i.v. vitamin supplements because of his poor nutritional status and to decrease the likelihood of cognitive impairment.

3. In the long term, he requires treatment for his alcohol dependence and a stable social environment. As he has no family or friends, the most likely option would be a hostel. While in hospital (or a specific unit for detoxification), he will be counselled about his drinking and offered treatment and help.

History 2

1. The house officer failed to detect his high alcohol consumption because of two reasons. The house officer did not have a high enough index of suspicion, given the history, and he took at face value what Simon said about his drinking.

2. The alcohol counsellor will provide Simon with clear information about the amount of alcohol he is drinking and the risks for him if he continues to drink this amount on a regular basis. She will tell him that his fit was probably alcohol related and a clear sign that he is beginning to develop physical problems because of his drinking. She will tell him that the medical team will carry out further investigations to check his liver function while he is in hospital. She will explain to him that he does not have to be abstinent, but he must reduce his alcohol intake. She will advise him about the safe and sensible limits for drinking. She works out with him that if he does not drink on three days a week, he can go out in the evening and drink 3–4 pints (but not more than 14 pints in the whole week). He thinks he can cut out lunchtime drinking without too much of a problem. She asks him to start to keep a diary and says she will see him after he has left hospital. She will also liaise with his GP so she can also re-inforce the advice he has received from the counsellor.

History 3

1. The GP should not prescribe antidepressants. Her low mood may be caused by the excessive amount of alcohol she is drinking. He should counsel her about her drinking and advise her to stop completely in the short term. He should review her in one week. If her mood has not improved, he may then consider antidepressants.

2. After a period of abstinence, and provided she has not developed any major physical complications from drinking, she will be able to drink up to 14 units per week, with at least 2 alcohol-free days per week.

3. She is probably depressed because alcohol is a depressant if taken on a regular basis in excessive qualities.

OSCE answer

The categories that should be covered in your questions to elicit the alcohol history are listed below.

Name and age
Amount of alcohol per week

Amount of alcohol per day
Go through the week (i.e. how much each day of an average week)
Age first began drinking
Amount drunk during teenage years
Amount drunk in twenties, thirties
(*Identify that alcohol pattern became fixed 5 years previous*)
Ask about tolerance
When has first drink of day
Enquire about withdrawal symptoms: shaking, nausea, sweating
Enquire re withdrawal fits
Enquire re delirium tremens

Memory lapses: ask about palimpsests
Memory lapses: ask about short-term memory problems
Periods of abstinence
Effect on job
Effect on family
Effect on mood
Other physical symptoms: ask about common physical sequelae
Other social sequelae, e.g. finances
Forensic history
Previous treatment for alcohol abuse
Family history of alcohol-related problems
Self-appraisal
Motivation to stop drinking.

9 Sexual problems

Overview

Sexual dysfunction refers to sexual difficulties that have been present for more than 6 months, do not have a physical cause and result in psychological distress. They can be divided into problems with sexual desire and arousal, and problems with the execution of sexual activity. The latter includes premature ejaculation, orgasmic dysfunction, vaginismus and dyspareunia. Most sexual problems respond well to treatment, which is usually based upon behavioural principles. Most doctors should be able to take a detailed sexual history and make a diagnosis. They should be able to discuss sexual problems without feeling embarrassed and give simple advice regarding safer sexual practices. Paraphilias refer to intense sexual urges involving nonhuman objects, children or other non-consenting persons. At present, there is very little evidence for effective treatments for these conditions.

9.1 Sexual problems and taking a sexual history

Learning objectives

You should:

- be able to talk to patients about sex
- be able to take a detailed history of sexual problems

Sexual practices between consenting adults include a wide spectrum of different behaviours. Defining nor-mality and abnormality is, therefore, difficult. Individuals are considered to suffer from sexual dysfunction if (i) they are unable to participate in a sexual relationship as they would like; (ii) the problem has been present for more than 6 months; (iii) the problem cannot be account-ed for by a physical disorder or drug treatment; and (iv) the problem causes emotional distress or interpersonal difficulties.

Sexual problems can be understood in terms of problems with sexual arousal or desire, and problems with the execution of sexual activity (e.g. premature ejaculation). Most sexual problems that arise within the context of a two-person relationship are best under-stood in terms of a 'couple problem' rather than the 'problem' being attributed to one member of the part-nership. Occasionally, people who are not in a current sexual relationship will present for treatment on an individual basis. Relatively few people with sexual problems ever consult their GP, and a very small percentage of individuals are referred for specialist treatment.

Some forms of sexual behaviour are considered unacceptable within the context of our current society and legal framework. Most of these behaviours are considered unacceptable because they involve either children or non-consenting adults. Some behaviours may not involve harm to others but may cause distress to the individual who is performing them, who may then ask for help to stop or control them. These behaviours have been loosely classified together as *paraphilias*.

Taking a sexual history

Most couples who present for treatment should be interviewed together regarding their problems, but a detailed individual history should then be taken from each person, without the other present. The interview-er should be sensitive to each person's potential embarrassment and should conduct the interview in a sympathetic but 'down to earth' manner. It is import-ant for doctors to be familiar and knowledgeable regarding the diversity of sexual practice within the general population. An open and non-judgemental attitude is essential. The interviewer should use lan-guage that is appropriate to the individual's level of understanding and should avoid anatomical terms unless the person is familiar with these terms. A detailed understanding of the problem should be obtained, and sometimes it may be helpful to use diagrams or anatomical drawings. Box 50 shows the main topic areas that should be covered.

It is also important to carry out a physical examination, with appropriate investigations where indicated (Table 16). A record of the patient's medication should be noted, and any drugs that many impair sexual performance identified (Table 17).

Sexual problems are common in the general hospital setting but may be missed by doctors, as patients are reluctant or embarrassed about discussing such matters and some doctors do not routinely enquire about sexual function.

Box 50
Taking a sexual history

History of the presenting problem
Nature of problem
How it began and its course
Key life events or change in circumstances around its onset
Factors that alleviate or exacerbate the problem
Effect on the individual's relationship (if has steady partner)
Any previous treatment or advice

Current sexual relationship
Nature and duration of relationship
Previous experience of sexual function within current relationship
Frequency and variety of sexual activity within relationship
Level of communication between partners about sex
Quality of interpersonal relationship (warmth, rapport, communication between partners about non-sexual matters)
Overt problems or difficulties in the relationship

Sexual development
Method by which individual acquired knowledge about sex and different sexual practices

Onset of puberty
Overall awareness and degree of knowledge regarding own body and sexual matters in general
Childhood trauma (either physical or sexual)
Other adverse sexual experiences
Positive sexual experiences
Pattern of sexual activity during adolescence and adulthood prior to meeting current partner
Previous problems or difficulties in sexual relationships

Medical and psychiatric history
Take particular note of medical conditions or pharmacological or surgical treatment that could potentially cause sexual dysfunction
Note if there is a prior history of anxiety in relation to performance in other non-sexual activities

Drug and alcohol use
Make a careful record of the amount of alcohol the individual consumes
Check whether there is any evidence of an excessive intake or abuse
Check whether the individual uses alcohol or other drugs to aid sexual performance

---

Table 16 Physical examination and investigations for sexual dysfunction

Area	Action
Physical examination	Look for general signs of illness: diabetes, thyroid disorders, alcohol-related disorders, adrenal cortex disorders Look for hair distribution, gynaecomastia in men, blood pressure, peripheral pulses, reflexes, sensation
Genital examination	Penis: look for congenital abnormalities, size, symmetry, tenderness, signs of plaques, infections, urethral discharge Testicles: both present, size, symmetry, texture, sensation Vagina: lubrication, tenderness, ability to tolerate internal examination, discharge Clitoris: presence, any damage, receptive to stimulation (should ask woman to check this herself) General points: any other abnormality, evidence of infections, warts, etc.
Blood tests	Testosterone, luteinizing hormone, glucose-fasting prolactin
Specific investigations	Nocturnal penile tumescence Penile pressure Corpus cavernosography Arteriography of genital blood supply Sacral cord evoked potentials Visual stimulation and penile tumescence

Table 17 Drugs that affect sexual function

Specific action on sexual function	Drug
Decreased desire	Antihypertensive and cardiovascular drugs: acetazolamide, chlortalidone, clofibrate, digoxin, methyldopa, propranolol, reserpine, spironolactone, timolol Gastrointestinal drugs: cimetidine Hormonal drugs: Oestrogens (decreased desire in men)
Inhibited arousal	Antihypertensive and cardiovascular drugs: atenolol, betanidine, clonidine, disopyramide, guanethidine, methyldopa, propranolol, reserpine, spironolactone, thiazide diuretics, timolol, verapamil Antidepressants: all tricyclic antidepressants, citalopram, fluvoxamine, maprotiline, paroxetine, sertraline, venlafaxine Anxiolytics drugs: benzodiazepines Non-steroidal anti-inflammatory drugs: naproxen
Decreased libido	Antidepressants: citalopram, clomipramine, desipramine, doxepin, fluvoxamine, imipramine, maprotoline, paroxetine, sertraline, venlafaxine Anxiolytics drugs: benzodiazepines
Anorgasmia	Clomipramine, selective serotonin reuptake inhibitors (SSRIs), venlafaxine (less so than pure SSRIs) Anxiolytics drugs: benzodiazepines
Inability to ejaculate	Antihypertensive and cardiovascular drugs: guanethidine, methyldopa, phenoxybenzamine, reserpine, timolol Antidepressants: clomipramine, desipramine, imipramine Anxiolytics drugs: benzodiazepines Non-steroidal anti-inflammatory drugs: naproxen
Breast enlargement	Antihypertensive and cardiovascular drugs: reserpine
Decreased sexual activity	Anti-eplileptic drugs: phenytoin

9.2 Specific problems

Learning objectives

You should:

- be able to identify problems with sexual desire/aversion

- be able to identify problems with genital response in males and females

- be able to identify orgasmic dysfunction in males and females and recognize characteristics suggesting an underlying physical cause

- be able to diagnose premature ejaculation and dyspareunia in males

- be able to diagnose vaginismus and dyspareunia in females

- understand the term paraphilia and know the main types

- know the main features of gender identity disorders and be able to adopt a professional and non-judgemental attitude to individuals seeking help.

Problems of sexual arousal and desire

Lack of desire

Lack of desire is characterized by a reduction of, or absence, of sexual fantasies and desire for sexual activity. This is only a problem if the individual or his/her partner is distressed by it. The problem may be global or situational, that is limited to a specific person or sexual activity. For example, the individual may have no desire for sexual intercourse but may still enjoy masturbation. Loss of desire may be lifelong and commence at puberty, or it may start in adulthood, occurring either on a continuous or intermittent basis.

Lack of desire may coexist with other sexual problems as it will inevitably result in problems related to the initiation and completion of sexual activity. Lack of desire may also be caused by other sexual problems, as an individual may become less and less interested in sex if he/she experiences regular difficulties in performance.

Sexual aversion

Sexual aversion refers to the active avoidance of genital sexual contact with a sexual partner coupled with feelings of revulsion. The problem may be specific to a particular sexual practice, for example vaginal penetration, or may extend to a generalized revulsion to all sexual stimuli, including touching and kissing.

Problems of arousal or genital response

In the female, the arousal response consists of vasocongestion in the pelvis, coupled with vaginal lubrication and swelling of the external genitalia. Difficulties with arousal occur if this process cannot be initiated or maintained throughout the duration of sexual activity. Lack of arousal and lubrication may result in painful intercourse, which, in turn, may reduce desire and the ability to become aroused.

In the male, lack of arousal is characterized by difficulties in gaining and maintaining an erection. This condition may be primary (i.e. the man has never been able to maintain an erection) or secondary (i.e. the condition develops later in life). Usually the condition is specific to a particular situation or person, and the man is able to gain or experience erections at certain times (e.g. through self-stimulation, during the night or on wakening). Erectile failure in all circumstances is usually suggestive of an underlying physical disorder. The gradual onset of erectile failure in older men is also suggestive of an underlying physical cause.

In both males and females, it is important that any underlying physical disorder is detected or excluded.

Problems in the execution of sexual activity

Orgasmic dysfunction

Females

Orgasmic dysfunction in women is characterized by a persistent or recurrent delay in, or absence of, orgasm following a normal phase of sexual arousal. This is one of the most common sexual problems in women, and it is often caused by a lack of knowledge about female sexual response. Some women never achieve orgasm and are relatively unconcerned about this; in which case, it should not be considered a problem. Orgasmic capacity increases with age in females; therefore, female orgasmic disorder may be more prevalent in younger women. Chronic medical conditions, such as diabetes or pelvic cancer, are more commonly associated with problems of arousal than orgasmic capacity.

Males

In males, sexual excitement occurs but orgasm is delayed or does not occur at all, associated with an inhibition of ejaculation. Situational orgasmic dysfunction is most likely associated with a psychological cause, such as performance anxiety or guilty feelings about sex.

Premature ejaculation

Premature ejaculation is associated with an inability to delay orgasm and ejaculation long enough for both partners to enjoy the sexual experience adequately. The male achieves orgasm with a minimal level of sexual stimulation. Most males are usually able to delay orgasm during self-masturbation for longer periods than during penetrative sex.

Vaginismus

In vaginismus, penetration of the vagina is impossible or very painful because of a narrowing of the vaginal opening caused by spasms of the pelvic floor muscles, which surround the vagina. It is important to exclude a physical cause such as a growth or tumour. Psychological causes include strong beliefs that sex is wrong, sinful or dirty; a fear of sex following a previous painful experience; and previous sexual trauma including rape and sexual abuse.

Dyspareunia

Dyspareunia is painful sexual intercourse. In males, the condition most often indicates an underlying physical disorder. In females, the pain may be superficial (around the opening of the vagina) or deep during penile thrusting.

Paraphilias

Paraphilias are characterized by intense sexually arousing fantasies or urges involving non-human objects, children or other non-consenting persons, or the suffering or humiliation of oneself or one's partner.

It is important to distinguish paraphilias from the use of sexual fantasies, behaviours or objects as stimuli for sexual excitement and gratification. Such things are only paraphilic if they cause distress or serious injury, involve children or non-consenting adults, or injury or distress to animals. The main forms of paraphilia are described in Table 18. Paraphilias of any kind are extremely rare in women. Fetishism and aspects of sadomasochism are a part of the normal spectrum of human sexual behaviour. Such activities should only be considered to be disorders if they cause significant distress to the person who enacts them, or they involve coercion or non-consent of others.

Behavioural techniques have been used to treat exhibitionism and fetishism. There is little evidence, at present, that paedophilia responds to any form of therapeutic intervention.

Gender identity disorders

Gender identity problems involve a dissatisfaction with the individual's current gender and a wish to live life as

Table 18 Types of paraphilia

Paraphilia	Description
Exhibitionism	Exposure of one's genitals to a stranger, usually child or female; the penis may be flaccid or erect, and the individual may or may not masturbate There is usually no further sexual activity
Fetishism	Intense sexual arousal and fantasies in relation to non-living objects (e.g. female underwear); the condition causes distress to the individual
Frotteurism	Touching and rubbing against a non-consenting person to achieve sexual arousal. This usually occurs in crowded places. The individual rubs his genitals against the victim's thighs or buttocks This condition is most common in young males 15–25 years of age
Paedophilia	Sexual fantasies and activity with children. Some individuals are only attracted to children, while others can be attracted to adults as well as children. Activity can include undressing, touching and fondling the child, with associated self-masturbation. More extreme acts can include penetration of the child's vagina, anus or mouth with fingers or penis. Such activities are rationalized as having educational value for the child or as being pleasurable
Sexual masochism	Intense sexual pleasure from being beaten, humiliated, bound or otherwise made to suffer
Sexual sadism	Intense sexual pleasure from the psychological or physical suffering of the victim or sexual partner; in severe cases, the activities may include rape, torture and murder

a member of the opposite sex. This may or may not include a desire for corrective surgery. A clinical threshold is reached when concerns become so intense as to seem to be the most important aspect of a person's life. Such struggles are known to be manifested from the preschool years to old age and have many different forms. The prevalence of such problems are very difficult to establish, but the most recent information of the transsexual end of the gender identity disorder spectrum from Holland is 1 in 11 900 males and 1 in 30 400 females.

Medical support and help includes the following:

1. A diagnostic assessment should be carried out to identify the problem correctly, and any other comorbid disorders that may need help in their own right.
2. Psychotherapy or counselling may be offered. The aim of such treatment is not to alter the person's views regarding gender identity but to allow him/her an opportunity to explore any concerns or worries.
3. Most individuals are asked to spend a period of time living and dressing in the opposite gender role to try to clarify their wishes.
4. If this is successful, hormonal therapy may be instituted.
5. This may be followed by eventual referral for gender reassignment surgery (Box 52). Usually the individual must have lived for at least 12 months in a real life experience as a member of the opposite gender.

The evidence from follow-up studies suggest that most people who opt for gender reassignment surgery are pleased with the outcome, and psychological distress about gender identity is reduced.

Individuals with gender identity concerns are sometimes wary of consulting doctors as many have been treated in the past with ridicule and contempt. Such behaviour from doctors is unacceptable, and all patients, no matter their concerns, should be treated with respect and compassion.

9.3 Treatment of sexual problems

Learning objectives

You should:

- be able to give educational advice about sex and about safer sexual practices, where appropriate
- be familiar with normal sexual responses in males and females
- be able to give simple advice about treatment of specific sexual problems
- be able to recommend useful self-help guides for patients
- be familiar with the government guidelines for the treatment of erectile dysfunction.

Doctors should be able to answer patients' questions about sex, dispel any myths and address underlying fears. Many sexual problems with a relatively brief history can be treated quickly using simple advice, self-help guides and simple behavioural interventions. An important part of the treatment process is the provision of knowledge and education about sexual function. The aim of this is to normalize the individual's or couples' experience and to reduce anxiety or embarrassment about sex. Table 19 summarizes the male and female sexual response cycle, and Figure 2 shows the physiological response cycle in males and females.

There are a variety of specific interventions and techniques for different types of sexual problem, and some of these are listed in Table 20. If individuals are not helped by simple advice or specific suggestions, referral

Table 19 Sexual response cycle in males and females

Phase	Males	Females
Desire Excitement	Fantasies, thoughts and wishes about sex Penile erection associated with a pleasurable genital sensation. The length, diameter and firmness of the penis increases markedly and there is a retraction of the foreskin The scrotal sac contracts causing decreased movement of the testicles	Fantasies, thoughts and wishes about sex The labia minora increase in size and separate; there is a pleasurable sensation in the genital area Fluid is secreted on the inner vaginal lining; the vagina darkens in colour as there is increased blood flow to the region The clitoris enlarges in size; the uterus also becomes engorged and rises, increasing the length and width of the vagina
Plateau	The penis increases further in diameter and its colour may change to reddish-purple The testes increase in size and become more elevated	The labia minora deepen in colour The vagina deepens in colour and increases slightly more in length and width The clitoris retracts under its hood if stimulation is continued
Orgasm	Emission: the vas deferens, seminal vesicles and ejaculating ducts contract to place semen at the entrance of the urethra. The internal sphincter of the urethra contracts to prevent semen entering the bladder Ejaculation: involuntary rhythmic contractions of the penis cause seminal fluid to be ejaculated under pressure from the urethra; after three or four major contractions, the contractions become irregular and weak	Between 2 and 15 involuntary rhythmic contractions of the muscles and the vagina and pelvic region occur; the orgasm is usually longer in duration than the males. The orgasm may last for a few seconds or, if sexual stimulation continues, further orgasms can be experienced immediately, without a refractory phase Generally, masturbation, oral or physical stimulation, or a vibrator produce the most intense orgasms, while orgasms experienced during intercourse tend to be of a lower intensity
Resolution	The bodily changes reverse; the penis returns to its pre-ejaculatory state. This time period is very variable. There is decreased tension in the scrotal sac. The testes decrease in size and drop back to their normal position Re-stimulation cannot occur until the male's arousal level has decreased to the phase of low excitement. This may take a few minutes (in young males) or a much longer period in older males. Males are unable to have multiple orgasms in quick succession	There is a reversal of bodily changes. Within 5–10 seconds, the clitoris returns to its normal position and the labia minora return to their usual colour. The vagina and clitoris take about 10–15 minutes to return to their normal size and colour. If orgasm has not occurred, it may take longer, even hours, for these changes to return to normal
Other bodily reactions	Heart rate and blood pressure rises Hyperventilation begins in the plateau stage	The female breast increases in size and the nipples become erect; this is less obvious in women who have breast-fed A rash or flush may appear across the chest, neck and face Heart rate and blood pressure increases Hyperventilation occurs

to a specialist sexual clinic should be considered. Problems with sexual arousal in women and vaginismus often require specialist help. Before referral, it is important to exclude or treat any underlying physical cause. Sexual difficulties in the context of severe relationship problems, or alcohol abuse, are unlikely to respond to sex therapy unless these other factors are tackled first. Severe emotional problems arising from childhood sexual abuse and trauma, which may present as sexual dysfunction, should be addressed before considering sex therapy.

There are very few controlled evaluations of sexual therapies, but limited evidence suggests that behaviourally based interventions are extremely effective for many types of sexual problem. Response rates vary from 75 to 90% for problems with a relatively brief history. Patients with long and complex histories are less likely to show such a favourable response.

Most sex therapy clinics and self-help manuals focus upon sexual problems that arise within the context of a heterosexual relationship. Although homosexual couples are occasionally referred for treatment, relatively few

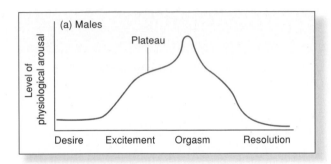

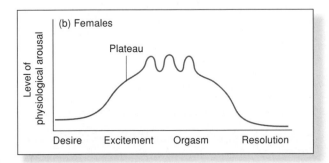

Fig. 2 Levels of physiological arousal during sexual activity for (a) males and (b) females. (Adapted from Masters and Johnson (1966) Human Sexual Response, Churchill, London.)

couples present for help. It is possible that homosexual couples experience fewer problems in relation to sex than heterosexuals as there are fewer taboos concerning sex within the homosexual community, and most individuals are comparatively knowledgeable and experienced.

There are relatively few physical treatments for sexual problems, but the recent development of sildenafil citrate (Viagra) for the treatment of erectile dysfunction has received a great deal of publicity. Sildenafil citrate treats impotence through the selective inhibition of an enzyme (phosphodiesterase V) that inactivates cyclic guanine monophosphate (cGMP), the mediator of smooth muscle in the corpus cavernosum. This allows a greater flow of blood into the penis when the man is excited, which aids erection. This drug is extremely effective for the treatment of erectile dysfunction. At present, GPs can only prescribe this drug on the NHS to men who are suffering from impotence and have a specified clinical condition, which includes diabetes mellitus, multiple sclerosis, renal failure, Parkinson's disease, prostate cancer, neurological disease and severe spinal or pelvic conditions. GPs can issue private prescriptions to men who do not have any these disorders. Men who are suffering from severe distress because of their

Table 20 Treatment strategies for different types of sexual problem in males and females

Problem area	Males	Females
Arousal		Sensate focus techniques (the giving and receiving of pleasurable caresses in a relaxed atmosphere) may help to stimulate arousal
Orgasmic dysfunction	Anxiety-reducing techniques Reduction of underlying psychological cause Increasing the level of arousal	Education Directed masturbation programme (initially carried out alone and then with partner participation) Increase methods of arousal
Premature ejaculation	Education Stop–start technique (stimulation of the penis until high arousal, followed by cessation of stimulation to allow arousal to subside, repetition of this 4–5 times) Squeeze technique (when the male indicates he is highly aroused, he or his partner applies a firm squeeze to the head of the penis for 15–10 seconds) Sensate focus techniques	
Vaginismus		Education Relaxation techniques Self-exploration Insertion of graded trainers Sensate focus Insertion of fingers or graded trainers by partner Gradual attempts at intercourse with the woman on top so she can control the rate and depth of penetration
Dyspareunia	Techniques to encourage full arousal Relaxation exercises Education about different positions for intercourse	Techniques to encourage full arousal Relaxation exercises Education

impotence can receive treatment from specialist services. Treatment, if prescribed, should be restricted to one treatment per week, according to government guidelines. Caution is required for men who have a history of ischaemic heart disease.

Other physical treatments, such as the implantation of a semirigid or inflatable penile prosthesis or self-administration of intracavernosal papaverine or prostaglandins prior to intercourse, have been somewhat eclipsed by the arrival of Viagra, but they may still be of benefit.

Safer sex

In the 1990s, there has been a particularly sharp rise in the diagnosis of acute sexually transmitted infections. During this period, diagnoses rose by 76% for genital chlamydial infection, 55% for gonorrhoea and 20% for genital warts. There are an estimated 30 000 cases of HIV-infected individuals in the UK, and about 2500 new diagnoses of HIV-infected individuals are made each year. The new inception rates for HIV are remaining steady, but the increased incidence in other sexually transmitted diseases in the 1990s suggests that unsafe sex practices remain common amongst young people.

Sexual intercourse between men remains the major route of infection for people who have been diagnosed as having HIV, but sex between men and women now accounts for one quarter of new HIV-infected individuals, and the number of people infected via this route is steadily increasing.

Box 51
How to negotiate safe sex

Points to remember
Talk about safe sex
Wait to have sex
Use a supply of condoms and discuss your sexual histories
Accentuate the positive
Get at least your partner's name (sex with strangers is risky)
Stay on topic (if your partner won't talk about safe sex then don't have sex)
Remember the kids (keep your future life in mind – you may want children at some stage and sterility is a real possibility with sexually transmitted diseases)
Get a check-up; if you are sexually active and not in a steady relationship, get regular check-ups
Stay in control (drugs and alcohol make you forget about safe sex)
Want more facts: contact http://starnews.webpoint.com/

Box 52
Gender reassignment surgery

Genital, breast, and other surgery for the male to female patient
1. Surgical procedures may include orchiectomy, penectomy, vaginoplasty, augmentation mammaplasty and vocal cord surgery
2. Vaginoplasty requires both skilled surgery and postoperative treatment. Three techniques are penile skin inversion, pedicled rectosigmoid transplant or free skin graft to line the neovagina
3. Augmentation mammaplasty may be performed prior to vaginoplasty if the physician prescribing hormones and the surgeon have documented that breast enlargement after undergoing hormonal treatment for 2 years is not sufficient for comfort in the social gender role. Other surgeries that may be performed to assist feminization include reduction thyroid chondroplasty, liposuction of the waist, rhinoplasty, facial bone reduction, facelift and blephoroplasty.

Genital and breast surgery for the female to male patient
1. Surgical procedures may include mastectomy, hysterectomy, salpingo-oophorectomy, vaginectomy, metoidioplasty, scrotoplasty, urethroplasty and phalloplasty
2. Current operative techniques for phalloplasty are varied. The choice of techniques may be restricted by anatomical or surgical considerations. If the objectives of phalloplasty are a neophallus of good appearance, standing micturition and/or coital ability, the patient should be clearly informed that there are both several separate stages of surgery and frequent technical difficulties that require additional operations
3. Reduction mammaplasty may be necessary as an early procedure for some large-breasted individuals to make the real life experience feasible
4. Liposuction may be necessary for final body contouring.

Patients also have general health concerns and should undergo regular medical screening according to recommended guidelines.

Doctors should be able to give advice about safer sex practices and counsel patients appropriately. Young people, in particular, should be encouraged to use condoms if they are, or are thinking of becoming, sexually active. The latex condom offers better protection against sexually transmitted infections than any other birth control method. Further details about contraception, how to put on a condom, how to advise women to say no to non-safe sex and persuade men to wear condoms are available from the website http://www.plannedparenthood.org/bc/condom.ht m Simple advice about safer sex, which can be given to patients, is shown in Box 51.

Further reading and sources

Hawton K 1985 Sex therapy: a practical guide. Oxford University Press, Oxford

Kaplan HS 1989 How to overcome premature ejaculation. Brunner/Mazel, New York

Pertot S 1994 A commonsense guide to sex. Harper Collins, Sydney

Sources

Department of Health website regarding current guidelines for GPs about the treatment of impotence. http://www.doh.gov.uk/impotencetreatment/index. htm

Useful websites for advice about safe sex: http:// www.safer-sex.org and http://www.gavilan.cc.ca.us/ health/safe.html

Self-assessment: questions

Multiple choice questions

1. In the normal human sexual response cycle:
   a. The excitement phase precedes the desire phase
   b. The penis increases in size in the plateau phase
   c. There is a refractory period in females following orgasm
   d. There is a refractory period in males following orgasm
   e. The resolution phase is characterized by a reverse of bodily changes

2. Premature ejaculation:
   a. Is characterized by an ability to delay orgasm
   b. Can be treated using the squeeze technique
   c. Occurs more commonly in older men
   d. Is usually more pronounced during masturbation than sexual intercourse
   e. Is an inability to achieve orgasm

3. Sildenafil citrate:
   a. Is an effective treatment for orgasmic dysfunction
   b. Is very effective for erectile dysfunction
   c. Works via decreasing the flow of blood to the penis
   d. Can be prescribed by GPs to all patients with erectile dysfunction
   e. Is available on the NHS for specific groups of patients with erectile dysfunction

4. Sex therapy techniques:
   a. Are predominantly based upon psychodynamic principles
   b. Have high response rates
   c. Always include a strong educative component
   d. Are unlikely to be effective if there are severe relationship problems
   e. Usually involve the treatment of both partners in a relationship

5. Frotteurism:
   a. Is the same as self-masturbation
   b. Involves intense sexual fantasies in relation to non-living objects
   c. Usually occurs in private
   d. Is more common in women than men
   e. Occurs more often in young people.

Case history questions

History 1

Mrs B visits her GP Dr Pria Kapur, who is new to a formerly all male practice, for advice about a recurrent ear infection. In the first few minutes of the consultation, Mrs B comments that she is pleased that the practice now has a female GP. As she is getting up to leave, she asks whether she can mention 'one other problem'. In a somewhat embarrassed fashion, she tells Dr Kapur that her sex life is not what it should be. She has always had a disinterest in sex, and this is now causing problems in her marriage.

What should Dr Kapur do?

History 2

Mr S was a 23-year-old man who presented to his GP with concerns about his gender. He had held a strong belief, since a boy, that he was female and should have been born a girl. He had tried to put these thoughts out of his mind but had become increasingly distressed over the last 5 years. He no longer felt that he could continue as a male and wanted to seek gender reassignment surgery. He had been living as a woman for the last year and had been taking female hormonal treatment for the last 6 months (which he had obtained illicitly). He had lived with a man for the last 2 years who was supportive of his wish to under go a sex change.

What would you do if you were this man's GP?

History 3

Mr J visits his GP with a request for 'Viagra'. He says he has read about it in the paper and would like to try it. He is 50 years of age and has noticed a decline in his sexual function in the last 2–3 years. He finds it difficult to reach and maintain an erection, and his penis is not as firm as it once was. He still experiences morning erections and is physically fit and well. He does not appear unduly distressed by the problem and has no history of mental illness.

What should be his GP's response?

Self-assessment: answers

Multiple choice answers

1. a. **False**. The excitement phase follows the desire phase.
    b. **True**. The penis undergoes a further increase in size during this phase.
    c. **False**. There is no refractory period in females following orgasm.
    d. **True**.
    e. **True**.

2. a. **False**. It is characterized by an inability to delay orgasm, so the male quickly achieves orgasm with minimal sexual excitement.
    b. **True**. Other treatments include sensate focus techniques, education and stop–start techniques.
    c. **False**. Is much more likely to occur in young men.
    d. **False**. Is less of a problem with self-masturbation than sexual intercourse.
    e. **False**. It is an inability to delay orgasm.

3. a. **False**. It is a treatment for erectile dysfunction.
    b. **True**.
    c. **False**. Sildenafil citrate increases the flow of blood to the penis.
    d. **True**. GPs can issue a private prescription for this drug to all patients with erectile dysfunction.
    e. **True**. It is only available to certain groups of patients with erectile dysfunction on the NHS (December 2000). Government guidelines may change over time.

4. a. **False**. They are predominantly based upon behavioural techniques.
    b. **True**.
    c. **True**. Provision of knowledge and education is an important part of therapy.
    d. **True**. Severe relationship problems need to be dealt with first.
    e. **True**. Most problems arising within a two-person relationship are best understood as a 'couple' problem.

5. a. **False**. Frotteurism involves sexual stimulation to arousal by rubbing against other non-consenting persons in crowded places.
    b. **False**. Intense sexual fantasies about non-living objects is termed fetishism.
    c. **False**. It occurs in densely packed, crowded places.
    d. **False**. It virtually never occurs in women.
    e. **True**.

Case history answers

History 1

Dr Kapur should arrange a specific time to see Mrs B to discuss the problem in more depth. She should ask whether Mr B could also attend the appointment.

At this 15 minute appointment, Dr Kapur established that they have been married for 5 years. They did not have sex before marriage and had only managed full intercourse on a few occasions since marriage. Both were sexually inexperienced and brought up in families where sex was not discussed. Their first attempts at sex were very hesitant and Mrs B found it more and more difficult to become aroused. Consequently, she found sexual intercourse painful and embarrassing. They both became more and more anxious about sex and gradually even became anxious about touching and caressing each other, as this raised the possibility of proceeding to sexual intercourse. Dr Kapur established that their relationship was good and there were no other psychosocial stressors or physical reasons for the problem. She suggested referring them to the sex therapy clinic at the local hospital.

History 2

Mr S requires a full assessment from a specialist in gender dysphoria. The GP may have to make enquiries from local psychiatrists as to who is an expert in this area. The GP should check that there are no other coexisting psychiatric problems, such as depression, which require urgent treatment. The GP should be supportive, advise against the use of illicit hormonal treatment but reassure Mr S that hormonal treatment may be offered after he has been formerly assessed. The GP should stress that assessment and progression through the various stages towards gender reassignment surgery may take some time, as it important to be absolutely clear that Mr S is certain he wants to pursue this treatment.

History 3

His GP tells Mr J that, under the current guidelines from the Department of Health, he is not allowed to receive the drug on the NHS, as he does not fit in to the category of any of the specialist groups who are eligible to receive it free of charge. His GP tells him that he would like to carry out some routine blood tests and a test of urine to exclude any underlying physical factors; however, his problem is unlikely to be caused by underlying physical illness. His GP recommends two options. First, he could refer Mr J to the local sex therapy clinic with the aim of being taught ways of improving his sexual performance. He would have to attend with his wife. Alternatively, he could be prescribed Viagra on a private prescription.

10 Personality disorder

Overview

Individuals with a personality disorder show an enduring pattern of inner experience and behaviour that deviates markedly from cultural expectations. These patterns are inflexible and pervasive across a wide range of social and personal situations and lead to clinically significant distress or impairment in social, occupational and other important areas of functioning. Published work on the treatment of severe personality disorders has largely been descriptive or qualitative, rather than quantative; comparatively few studies have quantified outcomes through the use of standardized inclusion criteria, randomized controlled trial design, standardized outcome measures or an adequate period of follow-up. A recent meta-analytic review of the effectiveness of psychotherapy for personality disorders reported on the outcome of 15 studies in which pretreatment and post-treatment effects were compared and/or recovery at follow-up. The studies included three randomized controlled trials, three randomized comparisons of active treatments and nine uncontrolled observational studies. The treatment interventions included psychodynamic/interpersonal, cognitive therapies, mixed and supportive therapies. All studies reported improvement in personality disorders with psychotherapy. Among the three randomized controlled trials, active psychotherapy was more effective than no treatment according to self-report measures. The current literature concerning the effectiveness of psychotherapy is, therefore, encouraging but inconclusive.

10.1 Definition and aetiology

Learning objectives

You should:

- be familiar with the main criteria for personality disorder
- understand the difference between axis I and axis II disorders
- be familiar with different ways of construing personality
- be aware of the importance of genetic, familial and environmental factors in relation to personality.

Personality

To understand the concept of personality disorder, one first has to understand what is meant by personality. This usually refers to the individual characteristics, behaviours and emotional qualities of a person, which the person knows to be themself. That people differ from each other is obvious. How and why they differ is less clear and is the subject of the scientific study of personality and individual differences. The study of personality includes multiple approaches to the question of who we are and how and why we are similar to and different from other individuals. One way in which personality and its extreme variations is studied is by developing descriptive taxonomies of individual differences. This approach emphasizes the similarities between different groups of people.

Why people develop certain ways of behaving and interacting with others is unclear. At least five different theoretical approaches have been used to try to address this question. *Evolutionary psychology* emphasizes universals of human behavior and attempts to explain individual variability in terms of alternative adaptive strategies. *Behaviour genetic* approaches analyse the variation in behaviour in terms of the complex interplay between genetic and environmental influences.

Systematic work in *biological theorizing* has emphasized the continuity of behaviour across species and searches for the biological underpinnings of temperament and complex behaviour. *Social cognitive theories* emphasize the importance of socialization and the effect of cognitive processes to create one's unique patterning of behaviour. Traditional *psychoanalytic techniques*, although not a major area of current personality theory, have had a major influence in the theories developed throughout much of the 20th century.

The possibility of personality disorder is only considered when aspects of the person's character cause repeated problems to him or herself or others. There is enormous diversity across populations, and many people with eccentric or odd behaviours would not be considered to have a personality disorder.

The formal definition of a personality disorder is:

an enduring pattern of inner experience and behaviour that deviates markedly from the expectations of the individual's culture, is pervasive and inflexible, has an onset in adolescence or early adulthood, is stable over time, and leads to distress or impairment.

Key aspects of the definition are that:

- evidence of a problem must be present from an early age, as the adult personality is beginning to form
- the behaviour is persistent and resistant to change
- behavioural problems are evident in a variety of different areas of social functioning, e.g. disruptive interpersonal relationships, poor work record, antisocial behaviour, etc.
- the behaviour results in damage or distress to the individual concerned or others.

Type I and type II psychiatric disorders

There is a debate within psychiatry as to whether personality disorder should be regarded as a psychiatric illness at all, and as to whether it is a useful concept for understanding abnormal behaviour. One difficulty has been the pejorative way, in the past, it has been used in relation to certain individuals; another problem has been the inconsistency of its use. Some psychiatrists do not accept the use of the term and regard it as a way of labelling individuals who do not fit into the conventional patterns of society.

Modern diagnostic systems in psychiatry classify psychiatric disorders according to different dimensions or 'axes'. Psychiatric disorders that have discrete beginnings and endings and can come on at any time in a patient's life are termed *axis I disorders*. These are synonymous with what most psychiatrists would think of as psychiatric illness and include conditions like depression and schizophrenia. Personality disorders are classi-

fied separately using a different axis or dimension: *axis II*. Personality disorders can, therefore, coexist with psychiatric illnesses or occur independently.

Personality disorder is not considered to be a psychiatric illness that can respond to treatment so the person is restored to a normal state of functioning. Rather it is viewed as a characterological problem, which may be modified by intensive treatment.

Different ways of understanding personality

Categorical types

Categorical types are used to understand personality in psychiatric classification systems. Individuals are grouped together according to particular characteristics; for example, someone with a schizoid personality would have the following characteristics: difficulty in making close social relationships, a preference for spending time alone, a cold and distant manner and a tendency to spend a lot of time day dreaming or thinking about abstract concepts rather than engaging in the real world. The different types of personality disorder are described later, but all are based upon extreme forms of what are essentially normal personality variations.

Dimensions

Instead of identifying characteristics that cluster together to form a personality type, this approach to personality focuses upon individual characteristics or so-called personality traits. Each characteristic is assumed to have a normal distribution amongst the general population, with small groups of people at the two extreme ends of each spectrum. Examples of personality traits include anxiousness, obsessiveness, neuroticism, introversion and extroversion.

Aetiology

Genetic factors

There is some evidence that particular characteristics of personality have a strong hereditary component (e.g. anxiety traits). Most of the evidence comes from twin studies, where monozygotic twins have a much greater probability of shared personality characteristics than dizygotic twins. However, the nature versus nurture argument is very difficult to untangle, and both are probably important.

Familial and environmental factors

There is very little hard evidence to confirm a general assumption that important components of personality are developed by learning from parental guidance or behaviour. Childhood neglect or abuse, however, is strongly associated with the development of certain forms of personality disorder as an adult. Therefore, it is easier to demonstrate the influence of negative childhood events or experiences on personality than it is to show the subtle effects of normal or mundane experiences.

Research in relation to patients with antisocial disorder (see below) has shown a strong association with some form of brain injury or insult as a child. This could result from birth trauma, a head injury or an infection such as meningitis or encephalitis. Adult patients with sociopathic disorder are more likely than controls to have abnormal computed tomographic (CT) scans, although it is difficult to be clear whether their brain abnormalities are primary or secondary to the condition. This is because patients with sociopathic disorder have a strong likelihood of getting into fights or injuring themselves in other ways.

10.2 Types of personality disorder

Learning objectives

You should:

- be familiar with the main types of personality disorder
- know which types of personality disorder are associated with certain forms of psychiatric illness.

The main types of personality disorder, with a brief description, are shown in Table 21. Fuller descriptions of the more common types of disorder are given later in this section.

Each category is based around a normal personality trait, which in the disorder is manifest in an extreme and pathological manner. Most personality traits convey some kind of positive advantage provided they are tempered by recognition of the needs of others and by some kind of balance within the personality itself. For example, moderate obsessional traits may be advantageous for individuals who have responsible jobs and have to carry out precise and meticulous work. Histrionic traits may be an advantage for individuals who wish to pursue an artistic career, and even antisocial traits may be useful for those in highly competitive industries where a certain degree of ruthlessness may be required.

Paranoid personality disorder

Characteristics of a paranoid personality disorder include suspiciousness, marked self-reference, feelings that other people are hostile or involved in conspiracies against the individual, a sense of injustice, preoccupation with imagined wrongs, litigious and aggressive behaviour, and holding of grudges.

Schizoid personality disorder

Individuals with schizoid personality disorder are aloof and isolative. They have little interest in others and prefer their own company. They are emotionally cold and may appear to be indifferent to others. They may develop interests in unusual hobbies or pastimes that do not involve human interactions.

This form of personality disorder has been associated with the later development of schizophrenia. However, it is unclear whether it is truly a risk factor or whether patients who appear to have schizoid personality disorder are actually in a long prodromal phase of the illness.

Antisocial personality disorder

Individuals with an antisocial personality disorder have a complete disregard for the thoughts of others. They

Table 21 Personality disorders

Type of personality disorder	Brief description of characteristic patterns of behaviour
Paranoid	Distrust and suspiciousness
Schizoid	Detachment from social relationships, plus restricted emotional response
Schizotypal	Acute discomfort in social relationships, perceptual distortions bordering on psychotic experiences, eccentric behaviour
Antisocial	Disregard and violation of others
Borderline	Instability in relationships, impulsivity and low self-esteem
Histrionic	Excessive emotionality and attention seeking
Narcissistic	Grandiosity, need for admiration, lack of empathy
Avoidant	Social inhibition, hypersensitivity to negative evaluation
Dependent	Submissive and clinging behaviour
Obsessive-compulsive	Preoccupation with orderliness, perfectionism and control

Based on DSM-IV (American Psychiatric Association (1994) Diagnostic and Statistical Manual of the Mental Disorders, 4th edn. American Psychiatric Association, Washington, DC)

are self-centred, selfish and sometimes cruel. They are cold and affectionless. They rarely form long-term relationships and usually exploit others with whom they are involved. They are unable to appreciate the needs or feelings of others or may even gain pleasure from the humiliation or suffering of others. They often have a criminal record, which may include violent or sexual offences. Evidence of antisocial or aberrant behaviour will be present from an early age. The disorder is more common in males.

Drug or alcohol abuse is common, which can result in the development of short-lived psychotic states or, in the case of alcohol, long-term brain damage. These individuals may also receive injuries to their brain because of frequent fighting or other kinds of reckless activity.

Obsessive-compulsive personality disorder

Individuals with an obsessive-compulsive disorder are extremely ordered, meticulous and pedantic. They find it difficult to express emotion or show feelings towards others, although inwardly they may ruminate and worry about social encounters. They are perfectionistic and often find it difficult to complete tasks because of such high standards. They are rigid and find it difficult to adapt to change. They often have conflicts regarding sex, which they may regard as messy or dirty. They find it difficult to develop long-term relationships as most others do not live up to their high standards. They rarely have a criminal record or drink excessively. They are at risk, however, of developing depressive or obsessional illnesses and are often socially isolated.

Histrionic personality disorder

Individuals are overdramatic in their behaviour. Minor troubles or events are perceived as major disasters. Individuals are overemotional and frequently moved to tears. They are self-centred and attention seeking and are rarely happy unless surrounded by admirers. They profess to be deeply moved but appear to be shallow and immature in relationships. They are at risk of developing depressive or anxiety disorders.

Dependent personality disorder

People with a dependent personality disorder are overly dependent upon others. They find it impossible to live on an independent basis and collapse emotionally whenever they have to fend for themselves. They often develop stable but imbalanced relationships with a very dominant partner, either a spouse or parent. They are at risk of depressive and anxiety disorders.

Borderline personality disorder

The borderline personality disorder is characterized by individuals who have explosive, short-lived emotionally charged relationships. They form intense relationships with others, which are initially idealized but then breakdown as disagreements develop. They view others as being either good or bad. Good people are those who support them and pander to their needs; bad people are those who frustrate them or do not provide enough nurturance. They are unable to tolerate frustration or disappointment; consequently, people whom they initially like and admire are soon perceived as being rejecting and unworthy as they inevitably disappoint or fail in some way. They often perceive themselves to be supportive and helpful towards others, but in reality are selfish and egocentric. They may drink heavily, take drugs or repeatedly self-harm. They are at risk of developing depressive disorders, anxiety disorders and eating disorders.

10.3 Assessment and management

> ### Learning objectives
>
> You should:
>
> - be aware of different methods of assessing personality
> - be able to assess personality from a clinical perspective
> - be aware of the specific treatment approaches that have been evaluated in the treatment of personality disorder
> - know the principles underlying clinical management.

Assessment

The diagnosis of personality disorder is difficult and often clinicians may disagree about the nature and severity of the disorder. Some psychiatrists believe that the term personality disorder should be discarded as it has been used in a pejorative way in the past to describe individuals who doctors do not like. There is also confusion as to whether individuals with personality disorder should be regarded as being ill. Finally, there is disagreement as to whether the condition is amenable to treatment (see below).

Various instruments have been developed to assess personality; some measure specific traits of personality in a dimensional form and others take a categorical approach. The most specific measures require in-depth standardized interviews, which can take several hours. Self-report measures are much less time consuming but are less precise and cannot generate diagnosis.

Clinical assessment

From a clinical perspective, the following areas of the clinical history should be paid particular attention.

1. Birth history: any evidence of birth trauma that may have lead to brain injury
2. Childhood brain illness (e.g. meningitis), epilepsy or head injury
3. Behavioural difficulties at school (expulsion, referred to educational psychologist)
4. Evidence of failure to form long-term friendships (describes self as loner at school, was bullied or was a school bully)
5. Cruelty to animals or other children (torture of small animals or younger siblings)
6. History of childhood physical or sexual abuse
7. Childhood neglect (foster care or parent alcoholic)
8. Criminal record (e.g. history of petty offences from an early age or serious offences such as arson or assault)
9. Evidence of an inability to sustain employment (e.g. never worked or no long-term work; history of conflict with employers)
10. Drug or alcohol problems
11. Disruptive and unsettled interpersonal/sexual relationships.

In addition to a history from the patient, it is important to gain a detailed history from an informant who has known the patient for a long time. If possible, childhood details should be checked for accuracy.

In some cases, the patient may have a superimposed axis I psychiatric disorder. Accurate assessment of the patient's premorbid personality will enable the team to determine the level of functioning to which the patient is likely to return if the psychiatric disorder is treated.

Management

There is little consensus within psychiatry regarding the treatability of personality disorder, particularly patients with antisocial personality disorder. Brief treatments are unsuitable and most therapeutic interventions involve treatments of greater than 6 months in duration. Cognitive analytic therapy, dialectical behaviour therapy and psychodynamic interpersonal therapy have been shown to be helpful in patients with borderline personality disorder.

Intensive inpatient treatment programmes lasting months to years have been tried in patients with antisocial personality disorder. These therapeutic regimens have usually been implemented in prison settings for individuals who have committed serious sexual or violent crimes. There is some evidence that very intensive

---

Box 53 Ethical issues in the diagnosis of personality disorders

There are very serious ethical issues in relation to the concept of personality disorder as a diagnosis. Some psychiatrists are vehemently opposed to the principles underlying the process of categorizing certain individuals in this way. What is considered acceptable behaviour by society is partly dependent upon the individual's behaviour but also depends upon the degree of tolerance the society has towards variance. There are many examples of behaviour that has been considered 'deviant' at certains time in the past and is now considered part of normal variation. The more intolerant the society, the greater the number of people who will be classified as aberrant and likely to have a personality disorder. These issues are particularly important at present, as the government is seeking to provide psychiatrists with greater powers to detain patients with antisocial personality disorders. This is discussed further in the chapter on the medico-legal aspects of psychiatry. It illustrates the difficult balance between protecting the human rights of individuals versus society. The diagnosis of personality disorder is not an exact science and is dependent upon the judgement of individual psychiatrists. It is, therefore, impossible to exclude bias in this process, although all psychiatrists should strive to be as objective as possible.

---

treatment may be helpful for certain individuals, but all these treatments require further evaluation before any firm conclusions can be drawn.

A recent review of treatment interventions for personality disorder by Perry and colleagues (1999) found 15 studies reporting empirical data on the outcome of personality disorders after either short-or long-term psychotherapy. All studies of active psychotherapies of personality disorders reported positive outcomes at termination and at follow-up. The control conditions in the randomized, controlled treatment trials produced only small to medium change in comparison with the active treatments. Psychotherapies of longer duration had the best outcome.

There is some evidence that different kinds of personality may respond differently to treatment. With cognitive therapy, patients with obsessional or anxious personality types do better than those with borderline personality. Patients with schizotypal personality disorder and antisocial personality disorder are more difficult to treat with psychotherapeutic methods.

Management

Most general psychiatry services do not have the resources available to offer intensive psychological treatment for personality disorder. Instead the aim of management is to:

- treat coexisting axis I disorders
- liaise with social services to provide a stable social environment
- help with alcohol or drug addiction
- consider low-dosage neuroleptics to reduce impulsivity or aggressive outbursts
- take a long-term view (aim for slow improvement)
- expect setbacks and crises
- provide clear policy and guidelines regarding the role of hospital treatment
- try to maintain a good working relationship with the patient
- conduct frequent assessments of risk to others and self (risk assessment and dangerousness is covered in detail in Ch. 15).

Further reading and sources

Butcher JN, Rouse SV 1996 Personality: individual differences and clinical assessment. Annual Review of Psychology 47: 87–111

Clark LA, Watson D, Reynolds S 1995 Diagnosis and classification of psychopathology: challenges to the current system and future directions. Annual Review of Psychology, 46: 121–153

Perry JC, Vaillant GE 1989 Personality disorders. In Comprehensive textbook of psychiatry, Vol 2, 5th edn, Kaplan HI, Sadock BJ (eds). Williams & Wilkins, Baltimore, MD, pp. 1352–1387

Perry J, Christopher MPH, Banon E, Ianni, F 1999 Effectiveness of psychotherapy for personality disorders. American Journal of Psychiatry 156: 1312–1321

Plomin R and McClearn GE (eds) 1993 Nature, nurture, and psychology. American Psychological Association, Washington, DC

Sources

Mental Health Net–All About Personality Disorders. Presents details about ten different personality disorders. Includes symptoms, treatment and links to other resources. personality disorders.mentalhelp.net

The Personality Project. A guide to the academic research literature in personality and personality theory. Meant for those with a serious interest in current personality theory and research. pmc.psych.northwestern.edu

Self-assessment: questions

Multiple choice questions

1. Individuals with a diagnosis of personality disorder:
   a. Have an axis II disorder
   b. Will have shown evidence of disturbed behaviour from an early age
   c. Never suffer from an axis I disorder
   d. Show evidence of stability in most areas of their lives
   e. Have close and rewarding relationships

2. Individuals with an antisocial personality disorder:
   a. Are warm and empathic
   b. Are supportive and understanding
   c. Are emotionally cold
   d. Are self-centred and selfish
   e. Often have a criminal record

3. Personality:
   a. Can be classified according to dimensions of behaviour
   b. Usually forms before the age of 12 years
   c. Is a psychiatric diagnosis
   d. Is changeable and never fixed
   e. Can be classified according to typology

4. Individuals with an obsessional personality disorder:
   a. Are at greater risk than the normal population of developing a depressive illness
   b. Are meticulous
   c. Adapt easily to change
   d. Find it easy to socialize
   e. Often have a criminal record

5. Treatment for personality disorder:
   a. Is usually brief
   b. Has shown psychotherapy may be helpful
   c. Never involves psychological treatments
   d. Can be delivered in a prison setting
   e. Is never given to individuals who have committed sexual offences

Case history questions

History 1

Jean is a 44-year-old woman. She has a history of sexual abuse and spent several years in care as a child. She was returned home by social services to live with her mother when she was 15 years old. Her mother showed little interest in her and she was threatened and bullied by her stepfather. She ran away from home and spent 2 years living rough on the streets. She survived by working as a street prostitute. She has had little schooling and is unable to read and write. She became pregnant at the age of 17 and was housed in a small flat by social services. After her son was born, she suffered from postnatal depression and received a brief period of inpatient psychiatric care. During this period, she began to cut herself. By the time she was 21 years old she had three children, all by different fathers. She had begun to abuse alcohol and social services had placed one of the children on the at-risk register. She has never formed any close relationships or friendships in her life and finds it difficult to trust others. She began frequently to present at the local A&E department with cutting to her arms and chest. She said that cutting helped to relieve tension but also said that she wanted to die. On assessment, she did not have any biological symptoms of depression although she complained of feeling depressed and tired most of the time.

What is the immediate and long-term management of this woman?

History 2

A 43-year-old man with a 25 year history of depression and self-harm confides in his GP that he has been killing his family pets for the last 5 years. He tells his GP that he has drowned two cats and strangled three dogs. He did it because he did not like the way they looked at him. He told his wife the animals disappeared. He has two young sons, aged 6 and 8, who both live at home with him and his wife.

What would you do, if you were the GP?

History 3

A 25-year-old man is brought to the A&E department after he has been arrested by the police for threatening behaviour towards his ex-girlfriend. He has told the police that he has a history of psychiatric illness and suffers from schizophrenia. The duty psychiatrist is called to assess him.

The psychiatrist is able to access his old notes prior to the assessment. The man has a long history of violence towards women. He has attacked girlfriends in the past, but they have never brought charges against him. He was admitted 5 years previously with a drug-induced psychosis, which rapidly resolved. There is no evidence in the notes that he was ever given a diagnosis of schizophrenia.

On assessment, there is no evidence of any type I psychiatric disorder. He complains of hearing voices in his head but he is not experiencing auditory hallucinations. He was brought up by a violent and alcoholic father and spent many years in care. He has never worked and continues to abuse cannabis, amphetamines and alcohol.

What is the diagnosis and appropriate management?

Self-assessment: answers

Multiple choice answers

1. a. **True**. These are synonymous with what is usually termed psychiatric illness.
   b. **True**.
   c. **False**. Patients with personality disorder often have comorbid axis I disorders.
   d. **False**. They show evidence of instability.
   e. **False**. It is difficult for people with personality disorder to form close and rewarding relations.

2. a. **False**. They are cold.
   b. **False**. They are self-centred and exploitative.
   c. **True**. They have a disregard for the thoughts of others.
   d. **True**. They are also often cruel.
   e. **True**. This may include violent and sexual offences.

3. a. **True**. It also has emotional qualities.
   b. **False**. Forms by early adulthood.
   c. **False**. Personality disorder is a psychiatric diagnosis.
   d. **False**. It can be modified.
   e. **True**. The various types are based on characteristics in categorical types and can also be considered in terms of traits, with a spectrum of normal to abnormal distribution.

4. a. **True**.
   b. **True**. They are extremely ordered and pedantic.
   c. **False**. They are rigid in their behaviour.
   d. **False**. They have high standards that others fail to achieve and they find it difficult to show their feelings.
   e. **False**. They rarely offend or drink heavily.

5. a. **False**. Most interventions last longer than 6 months.
   b. **True**. Those of the longest duration had the best outcome.
   c. **False**.
   d. **True**. Treatment of antisocial personality disorder has been implemented in prisons for those who have committed serious sexual or violent crimes.
   e. **False**. See (d).

Case history answers

History 1

The immediate management should involve a risk assessment for suicide and an assessment of risk to her children, either through harm or neglect. It is also important to establish whether she has a depressive illness, which could potentially be treated. In the long term, she will require help with her alcohol abuse if she is motivated to stop drinking. Further support from social services with more intensive childcare is essential. Adult literacy classes could be suggested to improve her eventual prospects of finding work and also to improve her self-esteem. Some local councils operate befriending services, which involve the provision of low-key long-term support to particularly vulnerable individuals. Advice about contraception could be important and there may be local self-groups that provide support or help for women who have been abused. Finally, referral for moderate to long-term psychological treatment should be considered if it is available locally.

History 2

This man requires a detailed assessment from an experienced psychiatrist. He is likely to have a combination of axis I and axis II disorders. Before this can be arranged, the GP needs to make an assessment of his dangerousness, to judge whether it is safe for him to be allowed home given that he has two small children.

The GP asks him to wait until the end of the surgery and in the meantime phones the local psychiatric unit for advice regarding assessment. He then carries out a risk assessment for dangerousness. He finds out that the man has no current thoughts of aggression or killing. The family have no pets at present, and he has never experienced thoughts of wanting to harm or kill his wife or children. He has never thought his wife or children 'look at him in a threatening way'. He has no criminal record or history of violence. He has no thoughts of self-harm. His mood seems similar to usual. He is not hearing voices. He is distressed by what he is doing and would like help. The GP tells him that his wife will have to be informed and the man agrees to this.

The GP concludes that the risk of immediate aggression or violence is low. He suggests the man goes home and says that he will arranges for an urgent domiciliary visit from an experienced consultant psychiatrist.

History 3

This man has an antisocial personality disorder and drug and alcohol abuse. He has suffered from a drug-induced psychosis in the past, but there is no evidence of acute illness in relation to this current presentation. The psychiatrist carries out a detailed risk assessment. He concludes that the man continues to pose a potential threat to his ex-girlfriend, as he has shown no remorse for any of his actions to date and during the interview referred to her as 'that slag who he was going to do over'. He does not have any suicidal thoughts. The psychiatrist explains to the police that he does not have schizophrenia and is not currently acutely ill. The psychiatrist advises the police to proceed with charging him.

11 Psychological aspects of physical illness

Overview

This chapter concerns the detection and treatment of psychiatric disorder in the general hospital setting. It describes the range of normal psychological reactions to physical illness, and the types of psychiatric disorder that can develop as a consequence of physical illness or its treatment. It is particularly important to be able to diagnose depression in the physically ill and to know how to treat it. The detection and management of acute behavioural disturbance on general medical wards is described. Finally, common difficulties in patient–doctor communication are described, and a schema for being able to break bad news to patients regarding their medical diagnosis is included.

11.1 Psychological reactions to physical illness and its treatment

Learning objectives

You should:

- be aware of the common psychological reactions to physical illness and its treatment
- be able to support and help patients to adjust to serious physical illness
- be aware of the problems encountered by patients who undergo amputation.

It is important that every doctor is aware of the psychological impact of physical disease. Serious physical illness is associated with worry and uncertainty. Clinical practice may exacerbate the patient's anxiety, as the patient may see different doctors on each visit, or the doctor may be vague and ambiguous in the information that he/she gives. Other common reactions to physical illness are:

- a search for meaning: 'Why has this illness happened to me?'
- loss of control: 'What is going to happen to me?'
- sense of failure: 'I have failed or done something wrong'
- stigma: 'I am ashamed or embarrassed about my illness'
- fear: 'Am I going to die or be in terrible pain?'
- secretiveness: 'I musn't tell anyone, I must keep it to myself'
- isolation: 'I am the only person going through this . . . . no one understands'.

Relatives and friends of people who have serious physical illness often find it difficult to provide support and help. It is distressing to see someone you love deteriorate physically or mentally and suffer pain or other unpleasant symptoms. Relatives and friends do not know whether to talk about the illness or whether to avoid it altogether. The doctor is a key figure to whom the patient or his/her relatives may turn for advice. He/she can, therefore, play a pivotal role in helping the patient and the patient's close family and friends to adjust to the illness.

The doctor should try to explore with the patient how he/she feels about the illness. It can be very reassuring for patients to realise that the way they feel is not unusual, particularly if they have strong feelings of bitterness or anger. Wherever possible, the doctor should encourage the patient to share these experiences with close friends. The doctor should not, however, force the patient to talk about his/her feelings, if he/she does not want to or feels unable to do so. The doctor's role is to facilitate the patient's natural adjustment to the illness, not to make him/her do something that feels alien or strange.

People adapt and cope with illness in different ways. There is no right or wrong way. People often feel very low or anxious in the immediate aftermath of being informed of their illness. They may find it difficult to assimilate all the information they have received and their concentration and attention may be impaired. People need time to assimilate and adjust to illness, in the same way as they need time to adjust to other major changes in their life, such as loss. Eventually, a particular type of coping pattern will emerge, and it is important for doctors to be able to respond appropriately to the different kinds of coping strategies that people employ.

Some people cope with illness by trying to take control. They find out as much as possible about their illness and accumulate data files and information from the internet. These people need to be involved in all aspects of their treatment, and doctors should recognize the importance of allowing them to participate in the treatment process, for both their physical and psychological welfare.

Some people cope with illness by denial (see defence mechanisms in Ch. 16). They will want to know as little as possible about their illness and leave major decisions about treatment to the medical staff.

Other people cope with illness by trying to channel their energies and focus into helping others. Such a reaction is termed stoicism. They may start an appeal for a hospital scanner or become involved in charity work. They may need to feel closely involved with the medical team, and it will be important for doctors to recognize and acknowledge their efforts.

Psychological reaction to treatment

Specific treatments for serious physical illness may in themselves result in powerful psychological sequelae. For example, radical surgery, radiotherapy, or powerful drug treatments.

Surgery involving the loss of a body part

Approximately one quarter of people who undergo surgery involving the removal of a body part (e.g. breast or limb) fail to adapt to the loss. Four kinds of problem can occur:

- the patient cannot accept that he/she is physically whole, which results in feelings of emotional vulnerability
- the patient cannot adjust to the new body image and cannot look at the affected part or consider a prosthesis
- the patient may feel unattractive and feel unable to allow his/her partner to see him/her naked or engage in a sexual relationship
- if the surgery involves loss of function (e.g. a limb amputation or a stoma) the patient may feel overwhelmed and unable to participate in rehabilitation.

Other forms of loss include loss of fertility for women following gynaecological surgery, and loss of voice following laryngectomy.

Radiotherapy and pharmacological treatment

Aggressive pharmacological treatment regimens can have profound effects on patients' physical and psychological status. Patients can experience continuous nausea or vomiting with chemotherapy for cancer, and some forms of treatment can also produce sterility. Many drugs can contribute to the development of anxiety or depression.

Patients treated for recurrent painful conditions (e.g. pancreatitis) can develop dependence upon opiates. Patients whose treatment involves nasogastric feeding may find it difficult to re-instate normal eating when their condition is better.

Patients who require regular injections can develop needle phobias, making their treatment difficult to administer.

11.2 Psychiatric illness following physical illness or its treatment

Learning objectives

You should:

- be able to diagnose psychiatric illness that develops in the context of physical disorder and know how to treat it
- be aware of the major forms of psychiatric disorder that are caused by the treatment of physical illness
- be aware of the drugs most likely to cause depression.

Depressive and anxiety disorders are approximately twice as common in medical patients in the general hospital setting as they are in the general population. Table 22 shows the prevalence of psychiatric disorder in the general hospital setting according to gender. Alcohol problems are especially common in young males, and all doctors should take a careful alcohol history in males under 50 years of age admitted to the general hospital for whatever reason. The detection and management of alcohol problems is discussed in more detail in Chapter 8. Most patients with psychiatric disorder in the general hospital setting are not identified by hospital staff, and very few are referred on for appropriate treatment.

Depressive disorders in the medically ill

Depressive disorders that are comorbid with physical illness tend to be persistent, and the depression often continues following discharge without attracting treatment from the GP. Depression predicts readmission over the subsequent 4 years even after adjusting for the confounding severity of physical illness.

Depressed subjects also incur higher healthcare costs than non-depressed patients, even after adjusting for the effect of physical illness, and the remission of the depression is associated with reduction of disability. Amongst outpatients, depressive/anxiety disorders have been associated with persistent impairment of quality of life.

It is sometimes difficult to diagnose depression in the medically ill. Staff may construe the patient's distress as a normal reaction (it's understandable he's upset because he's got multiple sclerosis) and, therefore, miss the depression. Also common symptoms of depression (e.g. weight loss, poor appetite and tiredness) are often present in the medically ill, so the normal symptom pattern cannot be relied upon.

It is important to note that most people adjust psychologically to having a serious illness, but this process takes time. The different kinds of emotional reaction have already been described (see above). In addition for looking for key symptoms of depression, present at the time of interview, the doctor should also establish whether the patient's distress is diminishing with time and whether there is evidence of adjustment to the distress (e.g. the patient has taken steps towards adapting his life commensurate with the degree of disability caused by the illness). A useful question to ask in relation to adjustment is: 'Do things feel as difficult and as distressing for you as when you initially learnt you had xxxxxx?' If the patient says that things still seem difficult but not as bad as previously, then this suggests some adjustment has taken place. If the patient says that he/she feels just as bad, if not worse, compared with when he/she was told the diagnosis, this suggests no adjustment has occurred and the patient may have a depressive illness. Medical and nursing staff often try to put themselves in the place of the patient and imagine what it must be like to have, for example, an amputation or a colostomy. They, however, only imagine the immediate trauma and fail to understand that, no matter how awful the disability or condition, most individuals cope emotionally if they are given support and time to adjust.

Box 54 shows the symptoms of depression in the medically ill and excludes biological symptoms of sleep and weight disturbance. It is important to note that suicidal feelings should always be taken very seriously and are very rarely a normal reaction to physical illness. Some patients with terminal illness may decide they wish to die, but there is usually evidence of careful and

Table 22 Prevalence of psychiatric disorder in the general hospital setting (prevalence %)

Psychiatric disorder	Males	Females
Anxiety depression	12	16
Alcohol problems	18	4

From Feldman E, Mayou R, Hawton K (1987) Psychiatric disorder in medical in-patients. Quarterly Journal of Medicine, 63, 405–412.

Box 54
Depressive symptoms in the medically ill

Persistent low mood
Diurnal variation in mood
Loss of interest
Suicidal ideation
Thoughts of hopelessness
Failure for mood to vary according to social cues
Withdrawn and uncommunicative
Overt distress (e.g. tearfulness)

thoughtful deliberation over a period of months. This is very different from a patient on a medical ward who suddenly tells staff he wants to die.

Three symptoms of depression provide particularly good discrimination between depressed and non-depressed medical patients. They are *depressed mood*, *morning depression*, and *hopelessness*.

Most patients with depression in association with physical disorder will respond to antidepressant medication. It is important to minimize the possibility of drug interactions or an exacerbation of the physical disorder.

Anxiety states and panic disorder

Pure anxiety states are much less common than depression in the medically ill. Patients with ischaemic heart disease may present with episodes of panic and chest pain, which are difficult to distinguish clinically from angina; however, all investigations for the discrete episode will be normal. The aim of treatment is to try to help the patient distinguish symptoms arising as a result of heart disease from symptoms arising because of panic. If the patient meets the criteria for panic disorder (Ch. 4), treatment should be instituted with antidepressants. Cognitive therapy may also be useful.

Conditioned responses

Patients who require regular injections can develop a fear of needles and become anxious and panicky at the site of a syringe. Patients with type I diabetes mellitus and patients undergoing chemotherapy are at risk of developing such reactions. These conditions are best managed using desensitization techniques (Ch. 16) and relaxation training. Sometimes, a brief course of anxiolytics may be justified so that the patient can continue with medical treatment, particularly if stopping it would have severe adverse consequences.

Body image problems

Patients can become inappropriately preoccupied with the idea that his/her body is disfigured or revolting. This problem is common following disfiguring surgery. Treatments (Ch. 16) including graded exposure, desensitization and cognitive therapy can be useful. It is important, however, to check that there are not underlying problems in the patient's marital relationship. It is not unusual for a body image problem to develop in a relationship where there are underlying problems.

Sexual problems

Sexual problems are common in the general population but are particularly widespread in general medical and surgical patients. Certain conditions such as renal disease and diabetes are associated with very high rates of sexual dysfunction. In renal disease, 90% of males have erectile failure, and 80% of women are anorgasmic. Sexual problems are reported by 35–40% of diabetic males.

Sexual problems can be caused by:

- direct effects of the condition
- effects of drugs and other physical treatments
- psychological sequelae of the condition
- the presence of coexisting psychiatric disorder (e.g. depression).

The common drugs that can interfere with sexual function are described in Chapter 9, in which more details about the assessment and investigation of patients with sexual problems are provided. It is important to note that antidepressants also affect sexual function, and this should be explained to the patient if such treatment is required.

Alcohol problems

Alcohol misuse not only causes physical illness but can occur as a consequence of physical illness. The sick person can turn to alcohol to relieve anxiety or block out fear about the illness. Increased alcohol consumption can also occur in the context of depressive illness, which may start following a serious physical illness.

Post-traumatic stress disorder

Certain patients who are admitted to the general hospital or who are seen in the A&E department have been injured as a result of an accident or other trauma. Post-traumatic stress disorder is a well-recognized psychiatric complication of such experiences that occurs in 10–25% of cases. It is usual to feel shocked and very anxious following a traumatic event. Flashbacks or vivid dreams are also common and should not be regarded as pathological in the immediate aftermath of a severe trauma. These feelings and experiences, however, usually subside within 6 to 8 weeks.

Routine psychological debriefing following the trauma has not been shown to be of benefit and may even be harmful for some patients. If the patient's symptoms do not subside within the few weeks following the trauma, specific treatment using cognitive-behavioural therapy may be required. Chapter 4 gives a full description of the symptoms of post-traumatic stress disorder.

Other psychiatric conditions, such as phobic anxiety disorder, also occur following trauma and are sometimes more common than post-traumatic stress disorder. The same principles, however, apply in regard to management.

Immediate treatment should be avoided and efforts should aim to facilitate the patient's natural coping

1. You have suffered a serious traumatic event.
2. It is usual to feel shocked, numb or rather dazed for a period of time.
3. You may then experience some sleeplessness and increased worry or anxiety.
4. Memories of the trauma may be vivid but should fade or become less frequent within a few weeks.
5. Try to talk about the trauma and not bottle up your feelings.
6. Try not to avoid things that remind you of the trauma.
7. Try to continue with normal daily experiences.
8. If any of the following occur, consult your doctor:
   (a) you experience vivid memories of the trauma that do not diminish with time
   (b) you cannot face events or things that remind you of the trauma (e.g. unable to travel in a car following a road traffic accident)
   (c) you feel tense and on edge, all of the time
   (d) you start to feel constantly low, miserable and upset.

strategies. It is helpful to provide simple advice at this stage and many hospital departments provide information sheets with straightforward advice and contact numbers for helplines (Box 55). It is also helpful to liaise with the patient's GP so that the GP can check the patient 6–8 weeks following the trauma and arrange for treatment if necessary.

Psychiatric disorder following treatment

Depressive disorders

A wide range of drug treatments for physical illness can produce a lowering in mood and cause depression in the medically ill. A list of the most common drugs associated with causing depression are shown in Table 23.

Table 23 Drugs which may cause depression

System or drug groups	Drug
Cardiac system	Digoxin, procainamide, lidocaine (lignocaine)
Antihypertensives	Propranolol, nifedipine, clonidine, methyldopa
Antiparkinsonian drugs	Amantidine, levodopa
Endocrine agents	Corticosteroids, oral contraceptives, bromocriptine
Anti-inflammatory agents	Non-steroidal anti-inflammatory agents, e.g. ibuprofen
Drugs used in cancer treatment	Methotrexate, interferon, vincristine
Antiepileptic drugs	Benzodiazepines, carbamazepine, sodium valproate
Antibiotics	Penicillins

A clear association between implementation of the drug regimen and the development of depression should be demonstrable before consideration is given to altering the patient's treatment or the addition of antidepressant treatment.

Acute confusion

A variety of drugs, including antidepressants themselves, can cause confusion in the medically ill. (See the management of acute behavioural disturbance in the general hospital setting, below.)

Psychosis

Courses of steroid treatment are well known for producing psychological disturbance. Depression is the most common side effect but hypomania and acute paranoid states are also recognized. The condition usually subsides when the dosage of steroids is reduced or stopped.

Antiparkinsonian drugs used in the treatment of Parkinson's disease can cause a paranoid psychosis that mimics schizophrenia. The psychosis is caused by the dopaminergic effect of the drugs on parts of the brain other than the substantia nigra. Treatment is difficult as most conventional antipsychotic drugs cause an exacerbation of the movement disorder. It is advisable to use the more modern antipsychotics such as olanzepine, respiridone and clozapine, in as small a dosage as possible.

11.3 Psychiatric disorder resulting in physical illness

Learning objectives

You should:

- be aware of the main psychiatric conditions that can result in physical illness

- be able to detect alcohol abuse in patients who present with physical illness.

Alcohol

Individuals with alcohol problems rarely consult the medical profession about their difficulties until the advanced stages of disease force them to seek treatment. The general hospital is an ideal setting in which to detect patients at a relatively early stage of the disorder, as patients may present with a wide range of physical problems resulting from alcohol abuse. Table 24 lists some of the common presentations in the general

Table 24 Different ways in which alcohol problems can present in the general hospital setting

Type of presentation	Examples
Trauma	Head injury (via falling, fighting or being mugged)
	Burns (accidentally setting fire to home while drunk)
	Other injuries (caused by fighting)
	Sequelae of road traffic accident
Neurological	Fit (withdrawal), blackouts, movement disorders (ataxia, peripheral neuropathy, etc.)
Gastrointestinal	Peptic ulcer, pancreatitis, alcoholic liver disease
Other	Withdrawal from alcohol, delirium, cardiomyopathy, proximal myopathy
Coincidental finding	Unrelated to reason for hospital admission

hospital setting. Alcohol counsellors (specialist nurses trained to identify alcohol problems and provide brief treatment) have been shown to reduce alcohol consumption in problem drinkers admitted to the general hospital for physical illness. The intervention usually involves detection and counselling in hospital, followed by a further session of counselling at home. The counselling usually consists of the following steps.

1. Taking a detailed alcohol history (Ch. 8)
2. Informing the patient that he/she has an alcohol problem, supported by information obtained from the history and any relevant physical investigations
3. Advice regarding the consequences of excessive alcohol consumption
4. Exploration of current drinking pattern and lifestyle to identify ways in which the patient can reduce or stop drinking
5. Involvement of patient's family in the process with his/her permission
6. Close liaison with patient's GP and medical staff
7. If alcohol problems are very advanced, liaison with alcohol treatment agencies
8. Follow-up at home following discharge to re-inforce treatment intervention.

Drug abuse

The most common physical sequelae following drug abuse that are seen in the general hospital setting are the consequences of intravenous drug use rather than the adverse effects of the drug itself. Sequelae include abscesses, infected needle sites, septicaemia, emboli, infection with human immunodeficiency virus (HIV), and the acquired immunodeficiency syndrome (AIDS).

Deliberate self-harm

Deliberate self-harm is covered in detail in Chapter 6; it is one of the most frequent examples of psychiatric disorder resulting in physical illness.

Schizophrenia/hypomania

Patients with schizophrenia or hypomania may suffer severe injuries as a result of acting upon their voices or delusions. It is not uncommon for a patient with schizophrenia to be admitted to an orthopaedic ward with multiple injuries after jumping off a high building. Psychiatric management should involve rapid assessment with the aim of re-instituting antipsychotic treatment as soon as possible. Extra sedation may be required to help medical and surgical staff manage the patient on the ward. Input from psychiatric nursing staff who know the patient may also be of value.

Eating disorders

Patients with severe anorexia nervosa may need admission to a medical ward for the treatment of severe starvation. This may include the correction of electrolyte imbalance, rehydration as well as feeding with a nasogastric tube. There is a precedent that this kind of treatment can be given under the Mental Health Act (1983) if the patient refuses treatment (Ch. 15). Chapter 7 provides more details about eating disorders.

11.4 Management of acute behavioural disturbance

Learning objectives

You should:

● be able to detect acute confusion in physically ill patients

● be able to manage it.

All preregistration house officers in their first few weeks of work are summoned to manage an acutely disturbed patient on a medical ward. In theory, this should never happen, as the patient's condition should be recognized at an early stage and appropriate management implemented.

Mild confusion or slightly odd behaviour on the part of the patient is often missed by nursing staff, and the condition is only recognized after the patient has become acutely disturbed. Medical and nursing staff often think that the patient has a formal psychiatric illness, particularly if the patient appears to be responding to auditory or visual hallucinations. However, the sudden development of a functional psychotic disorder in an individual with no previous history is extremely rare, and visual hallucinations are relatively rare in functional psychoses but are strongly suggestive of an underlying brain syndrome.

The central feature of delirium is clouding of consciousness. In a mild form, the patient can appear virtually normal; however, on detailed examination, the patient will display an inability to attend to simple tasks and will be disorientated for time, place and person. In a severe form, the patient may be very drowsy or even unconscious. Typically, the level of consciousness varies, with the patient often more drowsy and disorientated at night time. During the day time, he/she may have lucid spells and appear relatively normal unless asked to perform detailed cognitive tests. The physical cause will be successfully found in 90% of cases. Older patients are most at risk. Surveys show rates in general medical wards to be 10–20%, rising to 50% in geriatric wards. Table 25 summarizes the main features of delirium.

Management

If the patient is very disturbed, and potentially at risk of harming himself or others, immediate sedation may be required. The use of sedating drugs, however, can lead to further confusion, worsening the clinical picture.

The most appropriate drug to use in such circumstances is haloperidol, either by oral or intramuscular route. Intravenous drug administration is best avoided because of the risk of collapse or arrest. In medical emergencies, intravenous drug use may be warranted, provided facilities for medical resuscitation are immediately available. Figure 3 shows the schema that should be followed in the management of acute confusion. As with any drug, the patient's notes should be checked for any evidence of allergic responses to medication. Advice should be sought from a senior doctor, at any stage of the proceedings, if there is cause for concern.

The most important part of the management of a patient with an acute brain syndrome is the identification and treatment of the underlying organic disorder. The most common causes are listed in Table 26.

It is important to be able to recognize an acute brain syndrome caused by withdrawal from alcohol as the treatment and management is slightly different. The main features of *delirium tremens* have already been described in Chapter 8. Alcohol withdrawal should always be considered in patients who appear very agitated, have a coarse tremor and are sweating profusely. Management includes rehydration with intravenous fluids, intravenous vitamin supplements and sedation with a reducing regimen of chlordiazepoxide (Ch. 8).

Patients who are acutely confused should be nursed in a side ward. The room should be well lit to reduce the chance of visual misperceptions. The patient will require intensive nursing care, with regular monitoring of the level of arousal, fluid intake and other relevant physical signs.

Elderly patients or those with underlying degenerative brain disease are more prone to developing toxic

Table 25 Mental state abnormalities in delirium

Aspect of mental state	Signs
Appearance and behaviour	Dishevelled, self-neglect Behaviour either overactive with restlessness, wandering and disinhibition or underactive with somnolence Stereotypies and perseverative behaviour (e.g. plucking at bedsheets), agitation
Speech	May be reduced or mute, or loud; usually disjointed; dysarthria
Mood	Labile: mood swings rapidly over minutes, irritable Fear and anxiety can occur in response to visual hallucinations
Abnormal beliefs	Often transient ideas of reference or persecution
Abnormal perceptions	Visual hallucinations and illusions frequent Tactile and olfactory hallucinations also occur
Cognition	The following are usually impaired: immediate memory (digit span); concentration (serial 7s); orientation for time, day and place; recent memory Remote memory is usually intact
Insight	Impaired

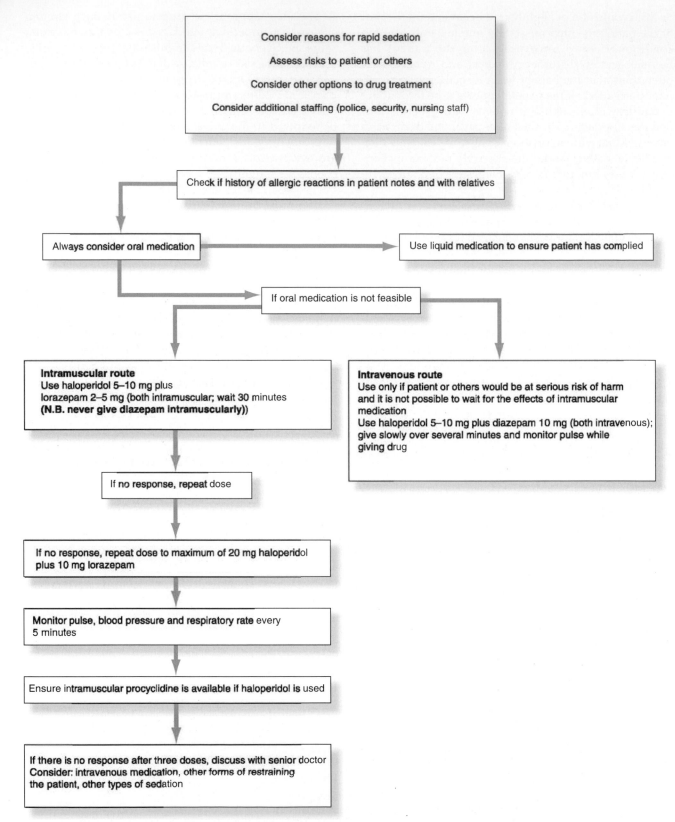

Consider reasons for rapid sedation

Assess risks to patient or others

Consider other options to drug treatment

Consider additional staffing (police, security, nursing staff)

Check if history of allergic reactions in patient notes and with relatives

Always consider oral medication

Use liquid medication to ensure patient has complied

If oral medication is not feasible

Intramuscular route
Use haloperidol 5–10 mg plus
lorazepam 2–5 mg (both intramuscular; wait 30 minutes
(N.B. never give diazepam intramuscularly))

Intravenous route
Use only if patient or others would be at serious risk of harm
and it is not possible to wait for the effects of intramuscular
medication
Use haloperidol 5–10 mg plus diazepam 10 mg (both intravenous);
give slowly over several minutes and monitor pulse while
giving drug

If no response, repeat dose

If no response, repeat dose to maximum of 20 mg haloperidol
plus 10 mg lorazepam

Monitor pulse, blood pressure and respiratory rate every
5 minutes

Ensure intramuscular procyclidine is available if haloperidol is used

If there is no response after three doses, discuss with senior doctor
Consider: intravenous medication, other forms of restraining
the patient, other types of sedation

Fig. 3 Algorithm for rapid sedation in acute behavioural disturbance.

Table 26 Common causes of a delirium

System	Examples
Drug toxicity	Complex treatment regimens involving polypharmacy, minor tranquillizers (benzodiazepines, anticholinergic drugs, tricyclic antidepressants), digoxin, lithium, anticonvulsants, selective serotonin reuptake inhibitors (SSRIs), antiparkinsonian drugs, diuretics, steroids, antihypertensives
Drug withdrawal	Alcohol, barbiturates
Deliberate self-harm	Many drugs taken in excessive quantities
Metabolic	Renal failure, hepatic encephalopathy, hypoglycaemia
Trauma	Head injury, subdural haematoma
Infection	Encephalitis, meningitis, septicaemia, chest infection, urinary tract infection
Vascular	Cerebrovascular accident (stroke)
Other	Cerebral tumour or cerebral metastases, post-ictal state, endocrine disturbance, AIDS, dehydration, any major systemic illness

confusional states than younger patients. Particular care is required when using sedation, and much smaller dosages should be used than those usually recommended for younger adult patients.

The basic investigations that should be carried out to find the cause of delirium are listed in Box 56. Specific further investigations may be required depending on the patient's physical condition.

Table 27 summarizes the main differences between the presentation of delirium and dementia.

Box 56
Looking for the cause of delirium

First-line investigations
Full blood, particularly white cell count
Urea and electrolytes
Liver function tests
Blood glucose

Second line, if clinically indicated
Chest radiograph
Urine culture
Urine street drug screen
Cardiac enzymes
Electrocardiograph
Plasma levels of drugs such as anticonvulsants
Arterial blood gases
Blood cultures
Electroencephalograph
Computed tomography

11.5 Pregnancy and postnatal disorders

Learning objectives

You should:

- know the main features and time course of postnatal depression

- know how to distinguish 'maternity blues' from postnatal depression

- know the main features of puerperal psychosis

- be aware of depression during pregnancy.

Maternity blues

Approximately half of all new mothers experience sadness, weeping and emotional lability on or around the fifth day postpartum. The condition is self-limiting and no treatment is required. The cause is unknown but is presumed to be related to biological and hormonal changes postpartum. 'Very severe blues' may herald the onset of a depressive illness.

Postnatal depression

Postnatal depression is similar to depression in other contexts. It usually begins within 6 weeks of delivery. It is

Table 27 Delirium or dementia?

Presentation	Delirium	Dementia
Onset	Acute, over hours or days	Insidious, over weeks or months
Consciousness level	Reduced and fluctuating	Normal
Visual hallucinations	Common	Rare except for Lewy body dementia
Physical cause	Present	Usually absent
Course	Transient; usually reversible	Chronic; usually irreversible and progressive

characterized by continuous low mood, anxiety, irritability, fatigue and poor concentration. Sleep is usually disturbed, but this may be difficult to assess if the mother's sleep is being disrupted by the baby. The mother may develop low self-esteem and feelings of inadequacy in relation to mothering. She may worry excessively about the baby, with repeated and unnecessary checking. She may also develop feelings of guilt and self-blame. Postnatal depression occurs in 10 to 15% of newly delivered mothers. However, it is much more frequent in those with chronic psychosocial difficulties. Box 57 shows the many psychosocial risk factors for postnatal depression.

Box 57
Risk factors for postnatal depression

Unwanted/unplanned pregnancy
Emotional disorder during pregnancy
Lack of support
Poor housing
Previous depression
Family history
Unemployed partner
No job to which to return

In most women (70%), treatment is successful, although one third of women may have chronic or relapsing depression. Treatment is usually carried out in primary care and can include:

- non-directive counselling
- cognitive-behavioural counselling, including advice on child care, enjoyable activities in relationships
- antidepressants.

Recent research has shown that antidepressants and brief cognitive-behavioural counselling delivered by health visitors are equally effective in the treatment of postnatal depression.

Caution is required when using antidepressants in women who are breast-feeding. It is important that the woman is made aware of all the relevant information before she comes to a decision about the most appropriate kind of treatment for her. Drug excretion in breast milk depends mostly on passive diffusion of the unionized unbound drug. However, the concentrations of drug in breast milk vary during the day in a complex and variable manner. Breast milk is composed largely of proteins and lipids, with the highest proportion of lipids being in the later portion (so-called hind milk). Antidepressant concentrations are higher in hind milk than in fore milk.

Most studies of selective serotonin reuptake inhibitors (SSRIs) in women who are breast-feeding report low or undetectable serum SSRI concentrations in their breast-fed infants. In addition, preliminary infant studies have not demonstrated alteration in growth or weight curves or in infant platelet serotonin concentration. No changes in infant neurodevelopment have been observed. There are, however, individual case reports of adverse effects in a small number of babies (Box 58).

Box 58
Antidepressants and breast-feeding

Nine antidepressants have been studied.
Amitriptyline, nortriptyline, desipramine: these have not been found in quantifiable amounts.
Dothiepin, sertraline: these have been found in breast-fed babies but no adverse reactions were noted.
Paroxetine, fluoxetine, doxepin, clomipramine: for these, adverse effects have been described in a small number of breast-fed babies.

Tricyclic antidepressants are found in very small quantities in breast milk and are probably safe to use, although caution is still required as metabolites can build up (Box 58). As in many clinical situations, the decision regarding which drug to use, will reflect the particular needs and circumstances of the individual patient. The prescription of an antidepressant for a breast feeding woman is a case-specific risk-benefit decision.

Puerperal psychosis

Postpartum psychosis is relatively rare, occurring in 0.2% of all deliveries. The risk is higher for a woman with a family history of bipolar affective disorder, a previous history of bipolar affective disorder, women with their first pregnancy and following a caesarean section.

The psychosis usually has strong affective component and begins within the first 2 weeks of delivery. It has a rapid onset, with fluctuating symptoms of depression or mania. Perplexity is a common feature. Less frequently, women can develop disorders that resemble schizo-effective psychosis or schizophrenia.

The mother may behave in a disorganized and chaotic fashion and may not be able to care for the baby. She may also develop florid delusional ideas concerning the baby; for example, the baby is going to die, although it is perfectly healthy, or the baby is the devil's child.

The ideal management is to admit the mother and baby to a specialized mother and baby unit of which there are a small number around the country. Many of these units now, however, refuse to accept women who are very psychotic and acutely disturbed, and they have to be treated separately from the baby until they are stable enough to be admitted to the special unit.

The treatment of puerperal psychosis usually consists of high doses of an antidepressant, lithium (if the mother is not breast-feeding) and neuroleptic drugs. In severe cases, short courses of electroconvulsive therapy (ECT) may be necessary.

In a mother and baby unit, in addition, the mother will receive help and support with baby care.

The prognosis is good, with most patients making a good recovery in 6 to 12 weeks. There is a risk of suicide in the first year following delivery, and a risk of infanticide.

The risk of further episodes of psychosis with subsequent pregnancies is 20–50% per pregnancy, and over 30% of women will have some kind of psychotic disorder (for example postpartum depression). Puerperal psychosis may also herald the beginning of bipolar affective disorder, as 40% of patients go on to develop further episodes of either mania or depression, at some time in the future, irrespective of pregnancy.

Psychiatric illness during pregnancy

It is becoming increasingly common for women to present with depression during pregnancy. Traditionally, pregnancy has been regarded as a time of good mental health for most mothers, and often mental illness actively improves in pregnancy. The following scenarios however are common.

Depressive disorder in pregnancy

Drug treatment should be avoided if at all possible during pregnancy, but in some cases the benefits of treatment may outweigh any potential harm to the fetus. Information is gradually accumulating about the use of SSRIs during pregnancy. To date, there is no evidence with fluoxetine (the most frequently prescribed SSRI) of an increased risk of congenital malformations; most SSRIs can probably be safely prescribed in the last trimester. Some clinicians would recommend they be stopped 2 weeks before delivery.

Schizophrenia in pregnancy

Drug treatment should be avoided if at all possible, but neuroleptics can be given in the last trimester. Prior to that, the schizophrenic patient may have to be managed on a drug-free basis, and this may involve admission to hospital. In individual circumstances, drug treatment may be indicated in earlier stages of pregnancy if the potential benefits to mother and child outweigh the risks to the baby. It is important to emphasize that discontinuing treatment because of pregnancy, or failing to treat during pregnancy, can also have substantial implications for the long-term welfare of the mother and infant.

Severe psychosocial problems and antisocial behaviour during pregnancy

Severe psychosocial problems are becoming increasingly common particularly in obstetric and gynaecology units that serve in deprived city areas. The prospective mother's behaviour during pregnancy is part of a pattern of long-standing difficulties; however, antisocial behaviour (for example hitting or spitting at people; getting into fights with other patients) is difficult to manage on an antenatal unit.

Drug treatment is usually inappropriate. The best management should involve the organization of a case conference to which the patient, obstetrician, ward sister, midwife, sister-in-clinic, social worker and community midwife should be invited. The aims should be to establish firm, structured support for the young mother during the pregnancy and for the perinatal period.

11.6 Psychiatric aspects of specific medical disorders

Learning objectives

You should:

- be aware of the common problems in ischaemic heart disease
- be aware of the common problems in epilepsy
- be aware of the common problems in cancer
- be aware of the common problems following frontal lobe damage
- be aware of the common problems following stroke
- be aware of the common problems in multiple sclerosis.

Ischaemic heart disease

There is strong evidence for an association between coronary artery disease and depressive disorders. The prevalence of depression in patients with coronary artery disease is 17–22%, about three or four times the rate in the general population. The depression tends to run a chronic course and has a detrimental effect on morbidity and mortality. Exactly how depression affects mortality is unclear, but there are several possibilities. Depression may:

- be linked to smoking and other addictive behaviours, which have a negative effect on outcome
- interfere with patient's compliance with treatment or rehabilitation
- affect heart rate variability and increase the risk of arrhythmias
- increase the risk of arrhythmias because of antidepressant drug treatment
- alter platelet aggregation, leading to thrombosis and vasoconstriction.

Anxiety is also common in patients with coronary artery disease or myocardial infarction (MI). It has been associated with readmission for unstable angina and recurrent MIs in patients who have a previous history of MI.

Treatment for depression and anxiety should be implemented quickly. It is advisable not to use tricyclic antidepressants following myocardial infarction, because they may cause prolongation of the Q-T and QRS intervals. They also cause orthostatic hypotension, particularly in the elderly, who may already be taking cardiac drugs, which also have a tendency to cause hypotension (e.g. diuretics, antihypertensives, nitrates). If a patient who is already taking a tricyclic antidepressant develops cardiac disease, abrupt withdrawal of the drug should be avoided and the patient should be tailed off treatment in a gradual fashion. The newer antidepressants, such as the SSRIs, venlafaxine, nefazodone and mirtazapine, do not effect the electrical conductance of the heart in normal doses and most do not cause hypotension.

Psychiatric aspects of epilepsy

Patients with epilepsy have higher rates of psychiatric disorder than the normal population. A variety of different and complex psychiatric disorders occur in epilepsy.

Psychosis associated with seizures

Psychosis is associated with seizures in two forms; postictal psychosis (PIP) and chronic interictal psychosis (CIP). Postictal psychosis is the appearance of psychotic symptoms, delirium or both within 1 week of a seizure in the absence of other obvious causes. PIP is more common in partial seizures than generalized epilepsy. CIP is slightly more common than PIP and occurs in about 7% of all epileptics. It has an insidious onset, beginning usually in the patient's twenties or early thirties. Many of the features are similar to schizophrenia and delusions are prominent. Affect, however, is usually retained, and the personality remains more intact.

Depression

Depression is common and the suicide rate is higher in people with epilepsy than other comparable physical disorders. Depression is more likely to occur in people with left-versus right-sided foci in partial epilepsy. Some antiepileptic drugs produce quite marked lowering of mood (e.g. phenobarbital), while others have a mood stabilizing effect (e.g. carbamazepine) and may be used as a treatment for bipolar affective disorder. Most antidepressant drugs lower the fit threshold, so caution is required when using them in epilepsy. Tricyclic antidepressants are best avoided. Citalopram, paroxetine, mirtazapine and nefazodone appear to be associated with low seizure rates.

Severe anxiety

Severe anxiety may occur in the prodrome of a seizure, which may go on for several hours or even days. Patients with temporal lobe epilepsy may describe extreme anxiety and fear during the actual seizure. Anxiety between seizures is also common. Patients may develop fears about going out in case they have a seizure, and they may begin to avoid travelling on public transport or going out alone. Such fears can rapidly develop into agoraphobia unless treated quickly.

Dissociative experiences

Dissociative experiences may occur during temporal lobe seizures and include déjà vu and jamais vu experiences. Usually patients are otherwise psychiatrically normal, although their experiences may cause worry and concern.

Violence and aggression

Violence and aggression is common postictally and usually occurs while the person is confused, particularly if some attempt is made to restrain him or her. Aggression does appear to be more common in people with epilepsy than the general population and may be caused by the combination of physiological factors (e.g. increased prevalence of head injury and brain damage) and social pressures caused by the stigma associated with the condition.

Pseudo-seizures

Pseudo-seizures are apparent seizures that occur without associated ictal activity in the brain. They commonly occur in patients with epilepsy, as well as in patients who do not have any evidence of epilepsy. They can take any form but most commonly resemble either complex partial or tonic-clonic seizures. Their cause is usually multifactorial. In patients who do not have any evidence of epilepsy, they are best understood as a variant of somatization, which is discussed in detail in Chapter 12. In patients with epilepsy, they may become more frequent at times of emotional distress, and they may be understood as a mechanism for eliciting more care or attention and avoiding certain difficulties in life.

In most cases, it is possible for medically trained staff to distinguish pseudo-seizures from epileptic seizures. However, caution is required in certain conditions. Frontal lobe epilepsy can result in bizarre seizures although there may be no ictal electroencephalographic changes.

Cancer

Depression is common in patients with cancer and in their carers. Those people most at risk are patients with a previous history of psychiatric disorder; a family history of psychiatric disorder; pancreatic, lung, head and neck cancers; advanced illness; poorly controlled pain; and those treated with drugs known to cause depression (e.g. vincristine, vinblastine, procarbazine, etc.). Although there are relatively few systematic trials of antidepressant treatment in cancer, detection and vigorous treatment of depression is important and can make a significant improvement to the patient's overall quality of life. Psychological treatment may also be helpful, but many patients feel too sick or too ill to cope with such an active treatment approach and may drop out of treatment.

Anxiety disorders, including simple phobias and post-traumatic stress disorder, are common. Some patients develop severe anticipatory anxiety before chemotherapy. Patients are often treated with benzodiazepines, in contrast with patients with anxiety disorders in other settings, as treatment response needs to be rapid, and many patients are too ill to learn psychological techniques to control their anxiety. Antidepressants are often used in conjunction with benzodiazepines for the treatment of panic disorder, obsessional-compulsive disorder and other psychiatric conditions comorbid with cancer.

Psychiatric aspects of frontal lobe damage

The frontal and temporal lobes are particularly vulnerable to contusions from closed head injury. Toxic effects of alcohol can result in a frontal lobe syndrome, as can specific disorders such as Pick's disease. Frontal damage can lead to a variety of problems including:

Dysfunctional executive syndrome

Dysfunctional executive syndrome involves an inability to integrate sensory information from multiple modalities, formulate goals with regard for long-term consequences, generate alternative responses and choose the most appropriate form of action. Memory can also be impaired as learning becomes inefficient because patients are easily distractable and have a tendency to make perseverative errors.

Disinhibition syndrome

Disinhibition syndrome is characterized by anosmia, disinhibited personality changes and amnesia with confabulation. The patient's behaviour is impulsive and socially unacceptable. A previously shy and mild-mannered person may become sexually disinhibited, irritable and uncaring. Emotional lability of mood is common, with a lack of regard for other people's feelings.

Akinetic syndrome

Akinetic syndromes most often occur following damage to the mesial–cingulate–supplementary motor system subserving drive and motivation. Lesions to the anterior cingulate gyrus can cause akinetic mutism in which the patient fails to respond to environmental stimuli. Akinesia can be persistent (with bilateral lesions) or transient (with unilateral lesions).

Psychiatric sequelae of frontal brain damage include depression, mania and aggression. Many patients are unable to live independently as their actions put them at risk of being exploited by others, and they are also unable to care for themselves adequately. Some can access young dementia services, while others are cared for by their families.

Psychiatric aspects of stroke

Cerebrovascular accidents or strokes are one of the most common causes of mortality and morbidity in the UK. About 40% of patients will develop a depressive illness following a stroke. Most depressive disorders come on within a few days or weeks of the event. Cortical lesions are more likely to be associated with anxiety in addition to depression, whereas subcortical lesions are more likely to be associated with retardation. Depression is more likely to develop if the site of the event is in the left hemisphere as opposed to the right (in a person who is right handed). Lesions involving subcortical structures on the left side are particularly susceptible to poststroke depression.

Poststroke depression results in increased morbidity following the stroke and poor functional recovery. Paradoxically, overcaring or very supportive families may impair recovery. Patients with overly solicitous and protective carers do less well than patients who are encouraged to take more responsibility for their own actions by their families. Depression should be treated with antidepressant treatment. The choice of drug will depend upon the individual patient's circumstances and comorbid physical conditions. The diagnosis of depression may be difficult if the patient has difficulty communicating because of an aphasic problem following the stroke. The presence of neurovegetative symptoms, non-verbal cues and impressions from the patient's family may help. Some patients, although not all, may be able to write down responses or complete a self-assessment depression scale.

Mania can also occur poststroke. Patients with a family history of mania or a prior history themselves of mania are at most risk. Several case reports indicate that patients make a good response to lithium, or other mood stabilizers. Schizophreniform psychoses are rare following stroke, although there are one or two case reports in the literature.

Some patients develop an apathetic state in which they lack motivation to participate in rehabilitation activities and distance themselves from family and friends. Although some patients with this syndrome may have depression that has not been identified, it is distinct from depressive disorder. There are no signs of appetite or sleep disturbance and no specific lowering of mood. The treatment of these states is extremely difficult, although there is some evidence that dopamine agonists may be helpful (e.g. amantadine).

Other organic complications of stroke can produce states of psychological distress in those affected and create an emotional burden for carers. Expressive aprosody means that affected patients have difficulty in producing non-verbal aspects of communication (e.g. variation in tone) and, therefore, speak in a robotic tone. This can be misinterpreted by others as not caring or being interested, thus leading to interpersonal difficulties and emotional distress. Affective disinhibition means that patients have an emotional incontinence that severely disrupts their ability to have normal interactions with people.

Multiple sclerosis

Psychiatric sequelae of multiple sclerosis (MS) are common. Depression and anxiety are common reactions to the illness. It is a particularly difficult illness to adjust to psychologically as the illness is often progressive, with a stepwise deterioration in function. Major depressive disorder occurs in about half of patients with MS and is more common in patients with more aggressive forms of the condition. Treatment with recombinant interferon beta may aggravate or precipitate depression. Bipolar affective disorder is also common and occurs in about 13% of patients. Both depression and bipolar affective disorder are associated with neural dysfunction; they appear to be a consequence of the disease, particularly in later stages. Cognitive impairment is present in about half of patients with MS and formal neurocognitive testing may be a helpful part of the assessment process. As the disease progresses, some patients develop confusion and a dementia-like state. Paranoid ideation can occur in the context of neurocognitive deficit.

Apathy and fatigue are common psychological reactions and it is often overlooked that nearly half of all MS patients suffer from significant amounts of pain, usually from muscle spasms or neurogenic dysethesia. Analgesics or muscle relaxants may not totally control the pain, which can be extremely distressing.

11.7 Communication between doctors and patients

Learning objectives

You should:

- be aware of the common problems in communication between doctors and patients
- be aware of your own difficulties in communicating with patients
- understand the main stages of breaking bad news.

Doctors and nurses find it very difficult to talk to patients about emotional matters. As a consequence, patients' psychological distress may be exacerbated and frank psychiatric illness may be missed (see below). Studies of doctor–patient interactions have revealed both professional-and patient-led barriers to communication. Much of the work characterizing the strategies doctors and patients use to avoid talking about feelings have been described by a psychiatrist called Maguire.

Professional-led barriers

Barriers can result from the actions of professionals in interacting with patients. These actions include:

- premature reassurance
- premature advice
- switching
- false reassurance
- jollying along.

Premature reassurance
Premature reassurance can often prevent the doctor from eliciting patient concerns. At an early stage of the interview, the doctor will suggest that everything is alright and the patient should have nothing to worry about.

Premature advice
A barrier to communication can occur when health professionals give advice or information to block the showing of emotional distress. Although this is a safe activity for the doctor, if the patient is distressed, he/she is unlikely to take in any information which is given.

Switching
Switching is when the doctor changes topics if the patient brings up emotional distress. For example,

Doctor   How have you been getting on since your operation?
Patient   It's this bag . . . I can't stand it
Doctor   And have you had any solid food yet?

False reassurance
False reassurance often occurs when the patient's prognosis is very serious but the doctor cannot bring him/herself to face this with the patient.

Patient   I'm not going to die?
Doctor   Of course not. We'll do the best we can for you.

Jollying along
Patients are often jollied along on hospital wards. They are encouraged to put a 'brave' face on things.

Nurse   Cheer up Mr Jones, you're going home at the weekend.

This discourages patients from showing their feelings and helps to prevent anxiety or depression from being detected.

Reasons for distancing

Doctors do not use these techniques because they are shallow or callous people. They are often concerned that by discussing emotional matters it will make the patient feel worse. Doctors also have fierce time constraints, maybe having to see 30–40 patients in a morning clinic. They worry that they do not have time to elicit patients' concerns, and if they did, they would not have time to deal with the emotional upset.

In fact, the failure to detect psychiatric illness or emotional upset results in increased hospital admission time and greater chronicity of symptoms.

Patient-led barriers

Patients also find it difficult to talk about their feelings. Below are some of the most common reasons for this.

Embarrassment

Patients may feel shame or embarrassment about feeling low or very anxious and they may regard it as a sign of weakness.

Misconceptions of the self

Patients may not think that psychological problems are an acceptable consequence of physical illness.

Misconceptions about medical staff

Patients may feel that doctors will not be interested in their problems or can do nothing about their problems.

Fear of repercussion

Patients may fear that if they disclose worry or depression, staff will think they are 'whingeing' or ungrateful, and this could jeopardize their treatment.

Disclosure is blocked

Patients may try to disclose their worries about their health on a trial basis. If their disclosure is met by blocking from medical staff, they will not disclose again.

Personality

Finally some patients, by their own nature, will find it more difficult to talk about their feelings than others. If someone has never discussed their feelings about anything in their lives, disclosure will be very difficult.

Improving recognition

The following points may help to improve the detection of hidden psychiatric disorders:

- inclusion of brief questions about psychiatric status in the systems review (Ch. 2)
- ask the patient how he/she feels, for example 'How do you feel about having to have the amputation?'
- pick up emotional cues: these are subtle ways in which patients may intimate they are upset without directly saying so (e.g. looks sad, looks worried, mentions feeling worried in the middle of a sentence and then changes the subject)
- stick with the patient's agenda if possible
- elicit concerns: only by eliciting the patient's concerns can you reduce anxiety, for example 'Are you worried about anything in particular?'
- ask how the patient is coping: 'How are you coping with all of this? It must be pretty hard'.

Reduction of anxiety

The following steps may help to reduce fear and anxiety, if present, and reduce the risk of psychiatric illness developing.

- Provide a clear explanation of the illness, its treatment and prognosis. This should be given in language the patient understands and may have to be repeated on several occasions.
- Give an optimistic but realistic outlook regarding recovery.
- Encourage expression of both positive and negative feelings.
- Allow the patient to reflect on loss and explore ways of coping with it.
- Involve the patient in decision-making.
- Involve the patient's family in rehabilitation before discharge.
- Liaise closely with the patient's GP.

Breaking bad news

One of the most difficult tasks a doctor can face is the breaking of bad news: for example to tell a patient that he/she has a life-threatening illness, such as cancer, or to tell the spouse of a patient that the patient has died. Until recently, doctors received no training how to do this, and as a consequence were often clumsey or inept, resulting in unnecessary additional distress for the patient or the patient's close family.

Although all doctor–patient encounters are unique, Box 59 is a guide to the general principles of breaking bad news and this can be summarized as a series of steps.

1. The doctor should arrange to see the patient in a private place and arrange for the nearest relative or close friend to be with the patient. The doctor

should give information in a clear and straightforward way. It is best to summarize the patient's symptoms to date (e.g. now the main problem for you has been this blood in your water for the past 4 months).

2. The doctor should then forewarn the patent that the diagnosis is serious by making a preparatory warning statement (e.g. 'We've got the results of the tests now, and I'm afraid it's quite serious').

3. The doctor should pause and give the patient time to take this in.

4. The doctor should then be guided by the patient's responses in as far as how much information is given. If the patient says, 'What do you mean, you think it's serious'? the doctor should slowly and clearly give as much information as the patient wants. The doctor should try to pause between information-giving to give the patient time to take it in.

5. The doctor should try to elicit the patient's concerns (e.g. 'now is there anything else you want to know, or is there anything you're particularly worried about?').

6. At the end of the interview, the doctor should allow the patient time to think of any other questions or concerns, and check that the patient has understood.

If at the beginning of the conversation, the patient indicates he/she wants to know very little (e.g. 'I'm very squeemish, I don't want to know the details'), the doctor should proceed with caution. It may be better to use a euphemism such as 'mass' or 'growth' instead of tumour. If the patient comes out and asks the doctor 'is it cancer?', the doctor should answer in a straightforward way. Boxes 60 and 61 give examples of breaking bad news. In Box 60, the patient intimates that he wishes to know the details of the problem. In Box 61, the patient cues the doctor not to discuss the details of the case with him.

Box 61
Breaking bad news when the patient cues that they do not want the details

Mr Gray and his daughter attend a follow-up outpatient appointment. He has had haematuria for 6 months. He has had a uroscopy and is returning for the results.

Doctor   Well, Mr Gray and Mrs Roberts, thanks for coming along today. Now . . . . . umh . . . . you know you've been having this trouble of blood in your water for a few months, but no pain when you pass water.

Mr Gray   Yes, that's right doctor.

Doctor   Well, and you've had the test where we put a camera into the bladder to see if we could find the cause.

Mr Gray   Yes.

Doctor   Well, I've got the results here and I'm afraid it's quite serious.

Mrs Roberts   Oh no.

. . . . *pause* . . . . . .

Mr Gray   Oh no . . . . I'm not very good with medical things.

Doctor   You have a mass in your bladder that is causing the bleeding.

Mr Gray   Well, can you operate doctor and get it out . . . . . ?

Doctor   Well, operating is one way we can help, the other is by using radiotherapy (X-rays) to shrink it.

Mr Gray   Right.

Doctor   Do you want to know more about it?

Mr Gray   No . . . . I'll leave it to you doctor.

Mrs Roberts   Dad, I think you should find out more, we need to know what it is.

Mr Gray   The doctor's said what it is . . . . . best let him get on with it.

Mrs Roberts   Look, Dad, can I talk to the doctor and you wait outside?

Mr Gray   That's fine . . . I'll get a cup of tea.

Doctor   Is that OK, Mr Gray?

Mr Gray   Yes, that's fine.

In this case the doctor continues the conversation with Mrs Roberts and answers all her questions. She only does this, however, after she has made sure that this is what Mr Gray wants.

Further reading and sources

House A, Mayou R, Mallinson C (eds) 1995 Psychiatric aspects of physical disease. Royal College of Physicians, London

Maguire P, Haddad P 1996 Psychological reactions to physical illness. In: Liaison psychiatry, Guthrie E, Creed F (eds). Gaskell Press for the Royal College of Psychiatrists, London, pp. 157–191

Royal College of Psychiatrists and Royal College of Physicians 1995 The psychological care of medical patients: recognition and need for service provision. Joint Report CR 35.

Stoudemire A, Fogel BS, Greenberg DB (eds) 2000 Royal College of Psychiatrists, London 2000 Psychiatric care of the medical patient, 2nd edn. Oxford University Press Oxford

Sources

American Academy of Paediatrics. Useful guide about the use of psychoactive medication during pregnancy. http://www.aap.org/policy/re9866.html

Self-assessment: questions

Multiple choice questions

1. Depression in the general hospital setting is:
   a. Rare
   b. Usually recognized by medical staff
   c. Results in prolonged hospital stays
   d. Adversely effects quality of life
   e. Is not treatable

2. Psychiatric disorder in the medical setting:
   a. Is higher than in the general population
   b. Never involves alcohol-related problems
   c. Is higher in the elderly (over 65 years) than younger patients
   d. Is more common in males
   e. Usually resolves spontaneously after discharge from hospital

3. The following symptoms are helpful when making a diagnosis of depression in the medically ill:
   a. Sleep disturbance
   b. Weight loss
   c. Persistent lowered mood
   d. Suicidal ideation
   e. Hopelessness

4. Professional-led barriers to communication between doctors and patients include:
   a. False reassurance
   b. Ducking
   c. Premature ejaculation
   d. Switching
   e. Jollying along

5. The following feelings are common psychological reactions to physical illness:
   a. Loss of control
   b. A sense of failure
   c. Fear
   d. Secretiveness
   e. A sense of isolation

6. The following factors may help to improve the detection of hidden psychiatric disorder in the general hospital setting:

   a. Elicit patient concerns
   b. Include psychiatric screening questions in the medical systems review
   c. Take a detailed drinking history from young male patients
   d. Never ask patients how they are feeling as it might upset them
   e. to cues of emotional distress

7. Patient-led barriers to communication include:
   a. Fear of repercussion
   b. Excessive confidence
   c. Embarrassment
   d. A belief that doctors will not be interested in their problems
   e. Blocking from medical staff following disclosure

8. Paranoid psychosis in patients with Parkinson's disease:
   a. Is best treated with chlorpromazine
   b. Can be treated with olanzapine
   c. Is usually caused by treatment with levodopa
   d. Never responds to treatment
   e. Is a good prognostic sign

9. Puerperal psychosis:
   a. Is usually affective in form
   b. Is more common in women with a previous history of pueperal disorder than women with no prior history
   c. Usually begins within the first 10 days postpartum
   d. Is usually obvious within a few hours of delivery
   e. Is the same as maternity blues.

10. The following factors are important when breaking bad news:
    a. See the patient alone
    b. Get the information out as quickly as possible to avoid keeping the patient waiting
    c. Get straight to the point
    d. Be guided by the patient's responses
    e. Elicit patient concerns

Case history questions

History 1

Mrs Jones is 59 years of age and has type I diabetes. She has been re-admitted to the medical ward because of a deterioration in her renal function. She has advanced periperal vascular disease and is partially sighted. Both her husband and ward staff notice a change in her during this admission. On previous admissions, she has seemed cheerful and sociable. On this occasion, she appears disinterested in the other patients and spends all of her time looking at the wall. She has told her husband that she is fed up with living and just wants to be left to die. She hasn't told the nursing or medical staff this as she doesn't want to trouble them. Things come to a head when it becomes clear that she will require continuous ambulatory peritoneal dialysis (CAPD) as her renal function deteriorates further. She refuses this treatment.

What would you do if you were the doctor in charge of her treatment?

History 2

Dr Ahmed, a preregistration house officer in orthopaedics, is called to one of the wards at 3.00 a.m. The nursing staff have become alarmed by one of the patients, Mr Jessop. Mr Jessop is not known to Dr Kapur, but he was admitted 2 days previously with a fractured neck of femur. He has become very agitated and aggressive. He has got out of bed and knocked over the drip stand of a fellow patient. Despite his facture, he is refusing to get back into bed and is lurching across the ward. The night sister has called for back-up and has also called security. Dr Kapur cannot get close enough to Mr Jessop to examine him but notices that he is very agitated, confused and frightened. He is trying to bat things off himself and is obviously visual hallucinating. He has a coarse tremor and is sweating profusely. The nursing cardex reveals that Mr Jessop had appeared odd all day and had been muttering to himself.

In the medical notes it is recorded that Mr Jessop is an average drinker.

What would you do if you were Dr Ahmed?

History 3

Mr Andrews was admitted to hospital 5 days previously following a road traffic accident. He was knocked down by a bus and his left leg became trapped under the wheel of the bus. The driver refused to move the bus in case his injury was made worse. He had to wait for over 1 hour before he could be freed. He sustained severe injuries to his left leg and at one point was told that it may have to be amputated.

The nursing staff have noticed that over the last 2 days Mr Andrews has become increasingly over familiar and loud on the ward. He is irritable and impatient at times. At other times he bursts into tears. He has upset one of the other patients by accusing him of 'looking at his goolies'.

The medical staff ask Dr Williams, the liaison psychiatrist, to make an assessment.

1. What are the possible diagnoses?

Dr Williams, the liaison psychiatrist, assesses Mr Andrews. He is able to remember the accident in detail and has been experiencing vivid flashbacks of the event. He has been unable to sleep and feels very irritated by the noise on the ward. He feels very angry towards the driver of the bus and tells Dr Williams that he intends to kill him when he gets out of hospital. He is emotionally labile throughout the interview and bursts into tears on occasions. He says that he misses his young son who is 3 months old. He cannot stand being in hospital and hates being unable to look after himself. He feels humiliated having to use the commode and has nothing in common with the other patients, who are at least 30 years older than him.

He is able to hold a rational conversation and is fully orientated for time, place and person. He is socially appropriate throughout the interview. He has no previous history of psychiatric illness and there is no family history. He denies any drug or alcohol abuse.

2. What is the likely diagnosis?
3. What is the management?

History 4

> Mrs A seeks advice from her GP. She has a little boy aged 3 and would like to have another child. Following her first baby, she developed a severe postnatal psychosis, which necessitated inpatient treatment. She has been well and off medication for 2 years. She has no other risk factors for psychotic illness.

What would you advise?

History 5

> A 15-year-old woman who is 32 weeks pregnant has had several admissions to the obstetric wards during the pregnancy. She has been admitted each time because of suspected bleeding post voiding, but she has never allowed any of the medical staff to perform a vaginal examination. On the ward, she is demanding and argumentative. She started a fight with another visitor and has been rude to staff and other patients.
>
> Her boyfriend is an intravenous drug addict who has recently been imprisoned. Prior to this, he used to beat her on a regular basis. Shortly before her most recent admission, she was sleeping rough.

What is the management?

History 6

> The GP is asked to visit Ms C at home. She is 10 days postpartum. She had a normal delivery and to date there have been no complications. Her partner became worried last night when she began to act strangely. She appeared confused and frightened. She became scared of the baby and told her partner that the baby's face looked evil. She has been very labile and at one time shook the baby excessively when he began to cry.

1. What is the most likely diagnosis?
2. What is your management?

Self-assessment: answers

Multiple choice answers

1. a. **False**. The prevalence of depressive disorder in the general medical setting is approximately 25%.
   b. **False**. Most cases of depression are undetected by medical staff.
   c. **True**. Depression causes an increased length of stay in hospital irrespective of the severity of the physical disorder.
   d. **True**. Quality of life is adversely effected by depression.
   e. **False**. Most cases of depression in the medically ill respond to treatment.

2. a. **True**. The prevalence is double.
   b. **False**. A large proportion of male patients have alcohol-related problems.
   c. **True**. Elderly patients in hospital have the highest rates of psychiatric disorder.
   d. **True**. Psychiatric disorder is more common in males than females in the general medical setting because of the high prevalence of alcohol problems in males.
   e. **False**. Psychiatric problems usually persist after discharge from hospital unless treated.

3. a. **False**. Sleep disturbance is not helpful as it is a common sequelae of physical illness, and most people find their sleep pattern is disrupted in hospital.
   b. **False**. Weight loss is a common factor in physical illness.
   c. **True**. Persistent low mood, which does not improve in relation to social events, is diagnostic of depressive disorder.
   d. **True**. Suicidal ideation is highly suggestive of a depressive disorder.
   e. **True**. Feelings of hopelessness are suggestive of depression.

4. a. **True**. False reassurance is a common blocking technique.
   b. **False**. Ducking is not a blocking technique.
   c. **False**. Premature ejaculation is a sexual problem!
   d. **True**. Changing the subject away from an emotionally charged one is powerful blocking technique.
   e. **True**. Encouraging patients always to be cheerful prevents the disclosure of psychological distress.

5. a. **True**. The patient feels things will 'happen to them'.
   b. **True**. Often, there is a sense of having done something wrong.
   c. **True**. There is fear of death, pain and the unknown.
   d. **True**. Patients often feel the need to keep things to themselves.
   e. **True**. All the reactions (a–e) are well-known reactions to physical illness.

6. a. **True**. Enquiring about patient worries may help to identify underlying psychological distress.
   b. **True**. The inclusion of psychiatric screening questions in the systems review improves detection of psychiatric disorder.
   c. **True**. A detailed drinking history should be taken from all young males who are general hospital inpatients.
   d. **False**. Opportunities should be provided to talk but patients should not be forced to do so.
   e. **True**. Commenting that a patient looks sad or worried is a helpful way to begin to explore how he/she is feeling.

7. a. **True**. Patients may fear that disclosing their worries will make staff less willing to treat them.
   b. **True**.
   c. **True**. Patients may feel that their fears are a sign of weakness.
   d. **True**.
   e. **True**. If an initial attempt to communicate is blocked by medical staff, the patient may be unwilling to try again.

8. a. **False**. Treatment with chlorpromazine will exacerbate the patient's movement disorder.
   b. **True**. Olanzapine is unlikely to provoke a deterioration in Parkinson's disease.
   c. **True**. The most likely cause of the psychosis is the dopaminergic effects of antiparkinsonian drugs on higher centres in the brain.
   d. **False**. Although treatment is difficult, most patients respond to antipsychotic treatment without a serious deterioration in their Parkinson's disease.
   e. **False**. It is not a good prognostic sign.

9. a. **True**. The most common form of puerperal psychosis is affective.
   b. **False**. Women with a history of puerperal psychosis are at higher risk of subsequent episode than women with no prior history.
   c. **True**. Puerperal psychosis usually begins within the first 10 days postpartum.
   d. **False**. The mother usually appears well for the first 2–3 days postpartum.
   e. **False**. Maternity blues is a temporary lowering of mood that occurs on the third day postpartum. It is unrelated to puerperal psychosis.

10. a. **False**. Try to see the patient with a relative.
   b. **False**. Take time, with pauses in between information gathering to allow time for the information to be assimilated by the patient.
   c. **False**. Prepare the patient by forewarning him/her beforehand.
   d. **True**.
   Always listen to the patient. Be aware how much information he/she wants.
   e. **True**. It is always important to elicit patient concerns. Do not assume the patient is worried about the things you imagine would worry him/her.

Case history answers

History 1

The most important aspect of this case is to understand why Mrs Jones has refused treatment. It appears out of character and not something that she has planned or discussed in detail with her husband. The medical team ask for an urgent assessment from a consultant liaison psychiatrist.

The psychiatrist sees both Mrs Jones and her husband. She initially denies feeling depressed, but it emerges that she has been feeling down for the previous 2 months. She has been unable to enjoy anything and has felt increasingly useless and hopeless about the future. In the last year, she has had to cope with the death of a close friend, the death of her beloved pet dog and the loss of her eyesight.

The psychiatrist diagnoses a depressive illness and explains to Mrs Jones that she has had one thing after another to cope with. Eventually it has got her down. The psychiatrist explains that this is a common reaction to severe and disabling illness and is not a sign of weakness. She persuades Mrs Jones to start CAPD and at the same time persuades her to start antidepressant treatment. She discussed the most appropriate medication with the renal team.

She reviews Mrs Jones a few days later. She has begun to feel a little better and has begun to socialize with other patients on the ward. She still feels low, but says she has got to get on with things for her husband's sake.

In a further 2 weeks, Mrs Jones is managing her own CAPD and has been home for a few hours. She has begun to enjoy things again and has started to think with her husband about getting a new dog. The psychiatrist advises that she remain on antidepressant treatment for at least 6 months and discussed her case in detail with her GP.

History 2

Dr Ahmed diagnoses that Mr Jessop is in acute alcoholic withdrawal. He is extremely agitated and, unless treated, could die from his condition. He is also placing other patients and staff at risk from his behaviour.

He is confused and lacks the capacity to consent to treatment. It is, therefore, possible to treat him under common law. A group of four nurses plus security officers, all trained in control and restraint techniques, wrestle Mr Jessop to the floor. An intravenous infusion of saline is started and he is given 10 mg chlordiazepoxide via the infusion. Dr Ahmed also requests intravenous multivitamins (parenterovite) to be given. He is given a further 10 mg chlordiazepoxide 15 minutes later and begins to settle. He is returned to bed, and his leg is immobilized. He is written up for further doses of chlordiazepoxide every 4 hours.

The next day, Dr Ahmed hands over to Mr Jessop's team. The ward sister has already contacted his wife, who says that he has been a heavy drinker for many years and sustained his current fracture by falling down the stairs at home while he was drunk. Mr Jessop's house officer realises that he should have taken a more detailed alcohol history when Mr Jessop was admitted.

Over the next 24 hours, he is stabilized on sufficient medication to control his withdrawal phenomena. His fluid intake is carefully monitored and his urea and electrolytes are regularly checked. He is then placed on a gradually reducing regimen of chlordiazepoxide and is referred to the hospital alcohol counsellor.

History 3

1. From the information in the referral, Dr Williams considers the following diagnoses:

- acute confusional state
- drug-induced psychosis
- hypomania
- acute stress reaction.

2. The most likely diagnosis now is that of an acute stress reaction. An acute confusional state can be

excluded as he is fully orientated and has good powers of concentration. Hypomania is still possible, as his mood is very labile but it is not elevated, and there is no evidence that the condition is progressing.

3. Dr Williams reassures Mr Jessop that he is not going mad and that his feelings are understandable. He suggests that over the next few days he will feel a little more relaxed and less distressed by the accident. He spends a lot of time talking with Mr Jessop about the accident and gently provides him with some advice on how to cope over the next few days. He advises that Mr Jessop contact his wife to see if she can spend more time with him in hospital. He advises Mr Jessop to talk to his wife about how he is feeling.

Dr Williams then liaises with the ward staff. He reassures them that Mr Jessop's behaviour will settle but will be more likely to settle if he can be moved to a side room. This way he can have more privacy. The staff agree to arrange this. Dr Williams prescribes haloperidol 5 mg three times daily on a 'as required' basis, in case Mr Jessop's behaviour does not settle, but asks them only to give this if he becomes very disturbed. Dr Williams says he will check on Mr Jessop tomorrow.

The next day Mr Jessop is visably more settled and relaxed. He has been moved to a side room and his behaviour has been socially appropriate. In a further week, his level of arousal has settled. He is still experiencing flashbacks but these are diminishing in frequency.

History 4

The doctor should give Mrs A as much information as possible so she and her husband can reach a balanced decision. The doctor should explain that the risk of another severe illness is 1 in 5 (20%), but that the risk of depression would be between 30 and 40%. It is possible to reduce these risks by the prophylactic use of either lithium or antidepressants after-delivery, but this would mean that she would probably not be able to breast-feed.

History 5

The obstetrician asked for a psychiatric opinion. The psychiatrist establishes that this young woman was sexually abused as a child and has been in care since 5 years of age. She has a history of disruptive and unruly behaviour and has frequently been involved in fights in the past. She has been moved from residential home to residential home as staff have found her challenging behaviour difficult to cope with.

She does not have any evidence of current depression, and there is no evidence of any other acute psychiatric disorder on mental state examination.

The psychiatrist asked the ward sister to arrange a case conference. At the conference, the young woman is treated in a sympathetic and supportive way. Accommodation in a hostel for mothers and babies is found. She is allocated a key worker and offered as much obstetric support from the community midwife as she wants. The obstetrician explains to her that while she is on the obstetric ward her behaviour must conform to certain limits, and if she goes beyond those limits she will be asked to leave. Staff agree with her programme of support for the next 8 weeks of her pregnancy and the follow-up period.

History 6

1. This young woman is developing a puerperal psychosis, although it would be important to rule out other possible differential diagnoses such as drug abuse.
2. She will require admission to a mother and baby unit, or some alternative safe environment. Her interactions with the baby need to be closely supervised and she should not be allowed any unsupervised contact with the baby. Intensive home treatment may be an option if there are very high-quality community services, and her family are willing to provide close support and care. The nature of her psychosis is as yet unclear.

12 Psychiatry and medically unexplained symptoms

Overview

The presentation of medical symptoms for which there is no underlying physiological cause is one of the most common scenarios in medicine. This chapter describes the prevalence of such problems, both in primary care and the general hospital. It reviews the pathogenesis of medically unexplained symptoms and in particular the role that doctors themselves have in exacerbating the patients' difficulties. The most common presentations of medically unexplained symptoms are described and their management is explained.

12.1 Definitions and prevalence

Learning objectives

You should:

- be familiar with the different terms for describing physical symptoms that have no apparent physical cause
- know the prevalence of somatization in the community and general hospital setting
- be aware of the strong association between medically unexplained symptoms and psychiatric disorder.

One of the most common scenarios in medicine is the presentation of a patient with medical symptoms (such as chest pain) for which there is no underlying organic explanation. In many cases, but not all, the presentation is associated with underlying psychiatric disorder, which often goes undetected. The terminology used to describe medically unexplained symptoms is confusing, but the most common terms and their definition are described below.

Somatization

Somatization refers to 'physical symptoms suggesting physical disorder for which there are no demonstrable organic findings or known physiological mechanism and for which there is positive evidence, or a strong presumption, that the symptoms are linked to psychological factors or conflicts'.

Illness behaviour

Illness behaviour is defined as the way in which individuals perceive and react to physical symptoms (whether they be organic in origin or have a strong psychological component). For most medical conditions, there are a range of illness behaviours, which are accepted as being normal. For example, it is usual to go to bed for a few days if one has influenza but unusual to go to bed for 6 months. The latter would be considered to be 'abnormal illness behaviour'. The reaction to the physical condition is out of proportion to the underlying problem.

In many respects, the concepts of somatization and illness behaviour overlap. Somatization usually refers, however, to the reporting of medically unexplained symptoms, whereas 'abnormal illness behaviour' refers to the patient's reaction to such symptoms, i.e. the degree of their disability. Abnormal illness behaviour can also be applied to a person who has organic illness, but whose response is out of proportion to the severity of the condition.

Hypochondriasis

Hypochondriasis is another term that is commonly used in connection with patients who somatize. Strictly speaking, hypochondriasis refers to illness beliefs that imply an overconcern or preoccupation with disease. For instance, patients can present to the doctor because they are worried that they might have cancer or may have caught AIDs (acquired immunodeficiency syndrome), when either of these possibilities is extremely unlikely. A feature of hypochondriacal thoughts is that they rarely respond to reassurance or explanation. The patient continues to worry that they have a serious disease despite clear evidence to the contrary.

Somatization, hypochondriasis and abnormal illness behaviour can occur together or separately. An example of a patient with all three processes is shown in Box 62.

Prevalence of somatization

Community

Somatization is relatively common in community samples, but the extreme forms, which warrant classification as psychiatric disorders, are rare. In a recent large American study, 4.4% of community subjects reported suffering from somatic symptoms (determined as at least four or more different somatic symptoms for men and at least six or more for women). These subjects reported greater disability and had made more use of medical services than 'non-somatizers'.

There is a strong association between the number of somatic symptoms people report and the likelihood of psychiatric disorder. The more somatic symptoms subjects report, the greater the likelihood of associated mental illness, regardless of the nature of the symptoms.

Primary care

GPs see large numbers of patients with somatization. Approximately one quarter of all patients who seek help from their GP do so because of physical symptoms that cannot be explained by underlying organic disease but are related to psychological distress.

General hospital

In the general hospital setting, somatization is common in outpatient clinics but relatively rare in the inpatient setting. Approximately 40% of new referrals to hospital outpatient clinics have unexplained medical symptoms, with no organic cause found for their symptoms despite investigation. Patients who are admitted to hospital, however, are often severely ill and usually have overt organic illness.

Box 62
An illustration of somatization, hypochondriacal beliefs and abnormal illness behaviour

A 35-year-old man develops headaches and he goes to his GP for treatment (somatization). The headaches consist of a band-like feeling around his head, which becomes tighter and tighter. He begins to worry that he may have a brain tumour. His headaches get worse and he becomes more and more convinced that he has a tumour and is going to die (hypochondriacal belief). He begins consulting his GP on a weekly basis and spends the interim in bed in a darkened room (abnormal illness behaviour).

12.2 Aetiology and consequences of somatization

Learning objectives

You should:

- be aware of the importance of childhood experience in the development of somatization
- be aware of the factors that exacerbate or prolong somatization in adults
- be aware of the long-term consequences of somatization.

Aetiology

Genetic studies in relation to somatization have not produced any conclusive results. Childhood experience, however, appears to play an important role. There are several studies that suggest that adults who somatize frequently report childhood experiences of illness in significant others (usually their parents). Equally, children who report somatic symptoms, compared with those who do not, are more likely to have mothers who somatize.

Experiences of childhood illness or symptoms during childhood appear to have a particularly powerful effect when they are coupled with parental lack of care, either because of the loss of a parent through death or because of a physically or sexually abusive relationship. It is hypothesized that parental lack of care sensitizes an individual to emotional disorder, while exposure to physical illness predisposes that person to misinterpret normal bodily experiences as signs of illness. Another important factor may be that children whose emotional needs are neglected by their parents may learn that physical illness triggers care and attention, either from their parents or others (e.g. admission to hospital) which otherwise they would not receive. Consequently, in later life, illness becomes a powerful, but inappropriate, method of meeting emotional needs.

A variety of factors can increase the likelihood of symptom severity or chronicity in adulthood.

Cognitive attribution

Individuals may misinterpret bodily symptoms attributing them to physical disease. This leads to an increase in worry about their symptoms, which in turn increases their attention towards the symptoms, which increases the severity of the symptoms and results in further worry. This cycle is shown in Figure 4.

Family re-inforcment

Family members may unwittingly exacerbate the situation by re-inforcing the patient's belief that he/she is

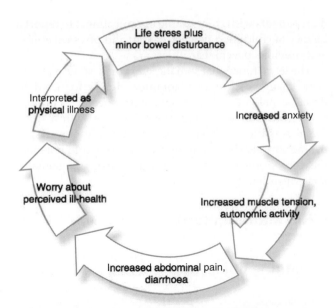

Fig. 4 The cycle of worry and symptoms leading to cognitive attribution. The aetiology of the development of symptoms is illustrated with functional bowel symptoms as an example.

ill. They may advise rest or tell the patient that 'you don't look well'. They may relieve the patient of certain tasks, like housework or shopping. They may encourage the patient to take time off work or may increase the patient's anxiety by reminding him that 'uncle Joseph dropped dead from a heart attack at the age of 38'.

Iatrogenic causes
Medicalization of the patient's symptoms by doctors by overinvestigation and inappropriate treatment reinforces the patient's illness beliefs. Failure to provide a clear explanation of the patient's symptoms and appropriate reassurance results in uncertainty and increased anxiety in the patient. Failure to recognize important emotional factors underlying the symptom presentation means treatable mental illness is neglected, and the patient's physical complaints become more chronic.

Lack of social support and confiding relationships
Failure to express emotion and the lack of a confiding relationship may increase physiological arousal and preoccupation with somatic symptoms. Although family members can re-inforce maladaptive patterns of coping with physical symptoms, a close confiding relationship in which the patient's emotional needs are met, and somatic symptoms are attributed to their emotional source, may protect against somatization.

Long-term consequences of somatization

In the long term, failures in the management of somatization can result in a variety of deleterious effects for the patient, the family and the health care system. These are:

- unnecessary and expensive investigations
- repeated admissions to hospital
- prescribed drug misuse with dependence
- untreated psychiatric illness
- iatrogenic illness, e.g. polysurgery
- disability and loss of earnings
- social disability payments
- poor quality of life
- secondary impact on family and social network.

12.3 Somatoform disorders and functional somatic syndromes

Learning objectives

You should:

- be aware of the psychiatric conditions termed somatoform disorders
- understand the difference between somatization and somatization disorder
- be aware of the main functional somatic syndromes.

Somatoform disorders

The term somatoform disorder was introduced in 1980 to describe a new diagnostic class of psychiatric disorder where the predominant symptoms were somatic as opposed to psychological. In order to warrant a psychiatric diagnosis of 'somatoform disorder', an individual has to be at the extreme end of the somatization spectrum. These disorders are quite rare. Their prevalence in the community is approximately 0.03%. Although rare in number, however, the individuals who warrant such diagnoses are likely to be high utilizers of medical services. The specific conditions are listed below.

Somatization disorder
Somatization disorder involves many physical complaints, beginning before the age of 30 and lasting for many years. At least eight different somatic symptoms should be shown, in different sites of the body or bodily systems. Symptoms are medically unexplained or out of proportion to underlying organic disease. The symptoms are not intentionally produced or feigned.

Psychogenic pain disorder
In psychogenic pain disorder there is a preoccupation with pain, which causes significant distress or impairment. Psychological factors are judged to play an important role in the onset and maintenance of the pain. The

pain is not feigned or accounted for by a mood or anxiety disorder.

Body dysmorphic disorder

In body dysmorphic disorder, there is excessive concern about a trivial or non-existent bodily abnormality.

Hypochondriasis

Hypochondriasis is a preoccupation with the fear of having or the belief that one has a serious disease. This preoccupation causes significant distress or impairment. The duration of disturbance is at least 6 months and the belief cannot be better accounted for by other psychiatric conditions.

Functional somatic syndromes

It is not uncommon for patients' symptoms to cluster around a particular bodily system. Patients with medically unexplained symptoms suggestive of disturbance in a particular system are likely to be referred to medical specialists within that system for further investigation. Psychological factors are rarely identified at this stage, and, unfortunately, are usually only considered when all other investigations and treatments have failed.

Because of the emphasis on physical factors as opposed to psychological issues, a variety of so-called functional somatic syndromes have been described (Table 28). Within individual specialties they are treated as discrete entities, whereas in reality there is a great overlap between the functional somatic syndromes. It is common for patients diagnosed as suffering from one of the conditions to have symptoms suggestive of other syndromes. It is also common for patients to develop different functional somatic syndromes over time. Psychological factors are significantly more common in patients in these conditions than patients with comparative organic illnesses (e.g. patients with irritable bowel syndrome have double the rates of psychiatric illness compared with patients with Crohn's disease or ulcerative colitis). The more severe the condition, and the longer its duration, the more likely patients are to suffer from psychiatric problems. Patients with functional somatic syndromes are also significantly more likely

than patients with comparable organic illness to report a history of childhood neglect, sexual and physical abuse, and previous psychiatric illness.

The term 'functional somatic syndrome' is not a psychiatric diagnosis but is a common descriptor used to describe patients who present with specific symptom clusters (e.g. bowel symptoms). Patients with a functional somatic syndrome such as irritable bowel syndrome may also be somatizers, but most would not meet the very stringent criteria for a diagnosis of a somatoform disorder.

12.4 Management

Learning objectives

You should:

- know how to take a history from a patient with medically unexplained symptoms
- be able to elicit relevant psychological details
- be able to link physical and psychological issues for the patient
- be aware of the main treatments available for patients with medically unexplained symptoms
- know the main prognostic indicators of outcome.

Mild-to-moderate symptom severity

The type of treatment and management used for patients with somatization is dependent upon the severity and chronicity of the patient's symptoms. In primary care, the appropriate management of patients presenting with somatic symptoms for the first time may not only lead to resolution of their symptoms but also to prevention of long-term problems. The aim should be good medical management provided by the GP. This includes:

1. Taking a clear history of the patient's symptoms
2. Taking a history of psychological symptoms and enquiring about social stressors
3. Picking up cues of emotional distress during the interview
4. Carrying out a physical examination with appropriate investigations
5. Summarizing the patient's physical and social problems
6. Helping the patient to understand links between physical symptoms and psychological state
7. Providing a coherent explanation for this link, which makes sense to the patient

Table 28 Common functional somatic syndromes

System	Syndromes
Gastroenterology	Irritable bowel syndrome, functional dyspepsia
Cardiology	Atypical chest pain
Neurology	Chronic fatigue syndrome, common headache
Rheumatology	Fibromyalgia
Gynaecology	Chronic pelvic pain
Orthopaedics	Chronic back pain

8. Being able to treat the patient's psychological symptoms or give advice about social stressors.

For this process to be effective, the doctor has to make the patient feel understood and that the symptoms are being taken seriously. The doctor must collect information about both the patient's physical symptoms and their psychological symptoms before a link can be made. The process will fail if the doctor makes the link too early or tries to make a link when he/she has not acquired all the relevant information.

An example of how a doctor may conduct such a consultation is shown in Table 29, together with the key points of such a consultation. It is important that the doctor takes a history of the physical symptoms first, before he enquires about psychological issues. It is important to examine the patient and provide clear feedback about the results of the examination. The doctor suggests a link between physical and psychological symptoms in a tentative manner, which allows the patient to accept or reject the idea.

After the doctor has made the link between physical and psychological factors, he should listen to the patient's response and try to facilitate further exploration of the patient's emotional problems. It is important that the doctor acknowledges the reality of the patient's pain and does not imply that 'it is all in the mind'. An explanation of how anxiety or tension may create muscle spasm, which in turn produces pain, may be helpful.

Moderate-to-severe symptom severity

For patients with chronic or severe symptoms, specific psychological treatments may be required. However, before any psychological treatments can be implemented, patients need to be engaged in the treatment process. They may be wary or frightened of referral to psychiatric or psychological services, and the referring doctor needs to prepare the patient for psychological treatment. This will include giving the patient a clear explanation of the cause of their symptoms, and providing a rationale for psychiatric intervention.

Cognitive therapy

Sessions usually last for 1 hour and number between 10 and 20 over a course of treatment. Assessment focuses on the patient's symptoms and associated cognitions and behaviour. The aetiological model takes into account both psychological and physiological mechanisms. The patient may be asked to keep a diary of these and then a formulation is constructed to explain how the patient's thoughts, behaviour and physiological responses are interlinked and are perpetuating his/her symptoms, distress and disability. The therapist tries to help the patient to become aware of particular cognitions that may exacerbate the symptoms (e.g. this chest pain means I'm going to have a heart attack), or behaviour (e.g. such as avoiding going out). The therapist encourages the patient to challenge maladaptive thoughts and to overcome avoidant behaviour.

Table 29 Linking physical and psychological symptoms (Adapted from Goldberg et al., 1989)

Consultation	Key points
A 29-year old woman goes to her GP with recurent pains in her chest	Take history of physical symptoms
The pains are sharp, and occur mainly when she is in bed at night. She is worried that she may have something wrong with her heart. The GP establishes that she has no other symptoms suggestive of ischaemic heart disease.	Picks up non-verbal cue
He notices that she appears very tense during the interview. He gently points this out and goes on to enquire how she has been feeling.	
She says that she has been feeling very stressed and harrassed at work, can't sleep and feels on edge all of the time. Her marriage has recently broken up.	History of psychological symptoms and social stressors
The GP asks to examine her. He takes her pulse, blood pressure and listens to her chest. At the end of the examination, he asks her to sit down and begins to discuss things with her.	Examine the patient
GP Well, first of all let me tell you what I've found; your pulse and blood pressure were normal, and your heart sounds were normal when I listened. You were a bit sore over your chest, where you're feeling the pain, and the muscles in your chest wall felt very tight when I examined that area.	Clear feedback of examination
First of all let me reassure you that I don't think that you have anything the matter with your heart. I'm going to do a couple of blood tests and get a tracing of your heart to make sure, but I'm absolutely convinced that your heart is fine.	Appropriate reassurance
The pain, I think is being caused by a kind of tension and spasm in the muscles over your chest. I'm wondering if it's being made worse by all the tension that your feeling generally in your body. You've said that you've been feeling very tense recently, you've not been sleeping, not been able to relax, and you've had a big upset in that your marriage has broken up.	Feedback of psychological symptoms
I'm wondering if there's connection between theses things. A connection between your emotional tension and the tension in your body which is causing this pain (tentative manner). And I know that it's a very bad pain at times.	Making the link and acknowledging the pain

Psychodynamic-interpersonal therapy

A course of psychodynamic-interpersonal treatment usually lasts between 6 and 12 sessions. Sessions usually last for 1 hour, except for the first session, which lasts for 3 hours. The aetiological model takes into account both psychological and physiological mechanisms. Emphasis, however, is placed upon resolving difficulties in the patient's life that may be exacerbating the symptoms, rather than focusing upon the symptoms themselves. In the first session, a long time is spent exploring the patient's physical symptoms. Gradually a link is made between the patient's physical symptoms and psychological status. Stressful factors and difficulties in relationships with significant others are identified. A formulation is developed that connects the patient's physical and psychological symptoms and their interpersonal difficulties. The patient and therapist agree to focus upon one specific problem area and explore and test out problem solutions.

Severe symptom severity

For patients with severe and intractable symptoms, an intensive treatment package may be required with admission to an inpatient unit or attendance at a day-hospital. Most treatment packages for severe somatization or chronic pain have a common set of components, which are summarized in Box 63.

Predicting response to treatment

Psychological treatment approaches are more likely to be successful if the patient accepts that psychosocial factors are contributing to the clinical problem, and the patient does not have a strong belief that his/her symptoms are caused by an underlying organic problem (e.g. a virus). They are also more likely to be effective if the symptom duration is less than 2 years in length. The main factors predicting a poor outcome are:

- strong belief in the physical nature of the symptoms
- inability to accept the importance of psychological factors
- long symptom duration (more than 2 years of continuous symptoms)
- strong support from a family member who looks after the patient and treats the patient as an invalid
- receiving state benefits for disability
- refusal to accept referral to psychological services
- hostility
- litiginous behaviour
- previous invasive medical/surgical treatment for symptoms.

Summary

Somatization is the most frequent form of presentation of psychiatric illness in the general hospital and primary care setting. It is the most common kind of psychiatric disorder that physicians, and surgeons encounter. If long-term problems are to be prevented, it is important that doctors are aware of the high prevalence of psychiatric disorder in patients with medically unexplained symptoms. Referral to psychiatry or psychology services should not be regarded as a last ditch option after all else has failed. A psychological assessment should be an integral part of the investigation of any patient with medically unexplained symptoms.

Further reading and sources

Barsky AJ, Borus JF 1999 Functional somatic syndromes. Annals of Internal Medicine. 130: 910–921

Bass C (ed) 1990 Somatization: physical symptoms and psychological illness. Blackwell Scientific, Oxford

Goldberg D, Gask L, O'Dowd T 1989 The treatment of somatization: teaching techniques of reattribution. Journal of Psychosomatic Research 33: 689–695

Wessely S, Nimnuan C, Sharpe M 1999 Functional somatic syndromes: one or many? Lancet 354: 936–939

Sources

International Foundation for Functional Gastrointestinal Disorders (IFFGD). Provides membership details and information on services. A useful website and organization for patients with irritable bowel syndrome. www. iffgd.org

---

Box 63
Common components of treatment packages for chronic pain or severe somatization

Identification of specific limited goals
Signed contract giving details of agreed goals and commitments
Activity programmes aimed at encouraging appropriate behaviours and reducing inappropriate behaviours
Physical exercise and activity
Marital and family interventions to prevent inappropriate re-inforcing of abnormal illness behaviour
Close liaison with other involved agencies
Cognitive strategies to challenge inappropriate beliefs about pain and illness
Relaxation training
Problem solving

Self-assessment: questions

Multiple choice questions

1. Somatization:
   a. Is a common way patients present with psychological problems in primary care
   b. The same as depression
   c. Is characterized by a fear of illness, e.g. fear of a brain tumour
   d. Is untreatable
   e. Describes the reporting of medically unexplained symptoms that have a strong possibility of having an underlying psychological basis

2. The management of somatization includes:
   a. Making the patient feel understood
   b. Helping the patient make a connection between his/her physical and psychological symptoms
   c. Telling the patient the symptoms are all in the mind
   d. Ordering extra investigations to reassure and allay the patient's fears
   e. Providing a clear explanation of the patient's symptoms and an explanatory model

3. Cognitive therapy for somatization:
   a. Involves asking the patient to keep a diary of his/her symptoms and thoughts
   b. Identifying inappropriate thoughts that may intensify anxiety
   c. Helping the patient with relationship difficulties
   d. Telling the patient to pull himself together
   e. Encouraging the patient to be more active

4. Somatization disorder:
   a. Is common
   b. Is one of the somatoform disorders
   c. Is a psychiatric diagnosis
   d. Only comes on in the elderly
   e. Requires the patient to complain solely of pain

5. Patients with irritable bowel syndrome:
   a. Are more likely to suffer from psychiatric disorder than patients with organic gastrointestinal disease
   b. May have a history of childhood sexual or physical abuse
   c. May complain of many non-bowel related symptoms
   d. Never improve following psychological treatment
   e. Always have psychological difficulties

6. Psychodynamic-interpersonal therapy:
   a. Is an effective treatment for patients with somatization
   b. Works by changing peoples' cognitions
   c. Focuses upon difficulties in peoples' interpersonal relationships
   d. Ignores patients' concerns about their physical symptoms
   e. Helps patients by linking their physical symptoms to psychological problems

7. The following are good predictors of treatment outcome for patients with somatization:
   a. Duration of symptoms for less than 2 years
   b. A strong belief that the symptoms have a physical cause
   c. An understanding that psychological factors may contribute to the severity of the symptoms
   d. Encouragement from other family members to overcome the disability associated with symptoms and have a daily programme of activities
   e. No litigation

8. Important components of treatment packages to treat chronic pain or somatization are:
   a. Exclusion of family members
   b. Physical exercise and activity
   c. Relaxation training
   d. Long periods of rest and sleeping
   e. Identification of specific, limited goals

Case history questions

History 1

A 34-year-old woman presents to her GP with frequent abdominal pain, bloating and a change in bowel habit. She has no other bowel symptoms suggestive of an underlying serious organic illness. She also complains of feeling tired and is unable to sleep properly. She looks miserable and tense. After taking a careful history of her physical symptoms, the GP comments that she looks rather low. She bursts into tears.

What should the GP do now?

The GP establishes that she feels fed up and irritable some of the time, but she does not have a depressive illness and she does not have thoughts of self-harm. She and her husband have been trying to have a baby for the last 2 years. She is desperate to have a child, and they have both recently started investigations for infertility. The abdominal pain and discomfort has felt to her like the last straw, and the GP elicits that she is worried that it is a sign that she may have an underlying gynaecological problem which will mean she will be unable to have a child.

2. What should the GP do now?

History 2

A 25-year-old woman attends the neurology clinic with a history of 'falls'. This is her fourth referral in the last 6 years. She has had seven electroencephalographs (EEG), two brain scans, three 24 hour EEGs, and a variety of other investigations. She has had three brief admissions to hospital for investigation of her falls and has also attended the A&E department on five occasions after she has had a 'fall' while out. All investigations have been normal. She has also been assessed at the gastroenterology clinic for abdominal pain and has been seen at gynaecology outpatients for chronic pelvic pain and dysmenorrhoea. She feels tired most of the time and suffers from frequent headaches. She dislikes going out by herself in case she falls and for the last 6 months has been virtually confined to the home.

She is referred to the liaison psychiatry service, and arrangements are made to assess her when she attends the neurology clinic again for follow-up. The psychiatrist ascertains that she has had a difficult and troubling up-bringing. Her parents split-up when she was only 3 years old. Her mother was an alcoholic and at the age of 8 the patient was taken into care as her mother could no longer look after her adequately. She enjoyed being in care and remained in a group home until she was 18 years of age. She then had to leave and was moved into a flat in the community. She found this adjustment hard, as she had always been used to having people around her. She began to develop falls and was admitted to hospital for the first time.

She tells the psychiatrist that she feels anxious and panicky at times, especially if she thinks of going out. She is convinced there is something wrong with her that is causing the falls and is angry with doctors for not finding the answers. She has a boyfriend who has lived with her for the last 3 years. He suffers from asthma and is unable to work. He cares for her and she is unable to go out without him.

1. What is this woman's main diagnosis?
2. What is the most appropriate form of treatment?

History 3

A 46-year-old man presents to his GP for the tenth time in 6 months. He is worried that he has contracted AIDS. The worry started after he had visited a public toilet known to be frequented by gay men. He has never had a homosexual liaison and has no other risk factors for HIV. He lives alone and works as a librarian. He has always tended to worry about his health and has visited the GP, over the years, on a fairly frequent basis with relatively minor concerns. He has no overt symptoms of depression or anxiety, although he is clearly worried. He is unable to be reassured by his GP. He tells his GP that he has had an HIV test (on a private basis), which was negative, but this had failed to reassure him. He checks his skin each morning, as he had heard that people with AIDs get skin lesions. He feels that people do not take him seriously and he believes that his concerns are genuine. He asks his GP to examine him and to carry out another HIV test.

1. What is the diagnosis?
2. What is the most suitable form of treatment?

History 4

A 52-year-old man was admitted to hospital following an episode of acute chest pain. He described the pain as predominantly central and dull, like an aching feeling. But he also experienced frequent sharp shooting pains all over his chest and back. The pain began after an argument with his wife. He had told her that he had been having an affair with another woman, for the last 10 years, although the relationship had now ended. His wife had told him to leave, and he had walked out of the house, without a coat, saying that he would not return. He then began walking through driving wind and rain and continued walking for the next 6–8 hours. He began to experience pain and palpitations in his chest, became sweaty and shaky and eventually collapsed at the side of the road. A passer-by called an ambulance and he was taken to hospital. He was kept in hospital for 3 days. All the electrocardiographs were normal and his cardiac enzymes stayed within the normal range. He had no prior history of cardiac disease or any significant risk factors. He did, however, have a previous history of panic disorder and depression, which occurred after the death of his mother 15 years previously.

While in hospital, he continued to experience episodes of sweatiness and shaking, tightness in his chest and palpitations. At these times he became very frightened and thought that he was going to die. Cardiac monitoring at the time he experienced these symptoms was normal.

1. What is the diagnosis?
2. What is the most suitable management treatment?

Objective structured clinical examination (OSCE)

Topic: anxiety: atypical chest pain
You are this patient's GP. He/she has suffered from atypical chest pain for 6 months. The patient complains of sharp, stabbing pains in the chest, over the area of the heart. All investigations have been normal. The cardiologist has remarked in his letter to you that the patient appeared very anxious during the last consultation, and the patient may be experiencing panic attacks.

Please take a history specifically to elicit whether or not he/she has panic disorder (with or without generalized anxiety disorder).

If you have someone who can simulate the patient, let them read the card and then answer your questions. You have 5 minutes to do this. You would *not* be expected to present the history but would be marked on your question style and the content covered. If you do not have someone to act as the patient, read the card below and list the questions you would ask to elicit the history. There is no need to write a detailed history.

Instructions for simulated patient

1. You are 25–45 years old (either gender). You have had chest pain for the last 6 months. Sharp pain in your chest. Catches you like a knife. It can come on at any time, but often comes on when you are out of the house. Once it starts you feel very frightened. You are scared you are having a heart attack and are going to die. Although the doctors have told you that your heart is fine, you still worry that you are going to die. When you get the pain, you find you can't breathe and you get more and more panicky. You have to fight for air. You begin to feel light headed and faint.

2. You also get palpitations (heart beating very fast), and numbness and tingling in your fingers. You feel sick. You do not sweat excessively.

3. The attacks are becoming more frequent. You have them two or three times per week. You have been taken to hospital (A&E) three times in the last month. On each occasion, the heart test has been normal. On two occasions the doctor asked you to breathe into a paper bag: that seemed to help.

4. You are frightened of going out by yourself in case you get one of these attacks. You rarely now go out by yourself. Even thinking about going out by yourself makes you feel anxious. Sometimes when you get anxious, the pain starts, but not always.

5. In between episodes you feel tense, nervous and on edge. You cannot relax. Your muscles ache and you feel tired and exhausted. You worry constantly about minor problems and cannot stop worrying about your heart. You check your pulse several times a day. You also check for pain in your chest (*you can rub your chest if you want to*). You are irritable and feel people do not understand you.

6. You have no major worries in your life at present. Your father died from a heart attack when he was 55. Your mother is alive and well. You live alone. You have no other family or friends.

7. You have always been an anxious person and were treated for anxiety and agoraphobia when you were 21 years old. That episode was precipitated by worry and stress over examinations. In the last year you have felt very stressed at work, hate your job and feel you are being picked on by your supervisor.

8. You are not depressed. You have no suicidal ideas.

Self-assessment: answers

Multiple choice answers

1. a. **True**. Somatization accounts for approximately one quarter of new attendances in primary care.
   b. **False**. Somatization is not the same as depression.
   c. **False**. Hypochondriasis is the term used to describe a fear of illness.
   d. **False**. Approximately two thirds of patients with somatization respond to psychological treatment.
   e. **True**.

2. a. **True**. This is important as many patients feel doctors think that they are making up their symptoms or do not understand what they are experiencing.
   b. **True**. It is important that patients see a connection between their physical symptoms and psychological factors.
   c. **False**.
   d. **False**. Extra investigations will re-inforce the patient's concern about illness.
   e. **True**. It is important to provide a rational model for patients in relation to their symptoms, which makes sense to them.

3. a. **True**. Diary keeping and symptom monitoring is an important component of cognitive therapy.
   b. **True**. It is important to identify irrational thoughts which may increase patients' anxiety and make them worry more.
   c. **False**. Cognitive therapy does not help patients with relationship difficulties.
   d. **False**. Therapists will give patients advice and instructions but telling them to 'pull themselves together' is not helpful.
   e. **True**. Patients are encouraged to be more active.

4. a. **False**. Somatization disorder is rare. This term is applied to patients with very severe and long-standing symptoms of somatization.
   b. **True**. Somatization disorder is one of the diagnostic conditions that are termed somatoform disorders.
   c. **True**. It is a psychiatric diagnsosis.
   d. **False**. Somatization disorder has to start before the age of 30 years.
   e. **False**. This is somatoform pain disorder.

5. a. **True**. Patients with irritable bowel syndrome are twice as likely to suffer from psychiatric disorder as patients with organic gastrointestinal disorder.
   b. **True**. Patients with irritable bowel syndrome have high rates of childhood sexual abuse.
   c. **True**. There is great overlap between different functional somatic syndromes.
   d. **False**. About two thirds respond to treatment.
   e. **False**. Between one half to one third of outpatients with irritable bowel syndrome do not have diagnosable psychiatric illness.

6. a. **True**. Approximately two thirds respond to treatment.
   b. **False**. Psychodynamic-interpersonal therapy does not focus upon patients' cognitions.
   c. **True**. The therapy focuses upon relationship difficulties (e.g. death of a loved one, marital difficulties, lack of assertiveness).
   d. **False**. The therapy always begins with a long exploration of patient's physical problems, before discussing psychological problems.
   e. **True**. Patients are helped to understand how their physical symptoms may be exacerbated by psychological difficulties.

7. a. **True**. The shorter the symptom duration the better the treatment outcome.
   b. **False**. This is a poor prognostic indicator.
   c. **True**. Patients who can acknowledge a psychological effect on their physical status have a good outcome.
   d. **True**. Relatives who encourage patients to be active, as opposed to adopting a sick role, enable the patient to recover more quickly.
   e. **True**. Litigation can provide a strong ulterior motive for patients not to improve.

8. a. **False**. Families need to be closely involved in treatment so that they can continue to help the patient when he/she returns home.
   b. **True**. Physical exercise is important to combat disability.
   c. **True**. This helps to reduce anxiety.
   d. **False**. Inactivity increases the likelihood of invalidism and disability.
   e. **True**. It is important to set clear targets that are achievable and towards which the patient can work.

Case history answers

History 1

1. The GP should structure a consultation to cover the following five points.
   a. The GP should acknowledge her distress (e.g., 'I can see you're really upset')
   b. The GP should enquire about her mood state (e.g. 'perhaps you can tell me how you've been feeling recently?')
   c. The GP should assess whether she has a treatable psychiatric disorder (e.g. does she have symptoms suggestive of a depressive illness)
   d. If she is depressed, the GP should check whether she has any thoughts of self-harm or suicide
   e. The GP should identify any current stressor that may have precipitated her decision to consult.

2. The next stage for the GP should include the following steps.
   a. The GP should examine her and give her detailed feedback of the examination
   b. The GP should suggest that her symptoms are characteristic of a bowel problem rather than a gynaecological one
   c. The GP should state that the bowel problem is not serious and is likely to settle of its own accord in a few weeks; the GP should suggest that it is caused by a spasm in the bowel, which affects many people from time to time but never leads to serious complications
   d. The GP should give her a plausible explanation for the pain (e.g. the bowel is like a large tube, lined with muscles . . . . each muscle has to squeeze in synchrony with the next in order to squeeze the food down the bowel; this requires very fine coordination, which sometimes goes slightly wrong)
   e. The GP should make a tentative link to her current stress (e.g. the bowel often reacts to how we're feeling, so if you get anxious, it works more quickly . . . . what I'm wondering is whether the worry you've experiencing . . . . and it is a big worry for you . . . . is making the bowel problem worse . . . .).

The patient is able to accept this and acknowledges that she has been under a lot of pressure. She goes on to talk about some difficulties in her marriage caused by the strain of trying to have a child. The GP reassures her again that the bowel problems are likely to settle and that she does not require specific treatment. The GP suggests some simple measures like increasing fibre in her diet and taking regular exercise. The GP suggests that it may be helpful if she lets her husband know how she has been feeling, as she has been tending to bottle things up. The GP also suggests that if things do not settle she may want to talk to the practice counsellor in more detail and, *in confidence*, about some of her worries.

History 2

1. This woman meets the criteria for somatization disorder in that she complains of many different symptoms in a variety of different bodily systems. The symptoms have started before she is 30 years of age.
2. Her symptoms are of a moderate-to-severe nature. She will require specific psychological treatment (either cognitive therapy or psychodynamic-interpersonal therapy) on a one-to-one basis over several weeks. In addition, her boyfriend will need to be seen, either jointly with her or by himself, to help him stop re-inforcing her symptoms and her disability. She may require specific help from a community worker to encourage her to start going out by herself. This should be done in a graded and gradual way. Joint meetings with the neurologist, on occasions, will be required to allay her concerns and prevent further unnecessary investigation. Her GP should be kept fully informed of the treatment.

History 3

1. This man is suffering from hypochondriasis. This could have developed in the context of a depressive illness, but there is no evidence that he is depressed. Another differential diagnosis would be an obsessional disorder, but his thoughts are not obsessional in nature.
2. The most suitable form of treatment is cognitive therapy. He will require 12–20 sessions over a 6 month period. The aim of the therapy would be to get him to examine his thoughts about illness in a more rational manner and to come up with plausible alternatives. The therapist may also help him to distract himself from certain thoughts and to stop behaviours that re-inforce the thoughts (e.g. checking behaviour).

History 4

This man is suffering from panic disorder, which developed acutely in relation to marital difficulties. He is experiencing frequent panic attacks associated with chest pain, palpitations, sweating and shaking. In view of his age, the onset of the pain with effort and the ambiguous nature of his pain, detailed physical investigation is necessary in order to exclude underlying cardiac disease.

While in hospital, he requires detailed feedback from a senior doctor concerning the results of his investigations. He needs to be reassured that his pain is unlikely to be caused by heart problems. He needs to be given a plausible explanation for his pain, which will involve acknowledging his emotional distress and anxiety, helping him to recognize that he is experiencing panic attacks and explaining to him how sudden severe anxiety can cause increased muscle tension and pain.

He requires a detailed assessment from a liaison psychiatrist, who will also want to interview his wife. Before he can return home, both he and his wife need to discuss their immediate future, so contingency arrangements can be made. He will require treatment with antidepressants. SSRIs (selective serotonin reuptake inhibitors) should be used instead of tricyclic antidepressants, as antidepressants are the treatment of choice for panic disorder. He may require further psychological treatment (e.g. cognitive therapy) if his symptoms do not settle. He should be encouraged to be active and resume his normal activities as soon as possible. Outpatient follow-up should be maintained for several months to ensure that he makes a good recovery and does not develop avoidance of activities or overconcern about his physical symptoms. He and his wife should be encouraged to talk about their difficulties, which may take several months to resolve, and they may require professional guidance from Relate. A Relate counsellor would help the couple to decide whether they wanted to stay together or whether it was best to separate.

OSCE answer

The following structure should have been followed in your questioning. Initially open-ended questions should be used, moving on to closed questions.

1. Introduced oneself to the patient
2. Picked up cues
3. Began by asking how the patient had been feeling
4. Elicited that the patient had been suffering from panic attacks
5. Elicited symptoms of the attacks
6. Elicited the frequency of the attacks
7. Elicited that the patient had raised anxiety between attacks
8. Elicited that the patient had begun to develop fears of going out
9. Elicited previous history of anxiety and potential stressors
10. Excluded depression and suicidal ideation
11. Asked other relevant questions.

13 Psychiatry of old age

Overview

The psychiatric care of the elderly (those over 65 years) is a separate specialty within psychiatry. Patient problems fall into two groups: psychiatric illness similar to that seen in younger adults and psychiatric illness particular to the elderly. Depressive disorders are common in the elderly but may be complicated by underlying organic psychosyndromes. Conditions such as dementia are more specific to old age. The psychiatric assessment of an elderly person is usually conducted in the home environment. The assessment includes all aspects of function including a psychological, cognitive and physical assessment. In addition, the social function of the patient, including financial status, daily skills of living, current stressors and social support, are assessed. There are effective treatments for depressive and psychotic disorders in the elderly, and treatments are beginning to develop in relation to dementia.

13.1 Assessment

Learning objectives

You should:

- know how to conduct a psychiatric assessment in the elderly
- be able to screen for common physical diseases
- be aware of common psychosocial stressors in the elderly
- be aware of the difficulties faced by the carers of the elderly.

Psychiatric services for older people are organized on a community basis, and services have dramatically increased during the 1990s. Initial assessments are usually carried out in the patient's home rather than the outpatient setting. This enables the psychiatrist to assess the patient's current psychiatric status and also provides him/her with a detailed picture of how the patient actually functions in the home environment. The patient is also most likely to feel more secure and in control in a familiar setting.

Before visiting the patient, the psychiatrist should establish the reason for referral from the GP. It is helpful to speak to the GP in person, who may have known the patient and his/her family for many years. The psychiatrist will also be able to establish the urgency of the problem, and what the patient has been told about the referral.

An old-age psychiatrist will often conduct a domiciliary visit with another member of the community team. The patient should have been informed beforehand about the purpose and timing of the visit, and the psychiatrist should carry and offer some form of official identification. The structure of the psychiatric history is similar to that outlined in Chapter 2. The psychiatrist should begin by asking the patient about his/her main problems or difficulties and then move on to the other parts of the psychiatric history. People with memory impairment may be able to give only limited information, but this in itself will give the psychiatrist an indication of the severity of the patient's problems. In addition to the conventional history, the psychiatrist should also carry out a careful assessment of the patient's social circumstances, disabilities and daily skills of living (Table 30).

A detailed assessment of cognitive function is also an integral part of the assessment procedure and it may take several visits before a full assessment can be completed. Many old-age psychiatrists use the mini mental state examination (MMSE; Ch. 2) as a quick measure of cognitive function. This test is relatively crude and if there is any evidence of disturbance, the psychiatrist should perform more detailed measures of cognitive function. The Report from the MRC Alzheimer's Disease Workshop (1987) provides details of many useful tests for specific areas of cognitive dysfunction.

It is very important to interview an informant about the patient's problems and difficulties. Table 31 lists the

Table 30 Psychosocial assessment of the elderly

Functional area	Specific points
Eyesight	Degree of impairment; potential of treatment or aids to improve eyesight
Hearing	Degree of impairment; potential of treatment or aids to improve hearing
Mobility	Degree of mobility, either with or without aids; potential of treatment (e.g. hip replacement) or aids to improve mobility
Toilet use	Bladder and/or bowel continence; independent toilet use (on and off, dressing, wiping), needs help; potential of treatment to improve function
Transport	Ability to drive; access to a vehicle; availability of public transport
Social support	Patient lives alone or with others Degree of support and supervision: number of close relatives and degree of support they provide, number of close friends, day centres and other social activities
Financial situation	Pension, occupational pension, additional benefits, debts, ability to manage financial affairs
Daily activities of living	Cleaning the house, shopping, cooking
Self-care	Washing, dental hygiene, feeding
Dependents	Elderly children (e.g. with learning difficulties), pets
Other important social stressors	Victim of burglary or intimidation, recent bereavements
Hobbies	Level of support and interest provided by hobby
Sexual relationship	Difficulties or problems if relevant

Table 31 Information that should be elicited from the main carer

Areas of enquiry	Specifics
Presenting complaint	How the illness started and when
Past history	A detailed account of the patient's previous history if he/she has been unable to give it
Family	The current support structure for the patient; strength of relationships with other family members; stresses or conflicts that may have a deleterious effect on either the patient's illness or their ability to cope
Medication	Current medication; any side effects; compliance
Premorbid personality	Evidence of anxiety, obsessional or depressive traits; past ability to cope with problems or difficulties; skills in interpersonal relationships; degree of emotional expression
Insight	How the patient views the illness, both explicitly and implicitly
Daily living skills	How the patient manages daily activites: washing, dressing, managing finances, shopping, etc.; the degree of help required to perform each task
Behaviour	Any particularly difficult behaviours and their frequency
Statutory help	Help from social services or other health service or voluntary agencies
Future plans	Any impending changes (e.g. plans to move, hospital admission, etc.)

key areas of enquiry. The psychiatrist should also establish the burden of care and how the carer is coping. The overall welfare of the patient may depend upon the care they receive from this person, and the carer may need help in order to continue in this role.

Physical assessment in older people

Physical problems in the elderly may present indirectly. The first sign of any problem may be a reduction in function. Any increased need for social care should trigger both a physical and psychiatric assessment in older people.

The assessment should begin with a detailed history from the patient and an informant. This should follow standard medical guidelines. On some occasions, patients may present with psychological problems, which actually have an underlying physical cause. Heart failure can be missed as it does not always present with breathlessness. Instead, patients can present with vague symptoms such as tiredness or exhaustion. The early signs of Parkinson's disease may be confused with a psychiatric disorder, and the clinical signs of anaemia are very non-specific. Malignancy should be included in the differential diagnosis of almost all conditions presenting in late life. A careful check should be made for signs or symptoms of cerebrovascular disease. Severe constipation is common in old people and faecal impaction may present non-specifically with profound malaise or with urinary or faecal incontinence. Table 32 provides a brief summary of particular conditions that can present with psychological symptoms and which should be screened for in the physical examination. Table 33 lists some of the common investigations that should be carried out in an elderly person presenting with psychiatric illness.

Psychosocial factors which may precipitate or maintain illness

In the assessment of an older person, it is important to enquire about specific psychosocial stressors that com-

monly affect this group of the population. Individuals may not spontaneously divulge information about stressors, as they may be ashamed, embarrassed or feel they have to put a brave face on things.

Loss

Dealing with loss, in particular the loss of a spouse or life partner, can be the most painful life event in old age. It can be very difficult to adapt to living alone if the person has shared his/her life with someone else for many years. The fragmentation of the family system in Western culture has intensified this problem, as parents and their children have become increasingly estranged.

Table 32 Specific conditions to check for in the elderly presenting with psychiatric disorder

Condition	Action
Heart failure	Check for breathlessness on minor exertion and at night. Use auscultation of anterior chest wall to assess apex rate (atrial fibrillation); check for ankle oedema and sacral oedema. Jugular venous pressure can be difficult to assess. Basal crackles are common in old people so may not be useful
Infective endocarditis	Check for finger clubbing, splinter haemorrhages under finger nails and retinal haemorrhages
Postural hypotension	Check for sudden history of immobility, dizziness or falls Measure blood pressure after the patient has been supine for 10 minutes, and then standing for 2 minutes. A fall of 20 mmHg or more in systolic pressure is usually regarded as significant Check the patient's medication (diurectics, hypotensives, antidepressants, antiparkinsonian drugs)
Malignant disease	Check for loss of weight, examine breasts in female patients and axillary and local neck nodes; supraclavicular nodes may be a marker of intra-abdominal malignancy. Carry out further and detailed investigations if any other signs
Cerebrovascular disease	Carry out a careful neurological examination checking for sensory or motor problems
Parkinson's disease	Check for tremor, which may be unilateral at first and sometimes mild and intermittent; check for facial hypokinesia
Thyroid disease	Palpate thyroid, if enlarged, auscultate for bruit Check for signs of hypothyroidism (cold intolerance, alopecia, a puffy face, slow-relaxing relexes, cerebellar ataxia) Hyperthyroidism may be indicated by warm peripheries, fine tremor, tachycardia, atrial fibrillation, eye signs
Hip fracture	Proximal femoral fractures are common, yet are often missed, if the patient is confused; check for this if the patient suddenly becomes bedridden
Confusion	Check for renal failure, liver failure, hyponatraemia, hyper- or hypocalcaemia plus any of the above conditions

Table 33 Some common investigations in the elderly presenting with psychiatric disorder

Investigation	Reason
Full blood count	Anaemia, excess alcohol intake, hypothyroidism
Urea and electrolytes	Renal function, starvation
Calcium	Malabsorption syndromes, vitamin D deficiency, hypoparathyroidism
Blood sugar	Diabetes
Thyroid function	Hyper- or hypothyroidism
Liver function	Liver disease, alcohol problems
Vitamin B_{12}	Anaemia
Folate	Anaemia
Computed tomography (brain)	Only if clinical indication (rapid onset of psychiatric illness with associated neurological changes)
Electroencephalography	Only if clinical indication (helps to differentiate depression from underlying organic syndromes)

Often the bereaved person may be left isolated even though he/she has adult children.

In other cultural groups, such as Asian families, there is often more support provided by the family for elderly parents. In Western families, there is greater expectation that the state should provide care and welfare for the elderly, although with the increasing number of old people, this is becoming more and more difficult.

In addition to the loss of a spouse, older people also experience the loss of close friends and other relatives. If they live to a very old age, they may even have to cope with the death of their own children, who themselves will have died at a relatively old age. Many people will have experienced multiple losses, and sometimes the loss of an individual who was not a particularly close friend can rekindle deeper wounds and losses from the past.

Poverty

Many elderly people have to exist on their pensions and very little else. They may cut back on the amount of heating in the household or restrict the amount of food that they buy. Many fear getting into debt and may not mention financial difficulties unless there is a specific enquiry.

Role transitions

Individuals may have to adapt to painful and difficult role transitions. Retirement not only results in the loss of income but also in a loss of role for many people. Individuals who do not have well-developed social networks or interests and hobbies outside their work find it difficult to occupy their time when they no longer have a job. Work also provides a structure and routine, which many find hard to sustain in its absence. Following retirement, couples find they inevitably spend more time together. This can produce strain in a marriage if the relationship prior to retirement has been poor or fractious. Being married reduces the risk of depression in old age; however, the quality of the relationship is also important, and the lack of a confiding relationship is associated with increased depression.

Physical illness

Chronic and disabling physical illness is a strong risk factor for depressive disorder in older people. A previously active person can be devastated by the onset of ischaemic heart disease or a stroke. Blindness or deafness is a major loss that most people find difficult to deal with. It is not only important to assess the elderly person's physical status but also how they have adjusted to, or are managing, their physical problems. Many old people take a variety of different drugs for their physical status, which may in themselves result in unpleasant side effects (e.g. hypotension or confusion).

Crime

Elderly people, particularly those who are less well off, may become the victims of crime. They may not be able to afford to move out of crime-ridden areas and are easy targets for criminals. Burglary, fraud or even mugging are unfortunately not uncommon crimes against the elderly. Although the crimes may be perpetrated by young males who do not mean any physical harm, their effect can be devastating.

Abuse

In the last several years, it has become increasingly obvious that some elderly people suffer ill treatment and neglect from their own families. Elder abuse is defined as a repeated act against, or failure to act for, an elderly person that causes distress or damage and so prevents them living a full life. The forms of mistreatment of older people that have been recorded are shown in Box 64. It has been estimated that about 4% of elderly people in the UK suffer from abuse. In an average health district with 200 000 population and 30 000 elderly people, this approximates to 1 in 200. The typical victim tends to be:

- female
- over 75 years of age
- physically disabled
- cognitively impaired
- socially isolated.

The older person may not divulge the abuse, as they may afraid of retribution from the abuser, or they may fear the loss of what little support and care they are

---

Box 64
Types of abuse suffered by elderly people

Physical abuse
Physical assault, producing bruises, welts, sprains, dislocations, cuts, fractures, lacerations, burns, scaldings
Lack of food, producing starvation and malnutrition
Lack of medical care
Physical restraint: being tied to a bed or chair
Sexual abuse
Lack of heating or being deliberately placed in a cold room, resulting in hypothermia

Psychological abuse
Verbal threats
Shouting
Swearing
Intimidating
Isolation

Material abuse
Theft of money or misuse of money

Violation of rights
Forced from home
Forced from nursing home

receiving (even though it is abusive). If abuse is suspected, it is important to enquire about it in a sensitive manner.

Problems and strains faced by carers of older people

The major part played by families in providing community care for elderly people is widely acknowledged and has recently been formerly acknowledged by the government, which has stipulated that all carers, in addition to patients, must receive an assessment of their needs. Informal care of the elderly is provided by relatives, friends and neighbours. Formal care is provided by home helps, social workers, district nurses, etc. Families provide the greatest support, and within families it is usually a key female relative. Four out of five caring relatives are either spouses or adult children. The average age is between 60 and 65 years. These people provide care 7 days per week, each week of the year, unless some form of respite care is arranged. Most people with moderate or severe dementia are cared for in the community by their families. A relatively small percentage are actually cared for in residential settings.

Carers who look after elderly people with dementia, as opposed to other psychiatric conditions, report the highest number of problems and the greatest strain on their own emotional well-being. The problems and strain increase with the degree of dementia. Some carers develop psychological problems (mainly depression), which may need treatment in its own right.

The kinds of problem that carers face are summarized in Box 65. Physical dependence and disturbed behaviour appear to cause the most strain in carers, but the burden of looking after an elderly person with psychological difficulties should not be underestimated.

Statutory services should work in partnership with carers to provide the best care for older people with psychiatric difficulties. A range of community interventions are available that provide support and help for carers (Box 66). Eventually, the carer may be unable to cope any longer and the most appropriate option, in some cases, is permanent residential care. This does not suit all families and it needs to be carefully negotiated with the elderly person and the carer to find the right placement. It also has major financial implications as, in order to finance care, the elderly person may have to use up most of his/her savings.

Box 65
The different kinds of burden of care faced by carers of elderly relatives with psychiatric illness

Practical
Regular help with housework, getting up, dressed, toileting, making sure they eat

Behavioural
Dealing with repetitive questions, disturbed behaviour at night time, aggressive behaviour, wandering, unsafe acts (e.g. leaving the gas stove on), incontinence

Interpersonal
Sadness at the change in their relatives, loss of companionship, losing their temper

Social
Restrictions on getting out, seeing family and friends; not being able to have a holiday

Indirect
Additional burdens such as caring for other members of a family, being physically unwell themselves, loss of income as they may have had to give up work

---

Box 66
The kinds of statutory help available to carers of elderly relatives

Home helps
Provide cleaning services on a regular basis and usually provide unofficial social support and companionship

District nurses
Provide help with getting up, bathing, dressings, injections; gives advice about managing incontinence, plus incontinence supplies (pads etc.)

Community psychiatric nurses
Provide help and advice about managing difficult behaviour; give medication

Day care
The elderly person may attend a day care centre several days per week; they are usually picked up by official transport in the morning and returned home in the late afternoon. This enables the carer to have free time during the day

Psychiatric day hospital
Psychiatric day hospitals provided day treatment or patients with acute psychiatric or behavioural problems; patients are collected in the morning by ambulance and returned home in the late afternoon

Sitting services
Such services provide a regular weekly break so the carer can leave the house to see friends or carry out essential chores

Respite care
Short stays in hospital or homes provides carers with a longer break so they can go on holiday or have a weekend away

Permanent residential care
This can either be a residential home or a nursing home depending on the level of care that is required

13.2 Psychiatric illness similar to that seen in younger adults

Learning objectives

You should:

- know which psychiatric syndromes seen in younger adults also occur in the elderly

- know how depression may present in the elderly

- be able to treat depression in the elderly in primary care.

All the psychiatric conditions seen in young adults can manifest in older people. Certain conditions, such as illicit drug abuse and personality disorder, are rare. Alcohol abuse and abuse of prescribed drugs, however, are relatively common and can be easily overlooked.

Some patients with a recurrent affective (either bipolar or unipolar) disorder begin with the illness in young adult life and then progress to old age, with occasional exacerbations of the condition. Other individuals develop depression for the first time in old age. It is unusual for manic illness to begin in older people. Only about 14% of elderly patients who develop mania will not have had a previous history of affective disorder.

Depression

The most common condition is depression. In the community, the prevalence of significant symptomatology is around 15%, rising to about 33% in general hospital settings. Depression in the elderly has been found to impede physical recovery and is associated with an excess of mortality from medical causes. Concurrent physical illness worsens the prognosis of depressive illness in old age.

The clinical features of major depressive disorder in the elderly are similar to those in younger adults (Ch. 3). However, somatic symptoms, hypochondriasis and thoughts about death are more common in the elderly. Previous literature has emphasized a clinical picture of depression in the elderly characterized by agitation, poor memory and severe delusions. Recent research, however, has failed to establish evidence for this. In fact, younger adults with depression are more likely to complain of memory impairment than the elderly. However, major depressive disorder in the elderly can be complicated by an underlying *organic brain syndrome*, which can interfere with treatment and recovery. Also, the development of a depressive illness can be the first sign of a dementia (see below). Equally, depression in some elderly people can cause impaired concentration, result-ing in poor memory and disorientation. Depression can be mistaken for dementia (so-called *depressive pseudo-dementia*), but if treated correctly, attention and concentration will improve in most cases. If it does not, this may suggest that the elderly person has an underlying organic psychosyndrome.

Depression can also present with the development of neurotic symptoms, such as severe anxiety, obsessional symptoms or hypochondriasis. The development of such conditions in a person with no previous history of such problems should alert the psychiatrist to the probability of underlying depressive disorder.

In many respects, elderly people face far greater social and interpersonal problems than younger adults. On the one hand, this increases the risk of depression and can make the recovery from the illness much harder than in the young. On the other hand, individuals who have survived and coped with the vicissitudes of life without falling prey to depression until their later years may have a relatively low genetic component of the illness and quite a robust character. Both these two factors are good prognostic signs.

Management of depression

Management should be aimed at treating the depressive disorder and addressing the precipitating or maintaining factors. The latter can sometimes be the most difficult things to ameliorate or change. Recent research suggests that approximately 60% of older people who are successfully treated for depression remain well or have relapses that are successfully treated (Fig. 5).

Drug treatment Antidepressant treatment should be instituted but the dosage required may be lower than that usually prescribed for younger adults. Any coexisting physical disorders should be considered when selecting the appropriate drug.

Liver function deteriorates with age including a decrease in first-pass effects and a decrease in the overall metabolism of drugs. Renal clearance also declines with age, which may affect the excretion of the metabolites of several psychotropic drugs.

The lowest effective dosage of medication should be used in older people. Polypharmacy should be avoided and side effects should be closely monitored. Drugs that may induce sedation or falls should be avoided. Psychotropic drugs commonly cause confusion in older people and should be stopped if the patient presents with delirium.

Although newer antidepressants like the selective serotonin reuptake inhibitors (SSRIs) have fewer side effects than the more traditional tricyclic antidepressants, there is very little empirical data on their effects in the elderly, and many elderly patients are often excluded from drug trials. As many older people have coexisting physical disorder, tricyclic antidepressants are often

Box 67 Treatment of depression in older people in
primary care

Up to one third of elderly GP attenders are depressed,
yet only a small minority of depressed elderly patients in
the community are being treated for depression. GPs
are able to recognize depression in these patients but
seldom initiate treatment or refer for specialist
psychiatric evaluation. This may be for a variety of
reasons, including ageism and misconceptions about
the effectiveness of treatment and the potential danger
of antidepressants.

Worry about physical complaints (hypochondriasis) is
very common in older people, which often results in the
unnecessary treatment of physical symptoms.

Somatization (the presentation of psychological
distress in the form of unexplained physical symptoms;
Ch. 12) is also more common in older people than the
general population and may distract the GP's attention
from the individual's mental state. Feelings of guilt,
worthlessness, hopelessness and helplessness are
unusual in the non-depressed and should alert the GP
to the possibility of a depressive condition. The sudden
emergence of severe anxiety, obsessional symptoms or
severe hypochondriasis in an elderly person should be
taken very seriously. Patients presenting with anxiety
symptoms should be regarded as being depressed
unless proved otherwise. Phobic symptoms are more
likely to occur independent of depression.

Because of the greater prevalence of physical
morbidity, most elderly patients visit their GPs about
twice as often as the general population. This means
there may be a good opportunity to detect and treat
depression at a relatively early stage, provided GPs are
empowered to do this. There is evidence that
appropriate treatment for depression not only alleviates
symptoms in the short term but also can substantially
improve the medium-term prognosis and improve the
patient's quality of life.

A recent survey of GPs' views and habits regarding
the treatment of depression in the elderly suggested
that GPs were uncertain about treatment and
management. They were less familiar with using more
modern antidepressants than old-age psychiatrists,
were more likely to use drugs at subtherapeutic
dosages and were very unlikely to maintain patients on
treatment for the required period of time after they had
recovered. A high proportion of GPs said that they
would stop antidepressants after 3 months of treatment
instead of maintaining the patient on them for the
required 2 years. Only 1 in 12 GPs continued
antidepressants for over 6 months.

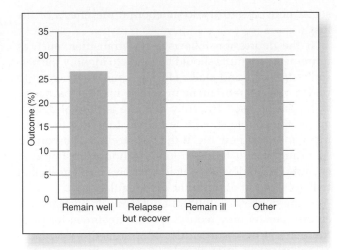

Fig. 5 Outcome in elderly patients treated for depressive
disorder.

who have been successfully treated for depression
should continue taking antidepressants for at least 2
years after recovery.

Psychosocial therapy Psychosocial therapies are
effective in late life, and both the efficacy of cognitive
behaviour therapy and brief psychotherapy have been
documented. Psychological treatments are best used for
elderly people with mild-to-moderate depression.
Elderly patients are less likely to be offered this form of
treatment than younger patients with depression. The
reason for this is unclear but may be related to a misperception that older people may not readily engage in this
form of treatment. There is also a shortage of therapists
trained to provide treatment. Psychological therapies
need to be adapted for use with older people; in this
group, therapy generally has a more structured
approach with a slower pace and more limited goals.
Emphasis is placed upon addressing issues relevant to
the particular needs of the older person and their individual circumstances.

Other treatment In many centres, electroconvulsive
treatment is used more frequently in older people than
in younger patients for the treatment of depression. It is
well tolerated by elderly patients. It should be considered if there is a high suicide risk, depressive delusions,
or refusal of food and drink. It has been shown to be an
effective treatment.

Management of precipitating or maintaining factors
Precipitating and maintaining factors need to be
addressed in addition to treatment of the main condition. If the depression follows bereavement, it is important to establish if the patient has grieved appropriately.
If not, specific grief work may be required to help the
person pass through the normal stages of grief. Help
may also be required to enable the person develop new

contraindicated because of their high side effect profile.
SSRIs and other new antidepressants (Ch. 15) should be
used in these cases. Drug treatment, particularly, if
using tricyclic antidepressants, should be started at
lower than usual dosages and increased slowly and cau-
tiously. Lithium can be used, but lithium toxicity may
occur at levels that would be considered therapeutic in
younger adults. Patients should be monitored on a regular basis. Recent evidence suggests that older patients

social networks to try to ameliorate the effects of the loss.

If the depression follows a role transition, such as retirement, attempts should be made to identify the person's strengths and skills. He/she should be helped to find a role in retirement in which his/her particular skills can be used fruitfully. If there is marital disharmony, the couple should be helped to adjust to retirement and their new life. If the wife feels the husband is spending too much time around the house, he should be encouraged to develop outside hobbies or interests that will get him out of the home on a regular basis.

If the depression follows an assault or burglary, the elderly person may require specific treatment for post-traumatic stress disorder (Ch. 4) or, sometimes, a practical intervention, such as help in moving to more secure accommodation (e.g. sheltered accommodation).

Successful suicide is over-represented in the elderly and accounts for about 20% of all suicides each year, when the elderly population accounts for about 14% of the total number of people living in the UK. Only 5% of deliberate self-harm is carried out by the elderly, but even relatively small overdoses in older people can result in a fatal outcome because of coexisting physical disease. Deliberate self-harm and thoughts of suicide should be taken very seriously in any older person, and it is very important to carry out a risk assessment for suicide in older people with depression (Ch. 6).

13.3 Disorders particular to older people

Learning objectives

You should:

- be aware of the signs and symptoms of chronic brain syndromes in the elderly
- be able to differentiate the different brain syndromes
- be aware of the treatment and management available
- be aware of other conditions that commonly occur in the elderly.

Chronic brain syndromes (dementias)

Although chronic brain syndromes occur in young and middle-aged adults, they are much more frequent in older people. Most psychiatric services for older people are specifically tailored to provide treatment and support to the elderly with chronic brain syndromes.

Chronic brain syndromes usually have an insidious onset and, unlike acute brain syndromes, the level of

consciousness is seldom impaired. Amnesia is the primary feature. Dementia is defined as: the development of multiple cognitive deficits that include memory impairment and at least one of the following cognitive disturbances: aphasia, apraxia, agnosia or a disturbance in executive functions.

By definition, the cognitive disturbance seen in dementia must reflect a decline from a higher premorbid level of functioning and be severe enough to interfere with social or occupational responsibilities. Prevalence estimates for dementia increase significantly with age, and approximately 6% of individuals over age 65 and 20% over age 80 suffer from a medically or socially disabling degree of dementia (Fig. 6).

The three most common forms in the elderly are Alzheimer's disease (or senile dementia Alzheimer's type (SDAT), Lewy body disease (LBD) and vascular dementia. Alzheimer's disease is the most common.

Alzheimer's disease

Alzheimer's disease (SDAT) has a slow and gradual onset. The individual may initially seem slightly more absent minded than usual. Forgetfulness becomes more prominent and the person may have problems in using appropriate words for certain objects. The individual gradually becomes more and more disorganized and unable to perform normal everyday tasks. At the beginning of the condition, the person is aware of his/her cognitive decline and may be very distressed or frustrated. As the condition proceeds, however, insight is lost as the person becomes unable to respond to or even recognize relatives.

The person may lose all ability to care for himself/herself and may need to be washed, dressed and fed.

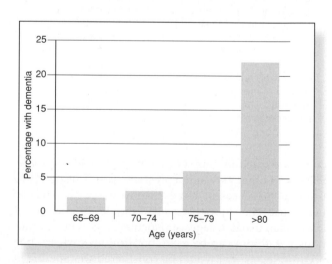

Fig. 6 The prevalence of chronic brain syndrome with increasing age.

Urinary and fecal incontinence is also common in the advanced stages of the disease.

The memory disorder associated with SDAT is typically characterized by poor learning and retention of information over time. SDAT patients fail to show learning over repeated testing and have a high passive learning style. Information is lost rapidly over relatively brief delays (e.g. within 10 minutes) and is evidenced by poor performance on both recall and recognition testing. The consistent finding of rapid loss of information even on tasks that have minimal retrieval demands suggests that the memory disorder in SDAT is one of information storage rather than retrieval (Ch. 1 describes types of memory loss).

In addition to the memory deficits described above, patients with SDAT also demonstrate marked memory deficits across all past decades of their lives. In earlier stages, however, there is evidence of a temporal gradient, in which remote events are remembered better than more recent events.

Focal neurological signs are not usually apparent in SDAT in the early stages of the disorder. In the later stages, patients usually show global neurological changes, including bilateral weakness and lack of power in limbs, poor coordination, tremor and dyskinesias. Some focal signs may be present, particularly if the person has a combination of SDAT and vascular dementia. Weight loss is common, sleep is often poor and the person's mood becomes labile, agitated or distressed.

Underlying pathology reveals widespread loss of neurones throughout the brain, especially in the limbic, temporoparietal areas and frontal areas. The cause of SDAT remains unknown, although a genetic component has been identified. Neuroimaging shows shrinkage of brain substance, with enlarged ventricles and widened sulci (Fig. 7). Histopathological examination shows neurofibrillary tangles and plaques of amyloid. There is also deficiency of cholinergic neurotransmitters.

There is mounting evidence of significant variability in the cerebral regions most affected by the neuropathological process of SDAT. Positron emission tomography indicates that SDAT patients show significantly more lateral asymmetry of brain glucose metabolism than age-matched normal subjects. Especially in the early stages of the disease, patients with greater metabolic dysfunction in one or the other cerebral hemisphere tend to demonstrate asymmetry of memory deficits consistent with the hemisphere most affected.

Lewy body disease

Dementia with Lewy bodies is the second commonest form of degenerative dementia, accounting for 10–23% of cases in the elderly. It is characterized by fluctuating cognitive impairment, spontaneous parkinsonism and

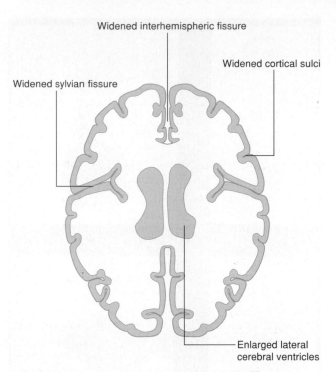

Fig. 7 Diagram showing the shrinking of brain tissue as visualized by a computed tomographic scan in a patient with Alzheimer's disease.

recurrent visual hallucinations (typically well formed and detailed). The fluctuation in cognitive function can be dramatic. Patients suffering from LBD can go from a coherent involved conversation to incoherent mumbling in a matter of minutes. Features supportive of the diagnosis are repeated falls, syncope, transient loss of consciousness, neuroleptic sensitivity, systematized delusions and hallucinations in other modalities. LBD is less likely if there is evidence of a stroke or any other physical illness or brain disorder sufficient to account for the clinical picture.

The nosological status of LBD is unclear, and opinion is divided as to whether it is a variety of SDAT, a distinct disease or a spectrum disorder related to both Parkinson's disease and Alzheimer's disease. Lewy bodies are intracellular inclusions composed of neurofilament proteins and various cell stress response proteins (e.g. ubiquitin and alpha-beta crystallin), suggesting that they are the result of a cytoprotective process (Fig. 8). The majority of patients with LBD have cortical and brainstem Lewy bodies in association with Alzheimer's type histological changes, which in about half fulfill the criteria for Alzheimer's disease.

Recognition of LBD is clinically important as patients with this condition have a high incidence of adverse and life-threatening reactions to antipsychotic medication. Patients initially develop sedation followed by severe rigidity with postural instability and falls. This is

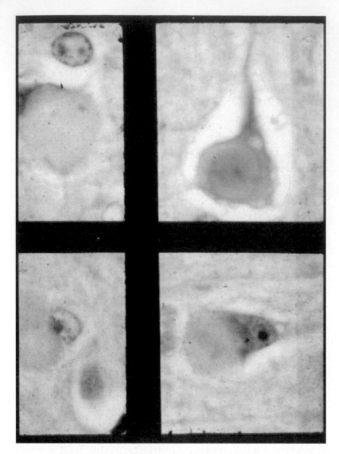

Fig. 8 Cortical Lewy bodies, stained with haematoxylin and eosin.

followed by rapid deterioration in the overall clinical state with increased confusion, immobility and reduced fluid intake.

Conventional neuroleptics are hazardous and are best avoided. Atypical antipsychotic drugs are less likely to induce extrapyramidal side effects. Clomethiazole can be effective in some cases although it can be very sedating. Agitation, which may be extreme, is sometimes helped by short-term use of benzodiazepines. Treatment of parkinsonian symptoms should be conservative, as there is a risk of exacerbating psychotic symptoms.

Vascular dementia

Vascular dementia has a different pattern of onset to SDAT and different pathology. Damage to brain cells is caused by repeated ischaemic episodes, which may be small or large. Onset is usually abrupt and follows an ischaemic episode. Focal neurological deficits are common and intellectual impairment is patchy.

It is very important with this form of dementia to identify any underlying treatable causes such as chronic hypertension. It is often difficult to distinguish SDAT and vascular dementia in a clinical situation, as they often coexist.

Frontal lobe dementia

Although frontal dementia often occurs in young individuals (i.e. below the age of 65 years) patients with this type of problem are increasingly cared for by services for the elderly, as they have particular expertise in the management of dementia.

The frontal lobes account for approximately half of the cerebrum and consist of the primary motor area (i.e. motor strip), premotor areas (i.e. Broca's area, supplementary motor area and frontal eye fields), and the prefrontal cortex. Given their size, the chances that the frontal lobes will be involved in any diffuse pathological process are high. However, some dementing disorders preferentially affect the frontal lobes. These include Pick's disease and Jacob–Creutzfeldt disease, both of which are relatively rare conditions. Recent evidence, however, suggests that a more common degenerative dementia specific to the frontal lobes may exist that is histopathologically distinct from these and other known dementing illnesses.

Although it may be too early to establish frontal lobe dementia as a distinct diagnostic entity, several features appear to be indicative of dementia associated with frontal lobe dysfunction. The patient with frontal lobe features typically presents with reports of a change in personality or adaptive behaviours that precede the onset of cognitive symptoms. When cognitive deficits appear, they typically involve disorders of planning, organization, mental flexibility and memory. The memory deficits associated with frontal lobe dementia typically reflect poor organization, use of inefficient learning strategies and increased susceptibility to interference. Ability to sustain attention is disturbed; however, there is no evidence of rapid forgetting of information, such as seen in SDAT. Errors in recall are quite common and include perseverations, intrusions and source memory problems (e.g. recalling words from an interference list when asked to recall the original target list).

Subcortical dementia

Certain conditions that affect subcortical structures and pathways, including Parkinson's disease, Huntington's disease, multiple sclerosis, Wilson's disease and brainstem–cerebellar degenerative disorders, are associated with the development of dementia. The predominant feature in all of these disorders is motor dysfunction (e.g. tremor, choreoform movements, and/or bradykinesia); however, significant cognitive disturbances are often present as well. Old-age psychiatry services may be asked to become involved in the management of these patients, even though they may be of a relatively young age.

Huntington's disease is autosomal dominant and presents with movement or psychiatric disorder in adult life progressing to dementia. Prenatal diagnosis and genetic counselling are available for affected families.

Management of dementia

The management of chronic brain syndrome involves five basic strategies:

- treatment of the disorder
- treatment of underlying disorders
- treatment of coexisting psychiatric disorder
- psychological interventions for cognitive impairment
- social support.

Treatment of the disorder itself

Recent developments in the study of SDAT have resulted in two new drugs, donepezil and rivastigmine, which delay the progression of the disorder in the early stages of the disease. They prevent the breakdown of acetylcholinesterase, thus increasing the availability of acetylcholine in the brain (Ch. 17).

Treatment of underlying disorders

A careful physical assessment and examination is required to identify any possible treatable underlying causes. The causes of chronic brain syndrome are shown in Box 68. Old-age psychiatry services usually work closely with geriatric services to provide comprehensive medical care.

Treatment of coexisting psychiatric disorder

Depression, acute paranoid psychoses and acute brain syndromes are all well-recognized psychiatric disorders that occur in patients with chronic brain syndromes and need treatment in their own right. Patients may receive brief inpatient or day-patient treatment for these conditions.

Psychological interventions to address cognitive impairments

In the early stages of the disorder, patients can be taught techniques to combat their memory difficulties. Some services run memory clinics, which patients and their spouses can attend. Patients are taught simple techniques such as rehearsal of important information, memory prompts and the use of lists.

Social support to prevent unnecessary deterioration

The majority of individuals with dementia live in the community, and only the most severe forms warrant

---

Box 68
Causes of chronic brain syndromes

Senile dementia Alzheimer's type
Lewy body dementia
Toxicity: alcohol
Ischaemia: hypertension, embolic disease, ischaemic heart disease, diabetes mellitus
Metabolic changes: thiamine deficiency
Subcortical changes: Parkinson's disease, Huntington's disease, multiple sclerosis, Wilson's disease, brainstem-cerebellar degeneration

---

Box 69 Ethical issues in the treatment of the elderly

In thinking through ethical dilemmas in relation to the elderly, it is important to guard against ageism, which is becoming an increasingly important issue in our society. A helpful way to do this, when confronted by a dilemma, is to imagine the elderly individual involved is middle aged or a young person, then consider whether this changes your way of thinking about the problem.

One of the most common ethical dilemmas involves the treatment of patients who lack capacity to make decisions about their own treatment. The way to determine capacity is described in Chapter 15, but it basically involves three key aspects. The patient must be informed, competent and not coerced. Capacity is not an all-or-none phenomenon and is often difficult to determine. If the patient clearly lacks capacity, the nearest relatives should be consulted. However, relatives may disagree with each other as to the best course of action, or the doctor may feel, on some occasions, they are not acting in the best interests of the patient. The doctor has to come to a considered opinion of what would be in the best interests of the patient.

Advanced directives are becoming more popular. An advanced directive is a written statement made by a person when competent about how he/she wishes to be treated in the future, should he/she become incompetent and in need of medical care. There are three main types of advanced directive: an *instructional directive* that states what specific treatment the person would want to refuse under clear specified circumstances in the future (e.g. 'If I were to become severely demented in the future and was unable to care for my own personal needs and hygiene, and I developed a chest infection, I do not want treatment with antibiotics or to receive intravenous fluids if I become deyhdrated'); a *statement of general values* that outlines broad management strategies (e.g. 'If I were to become severely demented, I would not want any treatment that would prolong my life'); or a *proxy directive* that authorizes another person to make decisions (e.g. next of kin) about treatment issues.

It is important to try to establish that the person was competent at the time the advanced directive was written. This is sometimes not easy. If the team are convinced the directive was made when the person was competent and was not coerced in any way, then the patient's wishes should be respected.

inpatient hospital treatment. Individuals tend to function at their best in familiar surroundings. The admission of an elderly person to hospital can actually result in a severe deterioration in their level of functioning because they cannot cope with the new environment. The aim of social intervention is to provide sufficient support so that the individual can continue to live in the community. A large number of elderly people with dementia are looked after by their spouse or children. These carers may require breaks from time to time, and many social services departments provide respite care. Other individuals may move into sheltered accommodation or residential homes. Social services may provide local day centres for the elderly or other forms of home support, such as home helps and meals on wheels.

Persecutory states

Although young adults develop persecutory states, these most often result from schizophrenia, alcohol or other drug-related conditions. In the elderly, a chronic delusional condition can develop for the first time after the age of 65 years. The condition is characterized by florid and systematized persecutory delusions. There may also be auditory hallucinations (voices talking to or about the person) and occasionally delusions of control (Ch. 1). It is unclear whether the condition is a delayed form of schizophrenia or whether it is related to subtle underlying organic change in the brain. It has been called *paraphrenia* in the past, but these days the most common term is *acute persecutory psychosis*. The condition may be more common in patients who are socially isolated or have impaired hearing. Those individuals with prominent premorbid sensitive and suspicious personality traits are at greater risk of developing the disorder. Treatment is with anti-psychotics and appropriate psychosocial intervention.

Further reading and sources

Baldwin B 1991 The outcome of depression in old age. International Journal of Geriatric Psychiatry 6: 395–400

Byrne EJ 1998 Dementia with Lewy bodies. Advances in Psychiatric Treatment 4: 360–364

Jackson R, Baldwin RC 1993 Detecting depression in elderly medically ill patients: the use of the Geriatric Depression Scale compared with medical and nursing observations. Age and Ageing 22: 349–353

Medical Research Council 1987 Report from the MRC Alzheimer's Disease Workshop. Medical Research Council, London.

Murphy E 1982 Social origins of depression in old age. British Journal of Psychiatry 141: 135–142

Stern S 1991 Depression in the elderly. Comprehensive Therapy 17: 40–45

Sources

The Alzheimer's Society. Founded in 1979, the society has 23 000 members in the UK. It provides information, help and support to sufferers and their families. It also supports research. www.alzheimers.org.uk

Mayo Clinic's information page on Alzheimer's disease. Provides up-to date and useful information about the disease. www.mayohealth.org/mayo/common/htm/alzheimers.htm.

Age Concern. Charity founded to help and protect the rights of the elderly. www.ace.org.uk

The British Geriatrics Society. Organization for physicians and other doctors interested in the care and treatment of the elderly. www.bgs.org.uk

Self-assessment: questions

Multiple choice questions

1. Depression in the elderly:
   a. Is the most common psychiatric illness
   b. Affects about 60% of elderly people at any one time
   c. Is detected reliably by GPs
   d. Is treated effectively by GPs
   e. Requires patients to remain on antidepressant medication for 2 years after recovery

2. The following are characteristic features of depression in the elderly:
   a. Agitation
   b. Delusions of wealth
   c. Memory impairment
   d. Somatic symptoms
   e. Neurovegetative symptoms

3. Depression in the elderly should be treated by:
   a. SSRIs (selective serotonin reuptake inhibitors) at higher than usual dosages
   b. Tricyclic antidepressants as a first-line option
   c. Electroconvulsive therapy if patients cannot tolerate antidepressant medication
   d. Addressing precipitating and maintaining factors
   e. Using as many different kinds of drug as possible

4. The following are important psychosocial stressors in the elderly:
   a. Poverty
   b. Occupational stress
   c. Physical illness
   d. Crime
   e. Role transition

5. Dementia is characterized by:
   a. Memory impairment
   b. Aphasia
   c. Apraxia
   d. Pseudo-dementia
   e. An acute onset

6. The memory impairment associated with Alzheimer's disease is characterized by:
   a. Poor learning and retention of information over time
   b. The retention of information for a relatively brief time
   c. A problem of information storage
   d. The demonstration of new learning with repeated testing
   e. Retrograde and anterograde memory impairment

7. Pathological changes characteristic of Alzheimer's include:
   a. Enlarged ventricles and narrowed sulci
   b. Focal loss of neurones confined to subcortical areas
   c. Plaques of amyloid
   d. Neurofibrillary tangles
   e. Increased cholinergic neurons

8. Lewy body disease:
   a. Is an uncommon form of degenerative dementia
   b. Has an unclear nosological status
   c. Is best treated with neuroleptics
   d. Is a dementia in which Lewy bodies are found only in the brainstem region of the brain
   e. Accounts for about one fifth to a quarter of cases of dementia in the elderly

9. Characteristic features of Lewy body disease include:
   a. Visual hallucinations
   b. A history of Parkinson's disease
   c. Continous cognitive impairment
   d. Syncope
   e. Systematized delusions

10. Vascular dementia:
    a. Is clearly distinguishable from Alzheimer's disease in most cases
    b. Is caused by repeated ischaemic episodes
    c. Presents with a gradual onset
    d. Should be considered if the patient has focal neurological deficits
    e. May be caused by underlying conditions that can be treated

Case history questions

History 1

A 75-year-old woman goes to the council to ask to be moved from her current home. She says that her neighbours are noisy and keep shouting at her. She has already been moved twice in the previous year because of similar problems. She says that her neighbours shout abuse at her all day. They are clever, however, and never let her see them actually doing it. They are pleasant and helpful to her face.

She thinks they are after her money and are planning to rob her. She has taken to sleeping with her purse in case they try and steal her money. She asks the council to involve the police.

1. What is the most likely cause of her concerns?
2. Would another move help?

History 2

A 69-year-old man is admitted to hospital with ischaemic heart disease. While in hospital, he makes a complaint to the hospital authorities that the physician looking after him has murdered his wife. He writes to his local MP and the local paper.

He is well known to his MP, who has received numerous complaints from him over the years about a variety of people he thinks have murdered his wife. The physician has never had any contact with his wife and asks a psychiatrist to review him.

It transpires that he has suffered from paranoid schizophrenia for over 30 years. He has no insight into his condition and usually refuses treatment. He is followed up at home by the old-age psychiatry team. It transpires that he is very lonely, socially isolated and has no friends.

What interventions may be of help?

History 3

A 74-year-old man was brought to casualty having tried to hang himself. He was found by chance and cut down quickly by a neighbour. He is admitted to hospital for observation. It transpires that his wife died 6 months previously from breast cancer. They had been married for over 50 years, and he had nursed her for several months before she died. They were a devoted couple but had few friends. He has two sons, one of whom lives in Australia and the other lives over 200 miles away.

When he is well enough to speak to a psychiatrist, he describes feeling devastated following his wife's death. He has had difficulty sleeping and has lost 2 stone in weight. He feels particularly bad in the early hours of the morning. His life feels empty and he misses his wife dreadfully. He says he wants to die and is sorry the attempt to kill himself did not work. He feels he would be a burden to his son and would be better off dead. He is visibly agitated and unable to relax.

1. What condition is this man suffering from?
2. What is his risk of suicide?
3. What treatment is required?

History 4

Mrs Jones is 72 and lives with her husband who is 75. Over the last few months, she has become increasingly forgetful. She cannot remember the name for many household items (e.g. she calls the fire a furnace and the vacuum cleaner a sweeper). She often forgets people she has met the day before or places she has visited in the past week. Her husband thinks she is no longer safe to drive a car as she easily loses her way and cannot remember where she is going. She is more irritable than usual and will burst into tears for no reason. Her husband has noticed she has begun to 'lie' about things. This distresses him, as she has never lied before. She makes up stories about where she has been and who she has visited. Her husband persuades her to see her GP and they both attend the appointment.

1. What is the most likely diagnosis?
2. What should her GP do?
3. What kind of treatment should she have?

Objective structured clinical examination (OSCE)

Topic: Mini mental state examination (MMSE)

In this OSCE, the candidate is asked to carry out a mini mental state examination on a normal volunteer. The candidate is asked to explain to the examiner what he/she is doing and what he/she is testing for in each part of the examination. The candidate is also asked to keep a score, add up the marks and tell the examiner at the end the total score. The candidate is told that there is 10 minutes to complete this task. If possible have someone simulate the patient. Otherwise, list the questions you would ask and the score you would expect from a normal volunteer. You may wish to use the cards (Fig. 1, p. 32) with two intersecting pentagons and the command 'close your eyes', which would be available at this station.

Self-assessment: answers

Multiple choice answers

1. a. **True**. Depression is the most common form of psychiatric illness in the elderly.
   a. **False**. The prevalence is 15% in the community at any one time.
   c. **True**. GPs can detect depression in the elderly.
   d. **False**. Many GPs fail to treat elderly patients with depression.
   e. **True**. Patients require treatment with antidepressants for 2 years after recovery.

2. a. **True**. Agitation is a prominent feature in many cases.
   b. **False**. Delusions of poverty rather than wealth may occur.
   c. **True**. Patients can appear to have problems with concentration and memory that mimic dementia, but they recover once the depressive disorder is treated.
   d. **True**. Somatic concerns and hypochondrical beliefs are common.
   e. **True**. Retardation, loss of weight and sleep disturbance are common in depression in the elderly.

3. a. **False**. SSRIs should be used at lower than usual dosages.
   b. **False**. SSRIs should be used in preference to tricyclic antidepressants because of fewer side effects.
   c. **True**. Electroconvulsive therapy should be considered if patients cannot tolerate antidepressant treatment, or if there is a high suicidal risk, delusions or refusal of food or drink.
   d. **True**. It is essential to change factors that have caused or maintained the illness.
   e. **False**. Polypharmacy should be avoided and the patient's treatment rationalized so that the minimum number of drugs at the lowest possible dosages are used.

4. a. **True**. Many elderly people have to manage on only the state pension.
   b. **False**. Most elderly people do not work.
   c. **True**. Physical illness is an important risk factor for depression in the elderly.
   d. **True**. The elderly are easy targets for criminals.
   e. **True**. Elderly people have to cope with major adjustments to their life, such as retirement.

5. a. **True**. Memory impairment is the main cognitive deficit in dementia.
   b. **True**. Aphasia is one kind of cognitive disturbance that can occur.
   c. **True**. Apraxa is one kind of cognitive disturbance that can occur.
   d. **False**. Pseudo-dementia relates to recoverable memory impairment in association with depression.
   e. **False**. Dementia has an insidious onset.

6. a. **True**. Patients are unable to learn and retain information.
   b. **False**. They are unable to retain information even over a brief period of time.
   c. **True**. The problem is with storage rather than retrieval.
   d. **False**. Patients fail to show new learning.
   e. **True**. Both anterograde and retrograde memory impairment is present.

7. a. **False**. The brain shows enlarged ventricles and widened sulci.
   b. **False**. There is widespread loss of neurones.
   c. **True**. Histopathological examination shows plaques of amyloid.
   d. **True**. Histopathological examination shows neurofibrillary tangles.
   e. **False**. There is a deficiency of cholinergic neurotransmitters.

8. a. **False**. Lewy body disease is the second most common degenerative dementia.
   b. **True**. It is unclear whether it is a separate disorder from Alzheimer's disease.
   c. **False**. Neuroleptics should be avoided because of the potential for severe, adverse side effects.
   d. **False**. Lewy bodies are found in the brainstem and cortex.
   e. **True**. 10–23%.

9. a. **True**. Well-formed and detailed visual hallucinations are characteristic of this disorder.
   b. **False**. Parkinsonism develops spontaneously; there should not be a previous history. A history of Parkinson's disease would be suggestive of a subcortical dementia.
   c. **False**. The cognitive impairment typically fluctuates.
   d. **True**. This is common.
   e. **True**. Patients develop complicated and connected delusional systems.

10. a. **False**. The two are often indistinguishable.
    b. **True**. It is caused by repeated ischaemic episodes.
    c. **False**. The onset is usually abrupt.
    d. **True**. Focal neurological signs may indicate an underlying ischaemic process.
    e. **True**. Certain underlying conditions such as hypertension may be amenable to treatment although the ischaemic damage caused to the brain cannot be reversed.

Case history answers

History 1

1. This lady is most likely suffering from a persecutory psychosis, and is experiencing auditory hallucinations.
2. Another move to a new house will not resolve her problems. She will develop the same ideas about new neighbours in a short space of time.

History 2

In addition to treatment for his condition, this gentleman needs a detailed psychosocial assessment. Although he has suffered from schizophrenia for many years, his condition could be being exacerbated by an underlying organic psychosyndrome related to his ischaemic heart disease. His score on the Mini Mental State Examination, however, is 20 (Ch. 2) and he has good daily skills of living. He is befriended by a community psychiatric nurse who, after several weeks, persuades him to take medication in the form of a depot. He is prescribed depixol 40 mg per month. Within a few weeks, many of his persecutory ideas subside. He is introduced to a day centre and arrangements are made for him to attend three times per week.

History 3

1. This man is suffering from a depressive disorder in the context of a serious bereavement. He has evidence of neurovegetative symptoms: agitation, sleep disturbance and weight loss, diurnal mood variation. His condition requires treating with antidepressant medication and, if this fails, electroconvulsive therapy should be considered.
2. He is at high risk of committing suicide.
3. He should be admitted to hospital for observation. In addition to treatment of depression, he will need a great deal of support and help to adjust to the loss of his wife. He may need specific grief work but will also need help to develop a social network of friends and support. This will not be easy.

History 4

1. The most likely diagnosis is senile dementia Alzheimer's type. She does not have a history of hypertension or any other risk factors for vascular dementia. The onset is slow and insidious. She shows problems with antergrade memory and has begun to confabulate. She may also be emotionally labile.
2. Her GP needs to examine her, check her blood pressure and exclude any possible physical conditions that could exacerbate her dementia.
3. Her GP needs to refer her to an old-age psychiatrist who will assess her at home, probably with another member of the old-age team. The psychiatrists will carry out a detailed psychosocial assessment, assess her mental state and cognitive function and will probably recommend that she attend a memory clinic so she can be taught ways to help her to manage her memory loss and that she is started on donepezil, which may delay the progression of the dementia. One of the team will also provide her husband with support and explain to him that her 'lying' (which he finds so upsetting) is part of the disease.

OSCE answer

An examiner would not prompt a candidate if they did not know how to carryout an MMSE. There would not necessarily be one mark per correct part of the examination. An overall mark would reflect the number of parts of the examination carried out correctly and the candidate's confidence and competence in conducting the examination.

The examination should take the following form.

1. Introduce self and explains nature of task to patient
2. **Orientation**
   Use a group such as

   - year, season, date, month, day (maximum 5 points)
   - county, city, part of the city, place, location of examination (maximum 5 points)

3. **Registration**
   Name three objects (e.g. apple, table, penny) taking 1 second to say each one. Ask the patient to repeat the names of all three objects.
4. **Attention and calculation**
   Use one of the following:

   - ask patient to spell 'world' backward (DLROW) (maximum 5 points)
   - serial 7s, if patient does the first five subtractions correctly the candidate should ask him/her to stop

5. **Recall**

Ask for the three objects repeated above

6. **Language**

a. Point to a pencil and asks the patient to name it. Do the same thing with a wrist watch. Asks the candidate to repeat 'No ifs, ands or buts'.

b. Give the individual a piece of blank paper and asks him/her to follow a three-stage command. 'Take the paper in your right hand, fold it in half and put it on the floor.' (marks are deducted if the candidate breaks up the commands)

c. Show the individual the CLOSE YOUR EYES message (but not the pentagons). Asks the patient to read the message and do what it says.

d. Ask the patient to write a sentence on a blank piece of paper. The sentence should contain a subject and a verb and must be sensible.

e. Show the individual the pentagons and asks him/her to copy the design exactly as it is. All 10 angles need to be present and the two shapes must intersect.

The total score in then rounded up (this should be 30 as the role player/volunteer should get it all right if they are carrying it out to the best of his/her ability).

14 Child and adolescent psychiatry

- be aware of the different ways of collecting and eliciting information
- be aware of the multifactorial aetiology of most childhood disorders.

Child psychiatry differs from other branches of psychiatry in many ways. Children themselves do not present for treatment but are brought for treatment by their parents or carer. Consequently, the parents' or carer's perception of the child's problems, their leniency or intolerance of certain behaviours, and their ability to tolerate concerns or anxiety about the child play an important role in the decision to ask for help.

Particular skills are required to carry out a competent psychosocial assessment of a child and his/her family, and several members of the child psychiatry team may be involved in different aspects of the assessment. Young children are unable to verbalize or articulate their worries or fears, and in very young children, their worries or concerns may emerge or be elucidated by play. Even in older children, it may be difficult for them to conceptualize or discuss their emotional problems, as they may never have learned to do this within the family. There may also be pressures upon the child from adult members of the family to keep secrets. This is often the case if the child is being physically or sexually abused.

Families consist of individuals but function as units, so not only do individual family members have to be assessed but also the way different family members interact with each other (family dynamics) needs to be understood. This complex process is sometimes helped by carrying out a family interview, with all the members of the family, in which their interactions with each other can be studied and understood. One or two members of the team may carry out the interview, with a third member(s) watching from behind a one-way screen. It is often easier to assess family interactions if one is not involved in the interview process, as the behaviour of all family members can be objectively observed. Although, the situation may seem somewhat artificial and the family may try to put on, 'their best behaviour', once the family begins to relax and is encouraged by the therapist(s) to interact with each other, the key relationship bonds and conflicts within the family become apparent.

Overview

Approximately 10–20% of young people at any one time have some form of mental disorder that is of sufficient severity to result in disruption and dysfunction in their own and their families' lives. Childhood disorders are usually grouped into three categories: emotional disorders, behavioural difficulties and developmental problems. Emotional disorders include conditions such as depression and anxiety, whereas behavioural disorders refer to conditions in which the behaviour of the child is the most salient feature of the disorder (e.g. conduct disorder or attention deficit hyperactivity syndrome). Problems with learning and developmental delay are usually identified in childhood, although the individual will continue to experience difficulties throughout life. Many children and adults with learning difficulties do not develop mental disorders, but in some conditions (e.g. autism) there is a close association between the two. Some conditions, such as eating disorders or schizophrenia, may begin in adolescence and continue into adulthood. These conditions are described in other chapters of this book.

14.1 Assessment and aetiology

Learning objectives

You should:

- know how to conduct a psychiatric assessment in young children and adolescents

Information should be obtained from a variety of other sources, including the child's GP, teachers and other professionals (e.g. social worker). Table 34 shows the different areas that need to be covered in a detailed assessment, in addition to the conventional areas of psychiatric assessment that have been described in Chapter 2 (e.g. past history or mental state examination).

Before being able to conduct a psychosocial assessment of a child, it is important to be familiar with the normal pattern of development in childhood including physical and psychosocial milestones. Some behaviours and emotional responses may be entirely normal and appropriate at one age but may give cause for concern if they are present at a different age. Table 35 shows some of the major physical and emotional milestones from birth to 5 years of age. From 5 years upwards, the developmental changes are more subtle although equally important. By 5 years, the child should have a sense of his/her own identity and gender. He/she will also understand the different roles assigned to gender by society. Although these roles are social constructions, and the boundaries between male and female gender stereotypes are beginning to blur, children who do not conform to such roles may still cause their parents concern. The child may experience extreme pressure from his/her parents to adopt a specific gender role (e.g. a boy may be discouraged from playing with dolls at this age and encouraged by his father to follow more 'manly pursuits'). These problems are best managed by working with the parents to reduce the pressure on the child to allow his/her natural development without censure or stigma.

Sexual feelings are present from an early age (at least 2 years upwards) and the child's natural intense curiosity may lead to sexual experimentation with other peers. Sexual interest and activities may be hidden from par-

ents, particularly if the child picks up a censorious attitude towards sexual matters from the family.

The child's social interactions become more complex as greater impulse control develops. He/she is more aware of the feelings of others, and his/her conscience and social and moral standards continue to develop throughout childhood. Numeracy, reading and writing skills are acquired, together with more complex use of language.

In adolescence, the youngster has to negotiate puberty. For girls this commences usually between 11 and 13 years; for boys, it is usually a little bit later, between 13 and 17 years. Adolescence is a period of time of heightened emotions and intense self-awareness. Peer group relationships are important and friendships of a deep and sometimes lifelong nature develop. Sexual attractiveness becomes an important issue for many adolescents and it can dramatically effect their self-esteem and sense of worth. The degree of actual sexual activity will be mediated by the adolescent's own values and those of his/her family and cultural background.

Box 70
Factors which contribute to depression in adolescence

Genetic factors
Early childhood neglect or abuse
Severe or chronic physical illness
Prolonged separation from parents
Parental death
Parental marital conflict
Parental demands to be a 'high achiever'
Bullying
Educational failure
Inability to form peer group relationships
Comorbid psychiatric disorders (e.g. eating disorders)
Concerns or fears about sexuality

Table 34 Important areas to include in the assessment of children and adolescents

Areas of assessment	Examples
Development milestones	Motor, speech, cognitive and social development
Emotional problems	Anxiety, depression, obsessions, suicidal ideation
Behavioural problems	Poor attention, impulsivity, hyperactivity, aggression, sleep disturbance
Relationships	With parents, siblings, peers and authority figures (evidence of separation anxiety or inability to form attachments, significant losses)
Trauma	Sexual or physical abuse, parental neglect
Physical symptoms	Physical illness, somatization (hospital inpatient treatment, chronic severe physical illness)
Significance of child's symptoms in appropriate developmental context	For example, bed wetting is normal in a child aged 2–3 years but abnormal at age 7
Schooling	Ability to learn, interact with others, conform to a routine, cope with separation from parent
Family dynamics and function as a unit	Ability to provide affection, support and appropriate limit setting; identification of specific conflicts between family members; attachment style; degree of parental concern

Table 35 Developmental milestones for young children from 6 months to 5 years

Age	Posture and movement	Hearing and speech	Vision and fine movements	Social behaviour and play
6 months	Can smile Sits with support Bears weight on feet	Turns to source when hears sound Laughs and chuckles in play Screams with annoyance	Eyes move in unison; stares at interesting objects within 15–30 cm Passes toy from one hand to another using palmar grasp If toy falls outside field of vision, searches vaguely for it or forgets it	Takes everything to mouth Friendly with strangers (becomes reserved with strangers from 7 months onwards) Early signs of separation anxiety from mother
12 months	Crawls on hand and knees Pulls to standing and sits down again Walks around holding on to furniture	Knows own name Babbles loudly Understands simple instructions May use a few words 'mama' etc.	Points with finger at objects of interest Recognizes familiar people approaching from distance	Likes to be in sight and hearing of familiar people Should have formed close, secure attachment with main carer(s)
18 months	Walks well; walks upstairs and downstairs with helping hand	Enjoys nursery rhymes Uses 6–20 recognizable words Obeys simple commands	Builds tower of three blocks Enjoys simple picture books	Assists with washing and dressing Imitates everyday activities (e.g. brushing the floor) Plays contentedly alone Dependent still on familiar adult
2 years	Walks up and down stairs Runs safely on whole foot Able to avoid obstacles	Uses 50 or more recognizable words Joins in nursery rhymes Indicates hair, nose, eyes, mouth and shoes on request	Good manipulative skills Recognizes familiar adults in photograph, but not self	Constantly demands carer's attention Resistive and rebellious when thwarted Tantrums Resentful of attention shown to other children by own carers Unable to defer gratification Special objects such as a blanket or teddy may afford comfort and help sleep
3 years	Walks alone upstairs using alternate feet Rides tricycle using pedals Can throw and catch a ball	Gives full names Still talks to self in long monologues Asks a lot of questions Can count to 10 by rote	Builds tower of nine or ten cubes Holds pencil Recognizes and names two or three primary colours	Shows affection for younger siblings Invented play including make-believe people and objects Behaviour is more amenable
4 years	Climbs ladders Expert rider of a tricycle Sits with knees crossed Can run up and down stairs	Speech grammatically correct Gives full name, address and age Enjoys jokes	Builds tower of ten or more cubes and several bridges Matches and names four primary colours	Eats skillfully Shows sense of humour Dramatic make-believe play Understands need for taking in turns during play with other children Shows affection and sympathy for others in distress
5 years	Walks easily along a straight line Plays ball games with skill	Speech fluent Loves to be told stories Enjoys jokes and riddles	Builds elaborate models Writes a few letters	Chooses own friends Protective towards younger children Dramatic play continues Behaviour more controlled and independent

When carrying out an assessment, it is important not to assume that the adolescent's sexual orientation will automatically be towards members of the opposite sex. Such an assumption may make it very difficult for a youngster who is unsure of his/her sexual orientation, or who is attracted to members of the same gender, to talk openly about his/her feelings.

Most youngsters manage to negotiate adolescence without major difficulties or problems. Rebellion or severe disturbance is unusual, despite the emotional traumas and tribulations of broken relationships or social alienation that many youngsters experience during this time. In other spheres of their lives, they have to begin to make choices about future careers, or whether to leave or stay at school. If they leave school, they will have to find paid employment and adjust to adult working practices, or they become involved in other training opportunities.

Some of the most common emotional and behavioural problems that occur in childhood and adolescence are listed in Table 36. In many cases, the problems can be resolved with simple reassurance and advice, if they are of a relatively mild nature and present relatively early.

Factors that contribute to the development of childhood mental disorders

Most childhood mental disorders have a complex multifactorial aetiology. As with other branches of psychiatry, aetiological factors should be considered according to biological and psychosocial factors. Important biological aetiological factors to consider include:

- genetic abnormalities, which can result in the development of specific syndromes or learning disabilities
- birth trauma, resulting in subsequent brain damage
- encephalitis or meningitis in early childhood, resulting in neurocognitive deficits
- the role of genetic factors in the development of the temperament or emerging personality of the child
- epilepsy, which is associated with high rates of psychiatric disorder in childhood through the direct effects of the illness and its treatment and the psychosocial effects.

Cognitive and emotional development is facilitated by a loving parental relationship, characterized by secure emotional attachments, consistency and limit setting. Important psychosocial aetiological factors for psychiatric disorders in childhood include:

- parental neglect or chaotic, inconsistent parenting, which can increase the likelihood of emotional and behavioural problems in children
- childhood physical or sexual abuse, which can cause severe emotional distress and long-term emotional and behavioural difficulties
- severe physical illness in childhood, which can result in considerable emotional distress and family disruption

Table 36 Common emotional and behavioural problems at different stages of childhood and adolescence

Developmental period	Type of problem
0–5 years	Difficulties with feeding
	Difficulties with sleeping
	Separation anxiety and clinging behaviour
	Temper tantrums
	Oppositional behaviour
	Hitting, biting or other kinds of minor aggressive behaviour
5–11 years	Nightmares and fears
	Fighting
	Disobedience
	Bullying or being bullied
	Other relationship problems with peers
11–16 years	School refusal
	Diets and faddiness with food
	Truancy
	Experimentation with illicit drugs
	Experimentation with alcohol
	Fighting
	Shop lifting or stealing
	Moodiness
	Rebellion
	Unwanted or unplanned pregnancy

- loss of a parent or significant other, resulting in both short-term and long-term emotional problems and vulnerability to depression
- parental mental disorder, which can have a variety of adverse effects on the parent–child relationship

Despite the relevant affluence of the UK, many children are brought up in poverty and have to face the constant stressors of social deprivation. These include:

- poor housing and overcrowding
- poor diet and malnourishment
- increased exposure to crime
- increased exposure to drugs and alcohol abuse
- high classroom sizes in inner city schools.

14.2 Emotional disorders

Learning objectives

You should:

- be able to diagnose depression in young children and adolescence
- be aware of the major treatments for depression in this age group
- be aware of the major features of separation anxiety disorder.

Depression

Depression is relatively infrequent in childhood and adolescence, although since the 1980s, there has been increasing concern about depressive disorders in young people. Adolescents who develop serious depressive conditions are at high risk of having another episode in adulthood and have an increased risk of both attempted and completed suicide. At the same time, the suicide rate in young men in the UK and USA has dramatically increased.

The diagnosis of depression in young people is based upon the same criteria as those applied to adults with depression (Ch. 3). However, irritability and social withdrawal are particularly common in depressed adolescents compared with their adult counterparts. About 20% of young people with depressive disorders also have a conduct disorder, and about one half have anxiety.

Most depressed young people have multiple psychosocial problems including educational failure, impaired social functioning and comorbid psychiatric disorders. In most cases, the cause of depression in young people is multifactorial. Box 70 lists the most common factors, and Figure 9 illustrates how different aetiological factors can interact with each other to produce depression.

During adolescence there is an increase in the incidence of depression, particularly in girls. By mid-teenage years, the prevalence of depression is 2–4%. The cause of this is unknown, but possible factors include development of cognitive maturity, changes in sex hormones, increasing exposure to adverse life events, and particular psychosocial stressors on young women to conform to certain stereotypical societal roles.

Severe depression with endogenous symptoms requires treatment with antidepressants. Selective serotonin reuptake inhibitors (SSRIs) are the treatment of choice, followed by tricyclic antidepressants plus/minus lithium if first-line treatment fails. As severe depression only accounts for less than one sixth of cases, most depression in young people is treated with psychosocial treatments.

Box 71 Ethical and legal issues in the care of children

Children have particular human rights, which should include the right to be cared for as part of a community that values their religious, racial, cultural and linguistic identity. Other examples of rights that might be assigned to children include the right to health, individuality, respect, dignity, opportunities for learning and socializing with adults and children, freedom from discrimination such as racism or sexism, and cultural diversity.

There are many complex ethical issues in relation to the psychiatric treatment of children, but their rights as outlined above should always be considered. Children themselves do not have the right to refuse treatment if they are under the age of 16. Consent for treatment is determined by their parents. The wishes of the child, however, should always be considered in relation to his/her age and ability to understand the intervention being offered.

If there are concerns about abuse or serious neglect of the child, health professionals may have to balance their responsibilities to the child with potential breeches of confidentiality in relation to the parents. It is not unusual for adult psychiatrists to be involved in the care and treatment of a parent, whose child is also receiving treatment from the child psychiatry team. In all circumstances, the welfare of the child is paramount and over-rides any other concerns regarding ethical dilemmas in relation to the rest of the family.

The main UK legislature in relation to children is The Children's Act (1989), which brought together most private and public laws about children, thereby replacing complex and fragmented legislation with a single statute. Part III of the Act gives local authorities a range of new duties, including identification of children who are in need, support of children's links with their families, provision of day care and setting up of procedures to consider representations about the provision of services.

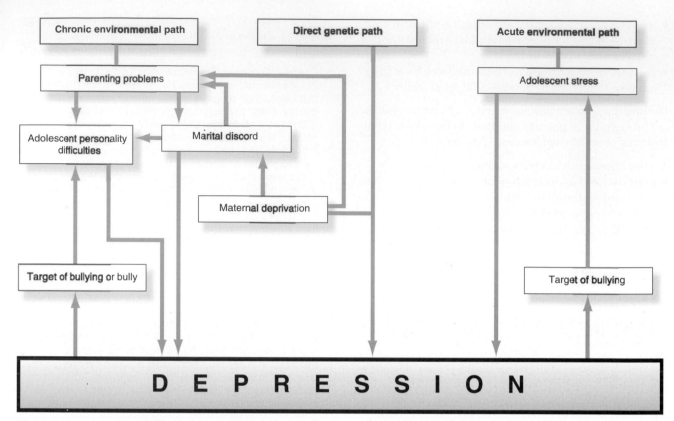

Fig. 9 The interaction of different aetiological factors in the development of depression in young people. (Adapted from Harrington, 1993.)

For mild cases of depression, simple interventions can be very successful, such as regular sympathetic meetings with the young person and his family, combined with practical advice and measures to reduce stress. For young people with moderate depression, the most appropriate form of psychological treatment is cognitive-behavioural therapy. Those with learning difficulties, are more likely to benefit from simpler approaches, which predominantly use behavioural techniques. Other treatment interventions, such as family therapies, interpersonal therapies or social skills training may be required for comorbid problems.

Adolescents who fail to respond to one form of psychological treatment for depression are unlikely to respond to a different psychological approach, and in these cases, pharmacological treatments should be considered.

The short-term prognosis is good, with most young people making good recoveries from moderate-to-severe depressive episodes. Those with severe depression, however, have a 50% chance of a further episode.

Separation anxiety disorder

Fears and anxiety are common in children and should be regarded as normal unless the anxiety becomes intense or pervasive and interferes with the child's psy-

chosocial function. The most common childhood anxiety disorder is separation anxiety disorder, which affects about 4% of all children and adolescents. This is characterized by severe anxiety whenever the child is separated from his/her parents. The young person may have difficulty in going to sleep at night and insist that the parent(s) stay with him/her. He/she becomes preoccupied that some harm will befall his/her parents whenever there is a period of separation, or that his/her parents will abandon him/her. The young person will try to avoid going to school and may develop physical symptoms and malaise to prevent attendance.

The condition is often triggered by a traumatic event but then takes on a life of its own; it can become chronic and extremely disabling. Parents can unwittingly reinforce the young person's symptoms by being oversolicitous or overprotective, so it is important to involve the family and help them to understand how their own concerns can actually be making the symptoms more severe. Treatment is targeted at reducing the young person's anxiety and returning him/her to school as quickly as possible.

Phobic anxiety disorders

Minor phobic problems in childhood are very common, such as fear of the dark or fears about insects. Severe and persistent phobias about animals or insects usually begin before the age of 5 years and usually decline with age, without specific treatment. Treatment is warranted only if the specific fear results in significant disruption to the child's life. Behavioural interventions are the most appropriate forms of treatment.

Obsessive-compulsive disorder

Ritualistic behaviour and magical thinking is common in childhood. Many children will repeat certain actions to bring them luck, e.g. avoid walking upon cracks in the pavement. However, these are not true obsessive-compulsive symptoms, as they do not cause distress to the child, are not resisted by the child and do not interfere with his/her life in a significant fashion. True obsessive-compulsive symptoms are rare in childhood but may develop in a small number of youngsters during adolescence. The symptoms are very similar to those seen in adults and may involve concerns about cleanliness, orderliness or contamination. The youngster may engage in repeated checking activities (e.g. school work) or hand-washing rituals. Obsessional-compulsive symptoms may be associated with other conditions such as tic disorders (see below) or developmental disorders (such as autism). The family's response to the youngster's symptoms is very important and may result in, either re-inforcement of the symptoms if there is overconcern, or secrecy concerning the symptoms if there is a hostile response.

Effects of childhood sexual abuse

Although childhood abuse is not in itself a psychiatric diagnosis, children who are the victims of abuse can develop a range of emotional and behavioural problems. In recent years, there has been a sharp increase in the number of children referred to child psychiatry services with a history of severe childhood abuse. In small children who have been sexually abused (below 5 years), a severely disrupted pattern of attachment can develop. The child may appear hypervigilant, guarded and fearful. He/she may be miserable and difficult to console and shrink away from physical contact. Other children can show the opposite kind of behaviour and are excessively overfamiliar and affectionate with strangers in a socially inappropriate fashion. Some may even show inappropriate sexual behaviour of a persistent kind towards other children or adults. Emotional disorders and behavioural disorders (see next section) can develop and there are significant long-term sequelae. Childhood adversity and sexual abuse are important risk factors for the development of emotional disorders, somatization and personality difficulties in later life.

Much sexual abuse occurs within the family and the offender is usually male, either a step-father, uncle or other male relative or friend. Girls are more likely to be sexually abused than boys. The prevalence is difficult to estimate, but between 10 and 30% of adult women retrospectively report some form of childhood sexual abuse. This can include a wide range of experiences from inappropriate touching and fondling to repeated penetrative intercourse.

Non-accidental injury

Physical abuse of children is relatively common. The most frequent types of injury include multiple bruising, cigarette burns, bites, bone fractures and head injuries. Small children and babies can be shaken violently or smothered with a pillow. This is often an attempt on the parent's part to stop the child crying.

Physically abused children may show a fearful response to the abusive parents and may be overly anxious or unhappy. They may be aggressive towards other children and find it difficult to establish normal peer relationships. The child may deny the abuse if questioned by doctors or social workers as he/she may be fearful of further abuse from his/her parents.

Adults who are abusive towards children are more likely to be young parents who live in stressful social circumstances, with little support from families or friends. They may have been victims of abuse or emotional neglect when they themselves were children.

The primary concern in any suspected case of abuse must be for the welfare of the child. The risk of allowing the child to stay within the family needs to be assessed, but this is the responsibility of child social workers. Depending upon the risk and the severity of the abuse, the child may have to be removed from the family to a safe environment or kept in hospital (if he/she has been admitted following injury) until a detailed assessment can be undertaken.

Suicide and deliberate self-harm

Suicide and deliberate self-harm are covered in detail in Chapter 6. Brief details, specific to children and adolescents, are discussed in this section. Suicide is exceedingly rare before puberty but becomes increasingly frequent through adolescence. Approximately 2000 US adolescents commit suicide each year.

The factors that predispose to completed suicide are many and include pre-existing psychiatric disorders and both biological and sociopsychological facilitating factors. The overwhelming proportion of adolescents who commit suicide suffer from an associated psychiatric disorder at the time of their death (more than 90%).

Stress events often precede adolescents' suicides, including a loss of a romantic relationship, disciplinary troubles in school or with the law, or academic or family difficulties. These stresses may ensue from the underlying mental disorder itself (e.g. trouble with the law) or they may be normative outcomes of uncontrollable events (e.g. a death in the family) with which the adolescent with a mental disorder may not be able to cope. An adolescent with an underlying mental disorder may be faced with a greater number of stressful events than the average adolescent or he/she may perceive the events that occur as more stressful.

Suicide is much more common in adolescent and young adult males than females (the ratio grows from 3:1 in the rare prepubertal suicides to approximately 5.5:1 in the 15- to 24-year-old age group); however, many of the risk factors are the same for both sexes. Mood disorders, poor parent–child communication and a previous suicide attempt are risk factors for suicide in both boys and girls, although a previous suicide attempt is more predictive in males. Substance and/or alcohol abuse significantly increase the risk of suicide in teenagers aged 16 years and older. Family pathology and a history of family suicidal behaviour may also increase risk and should be investigated.

Deliberate self-harm is more common in girls than boys (1.6:1). Mood disorders (particularly early-onset major depressive disorder), anxiety disorders, substance abuse and runaway behaviour independently increase the risk of deliberate self-harm in both sexes. A history of deliberate self-harm greatly increases the risk of eventual suicide in young males, but the predictive effect in females is less substantial.

14.3 Behavioural disorders

Learning objectives

You should:

- be familiar with the major features of conduct disorder and basic principles of management
- be familiar with the major features of attention deficit hyperkinetic syndrome and basic principles of management
- understand the terms enuresis and encopresis
- be familiar with the major features of Tourette syndrome and other tic disorders.

Conduct disorder

Conduct disorder is very unusual in young children and usually develops after the age of 10 years. It is charac-

terized by emotional and behavioural problems that result in an inability to function properly within the home, school and social society. The young people are often disruptive, rude, unruly and aggressive. They may be aggressive towards people or animals, destructive towards property, truant from school or run away from home, lie, steal and engage in deceitful behaviour. The condition is three times more common in adolescent boys than girls (6% versus 2%).

Many children with conduct disorder have coexisting psychiatric conditions such as mood or anxiety disorders, substance misuse, attention deficit and hyperactivity disorder, or learning difficulties. The aetiology of the condition is usually multifactorial with various combinations of the following being relevant: brain damage, genetic predisposition, child abuse, traumatic life experiences and inadequate parenting. All children with conduct disorder require a detailed assessment to identify possible coexisting psychiatric conditions and to identify factors that are exacerbating the child's aberrant behaviour.

Treatment can be difficult and challenging, as the child is usually uncooperative and distrusts adults. If the child has committed serious criminal offences, treatment may have to be implemented in a secure setting. In most cases, however, treatment involves individual work with the child to help them to control and express anger in a socially acceptable fashion. Parents often require expert guidance and help in carrying out special management and educational programmes in the home and school. Coexisting conditions require treatment, and the child may have special educational needs that need to be addressed. Pharmacological interventions usually produce short-term relief and are not recommended for widespread use. However, pharmacological treatments may be of benefit in particular circumstances (e.g. an inpatient setting, where treatment is strictly controlled and closely monitored), including methylphenidate, lithium and carbamazepine. Caution, however, is required when using these drugs.

About two thirds of children with conduct disorder grow up to become normal adults who behave appropriately. One third develop an antisocial personality. Poor predictors of outcome include onset before 10 years of age and learning difficulties. Good predictors include having a caring relationship with at least one adult, able to stay in school until the official school-leaving age and peer relationships with youngsters who do not have behavioural difficulties.

Attention deficit hyperkinetic syndrome (ADHD)

Attention deficit hyperkinetic syndrome is a rather clumsy term that refers to a condition in young children characterized by severe and excessive excitability and overactivity in most or all situations. The child usually has severe educational difficulties, with a short attention span, distractibility, and impulsive and reckless behaviour. Other features include depression, aggression, anxiety and tics. Some children have clear evidence of brain damage but most do not show evidence of cerebral dysfunction.

Behaviour management is the best validated psychosocial intervention and psychosocial education for the child and family is also important.

Pharmacological treatment, using stimulant drugs, results in significant improvements in behaviour in about two thirds of young people. Methylphenidate and dexamfetamine are first-line treatments, followed by pemoline and then antidepressants. All stimulant drugs should be prescribed judiciously and monitored carefully by specialists in close liaison with GPs.

Enuresis and encopresis

Nocturnal enuresis is persistent bedwetting at night after the age of 5 years. The child is usually dry during the day. It is more common in boys than girls, in children from a socially disadvantaged background and in children with developmental difficulties. Most children are never brought for treatment, and the condition usually spontaneously remits. There are a variety of good parental guides to bringing up children which give detailed advice about managing the problem (e.g. *Your Baby and Child* by Penelope Leach).

If the child is unable to keep dry in the daytime (diurnal enuresis) and has no other signs of developmental delay, the most likely cause is a physical abnormality of the genitourinary system.

Encopresis is faecal soiling after the age of 4 years. It is less common than nocturnal enuresis. It is more common in boys than girls and can have a variety of different causes. Psychological causes include toilet phobia, poor parenting (either rigid overcontrol, or lack of control) and severe emotional upsets (e.g. sexual abuse). Physical causes include faecal impaction and overflow or overly fluid faeces associated with gastrointestinal disease. The condition is usually treated by behavioural methods if it has a psychological cause. Appropriate behaviour is rewarded and soiling is ignored. One approach is to encourage the child to sit on a toilet for 10 minutes after each meal and with a reward if he/she manages this, plus a further reward if he/she passes a stool during this period. The parents may require a great deal of support and help to implement treatment, and to overcome any negative feelings they have about the child's behaviour. The prognosis is usually good and most children improve within 1 year.

Tourette syndrome and other tic disorders

Tics are involuntary, rapid, repetitive movements of individual muscle groups (Ch. 1). Several childhood disorders occur in which the most predominant feature is some form of tic. In all these conditions, boys are affected three times as commonly as girls.

Up to 15% of all children develop some form of tic during childhood, but most are short lived and are not associated with any other psychological or behavioural difficulties. Occasionally tics can become chronic and continue unchanged for many years.

Tourette syndrome was first described by Gilles de la Tourette and although once thought to be rare, it is now known to be quite common. It affects one person in every 2500 in its complete form and three times that number in its partial expression. It is characterized by multiform, frequently changing motor and vocal tics, and it usually starts before the age of 21 years. Approximately half of children with Tourette syndrome also have attention deficits, hyperactivity and a variety of challenging behaviours. Obsessions and compulsions are common and can be as disabling as the tics. Simple tics include eye blinking, grimacing, nose twitching, tooth clicking, and rapid jerking movements of any part of the body. Complex tics include hopping, clapping, picking scabs, writing over and over the same word, kissing, headbanging and writhing movements. In addition, children with Tourette syndrome show other motor and vocal abnormalities (Table 37).

Tourette syndrome appears to be a genetically inherited disorder that is autosomal dominant. If one parent is a carrier or has Tourette syndrome, there is a 50% chance that the child of that person will receive the genetic vulnerability for developing the disorder. There is a 70% chance that female gene carriers will express symptoms, whereas for males the penetrance is higher and 99% of carriers will develop some form of symptoms. However, 10–15% of sufferers do not acquire the condition genetically so other non-genetic factors are also important. The pathogenesis of the condition is unclear but the dopamine system has been implicated, in particular hypersensitivity of postsynaptic dopamine receptors. Other neurotransmitter systems may also be important. Stimulant medication increases the severity of tics in children who already have Tourette syndrome, and stimulants can precipitate the development of tics in children prescribed such treatment for attention deficit hyperkinetic syndrome.

The main treatment for tics associated with Tourette syndrome is haloperidol. This is usually prescribed in very small doses, which are gradually increased up to an average of 3–4 mg/day. Some children may benefit from as little as 1 mg/day. Although most children benefit from this treatment, some develop disabling side effects

Table 37 Motor and vocal abnormalities found in Tourette syndrome

Symptoms	Examples
Motor symptoms	
Simple motor tic	Eye blinking, frowning, finger movements
Complex motor tic	Biting the mouth, gyrating, rolling eyes upwards
Copropraxia	Making obscene gestures
Echopraxia	Copying gestures or movements of others
Vocal symptoms	
Simple tics	Coughing, gurgling, clacking, whistling, sucking sounds
Complex tics	'Blimey' 'shut up' 'be quiet' 'sit down'
Rituals	Saying something over and over
Speech atypicalities	Unusual rhythms, tone, accents
Coprolalia	Obscene, aggressive words or phrases
Palilalia	Repeating one's own words or parts of words
Echolalia	Repeating sounds or words

with long-term use. Other neuroleptics, such as pimozide (which has less severe side effects), have been used to good effect, and the newer atypical neuroleptics may be beneficial. Clonidine, which, in low doses, decreases the release of central noradrenaline (norepinephrine), has also been used although it is not as effective as either haloperidol or pimozide. Clomipramine and SSRIs are used to treat obsessions and compulsions in Tourette syndrome. Family therapy, behavioural interventions and psychotherapy are used to help the child and family cope and adapt to the illness. Children with attention and learning difficulties require specific educational help.

14.4 Learning difficulties

Learning objectives

You should:

- be aware of the causes of learning disabilities
- be aware of the stigma associated with such conditions
- be aware of the main features of Down syndrome
- be aware of the main features of autism and Asperger disorder.

Individuals with learning difficulties used to be described as being 'mentally handicapped'. This term came to be associated with stigma. The current preferred terms to describe individuals with low intelligence are 'people with learning difficulties or disabilities'. It is important to avoid stigma or prejudice in relation to people with learning disabilities and not use derogatory terms.

Difficulties with learning may not be detected until after the first year of life, unless there is an obvious cause (e.g. Down syndrome). Parents or health professionals notice that the normal developmental milestones (Table 35) are delayed. Causes include genetic conditions (Table 38), antenatal damage (fetal alcohol syndrome, intrauterine infection), perinatal damage, trauma or infection. In developing countries, malnutrition is a major cause of low intelligence, and in developed countries low intelligence is associated with poverty, poor housing and an unstable family background.

Down syndrome

Down syndrome is the most common genetic cause of low intelligence and occurs in 1 in every 1000 babies in the UK. Down syndrome is caused by a chromosomal abnormality: 95% of people with Down syndrome have trisomy 21 (i.e. three copies of chromosome 21 instead of two; Fig. 10). This is more common in babies of older mothers, and the risk increases from 1 in 1400 at 25 years, to 1 in 380 at 35 years, to 1 in 30 at 45 years. In 1 in 100 cases of Down syndrome, there is a translocation involving chromosome 21, and a rare form of the condition is caused by mosaicism.

The child with Down syndrome has a characteristic appearance, which includes a head that is flat at the back, eyes with oblique palpebral fissures and epicanthic folds, hands that are short and broad, with a single palmar crease, a small mouth, flat nose and a large tongue, which may protrude slightly. Joints are hyperextensible and there is decreased muscle tone. The child at birth is usually below average weight and length. Developmental milestones (Table 35) are delayed. The child is likely to sit alone at 6–30 months, start walking between 1 and 4 years and be toilet trained between 3 and 7 years.

Most children with Down syndrome have an IQ of 20–50; they are generally well behaved with a pleasant

Table 38 Genetic causes of learning disability

Type of disorder	Example
Chromosomal abnormalities	Down syndrome, Klinefelter syndrome, Turner syndrome
Dominant conditions	Neurofibromatosis, tuberose sclerosis
Recessive conditions	Inherited metabolic disorders
Sex-linked conditions	Lesch–Nyhan syndrome, fragile X syndrome

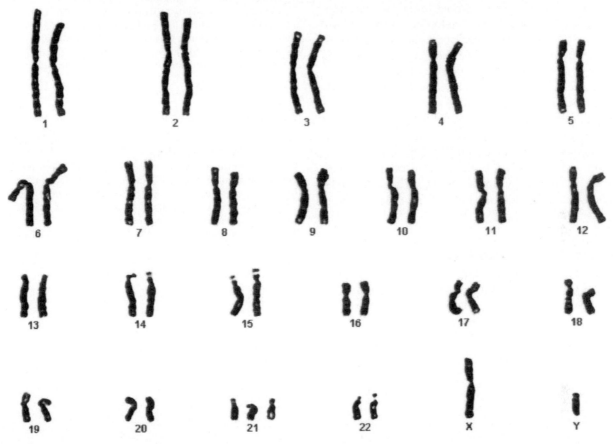

Fig. 10 Trisomy 21 in Down Syndrome.

and affectionate temperament. Congenital heart disease, hearing problems, intestinal abnormalities and early onset of Alzheimer dementia (at around 30 years of age) are common. Other genetic causes of low IQ are shown in Table 38.

Autism

Autism is a complex developmental disability that begins usually during the first 3 years of life. Autism or associated conditions occur in approximately 1 in 500 individuals, and it is three to four times as common in boys than girls.

The main problem areas include difficulties in verbal and non-verbal communication, social interactions, and leisure or play activities. Individuals with autism do not appear to understand normal human interactions and may seem distant and detached from significant others. They have poor comprehension of gesture and speech, lack imaginative play, have abnormal and delayed speech and avoid eye-to-eye contact. They may exhibit repeated stereotyped body movements and resist changes in routine. Although some autistic children may have remarkable specific skills, the majority are of low intelligence.

Approximately 60% of children with autism remain very disabled and are never able to live independently. A small minority are able to work and live independently, although social relationships remain impaired. A good outcome is predicted by high intelligence, stable family background, the early attainment of speech and good and appropriate schooling.

Asperger's disorder

Asperger's disorder is characterized by a qualitative impairment in social interaction; it is distinguished from autism in that there is no significant impairment in language or cognitive development. The child shows at least two of the following: marked impairment in nonverbal social behaviours (e.g. eye-to-eye contact), failure to develop peer relationships appropriate to the child's developmental level, a lack of spontaneous seeking to share enjoyment with others, or lack of emotional reciprocity. The child also shows restricted, repetitive patterns of behaviour (e.g. repetitive motor mannerisms or preoccupation with parts of objects). Although the child has normal cognitive development, there is significant impairment in social functioning, which results in social isolation and sometimes bullying from other children. Later on in life, individuals find it difficult to make friendships and find work because their social interactions are so impaired.

Further reading and sources

Cohen DJ, Bruun RD, Leckman JF 1988 Tourette's syndrome and tic disorders: clinical understanding and treatment. Wiley, New York

Department of Health 1989 The Children's Act 1989: Guidance and Regulations. HMSO, London

Harrington RC 1993 Depressive disorder in childhood and adolescence. In: Studies in child psychiatry, Rutter M (ed). Wiley, Chichester, UK pp. 1–249

Harrington RC, Fudge H, Rutter M, Pickles A, Hill J 1990 Adult outcomes of childhood and adolescent depression, I Psychiatric status. Archives of General Psychiatry, 47: 465–473

MTA Cooperative Group 1999 A 14 month randomized controlled trial of treatment strategies for attention-deficit/hyperactivity disorder. The MTA Cooperative Group. Archives of General Psychiatry 56: 1073–1086

Pelham WE, Wheeler T, Crimson A 1998 Empirically supported psychosocial treatments for attention deficit hyperactivity disorder. Journal of Clinical Child Psychology 27: 190–205

Sources

American Academy of Child and Adolescent Psychiatry (AACAP). www.aacap.org

Conduct disorders website. www.conductdisorders. com

Down's syndrome website. www.nag.com/downsyn

Leach P 1997 Your baby and child. The essential guide for every parent. Penguin Books, London (*Good self-help guide for normal childhood development*)

Tourette's disorder website. http://+mgh.harvard.edu

Self-assessment: questions

Multiple choice questions

1. Depression in young people
   a. Is less common than in adults
   b. Is rarely associated with anxiety
   c. Is usually associated with multiple problems in the young person
   d. Is more common in young men than young women
   e. Is associated with an increased risk of suicide and deliberate self-harm

2. The following symptoms are particularly common in depressed young people compared with adults:
   a. Low mood
   b. Irritability
   c. Agitation
   d. Social withdrawal
   e. Depressive delusions

3. In the treatment of depressed young people:
   a. Pharmacological treatment is the treatment of choice
   b. Pharmacological treatment is usually reserved for those with severe depression with endogenous features
   c. Cognitive therapy is the most commonly used focused treatment
   d. Those with severe depression, who do not respond to SSRIs (selective serotonin reuptake inhibitors) should be offered cognitive-behavioural therapy
   e. Focused treatments usually need to be combined with more general treatments such as family work or social support

4. Conduct disorder:
   a. Is characterized by severe and excessive excitability and overactivity
   b. Is more common in females than males
   c. Is commonly associated with other psychiatric conditions
   d. Usually begins at around the age of 5 years
   e. Is rarely associated with unruly or aggressive behaviour

5. Tourette syndrome:
   a. Is an autosomal recessive condition
   b. Is primarily treated using counselling
   c. Is treated using stimulants
   d. Is characterized by multiform, motor and vocal tics
   e. Occurs in about 15% of all children

6. Non-accidental injury is more likely to be committed by:
   a. Parents who themselves have a history of abuse
   b. Elderly parents
   c. Parents who are subject to great social pressures
   d. Parents who have little social support
   e. Parents from social class I or II

7. Children who have been sexually abused may show the following characteristics:
   a. Excessive familiarity with strangers
   b. Inappropriate sexual behaviour
   c. Fear of physical contact
   d. Misery
   e. Be victims of bullying

8. Phobic anxiety disorders in children:
   a. Begin after the age of 5 years
   b. Get progressively worse with age
   c. Should be actively treated from the outset
   d. Are best treated with psychodynamic therapy
   e. Often involve fears of snakes, spiders and other small creatures

9. Separation anxiety disorder:
   a. Is the most common childhood anxiety disorder
   b. Affects about 10% of children and adolescents
   c. Is sometimes triggered by a traumatic event
   d. Usually spontaneously improves if the parents reduce the child's fear by staying with him/her whenever he/she is upset
   e. Is treated by keeping the child at home until the fears spontaneously resolve

10. Autism:
   a. Is usually associated with normal intelligence
   b. Is the same as Asperger syndrome
   c. Spontaneously resolves in adulthood
   d. Is characterized by overfamiliarity and warmth in social relationships
   e. Is characterized by poor eye contact

Case history questions

History 1

A 14-year-old young woman was brought to the A&E department by her mother after she had taken an overdose of her mother's antidepressant pills (fluoxetine 30 tablets).

Describe how you would conduct an assessment

History 2

You are a GP. Mrs King comes to see you with her 5-year-old son David. David is of normal intelligence. She tells you that he repeatedly wets the bed at night and she has tried everything to get him to be dry. He was dry for a few months, but he has begun to wet the bed again in the last 6 weeks. She is wondering whether he may have a physical problem.

1. What questions would you ask to establish the likelihood of any underlying physical problem?
2. What advice would you give?

History 3

A 14-year-old boy is referred to child and adolescent psychiatry services. He has become pre-occupied with dirt and dust. If he sees any dirt or dust, he starts to panic and scream. He is difficult to console unless the dirt or dust is removed. He does not feel depressed but is very tense and anxious. His parents have tried to cope with his problems by keeping the house as clean as possible. His mother vacuums three or four times per day and dusts each room each day. His symptoms, however, have become worse and worse. He now gets upset if the family use the upstairs bathroom or come upstairs at all. Consequently, the parents have moved their bed downstairs and only use the downstairs toilet. The last time his father tried to go upstairs, the young lad screamed, and shouted for over 2 hours. He became overwhelmed with anxiety and the parents were unable to cope with him.

His problems began about 18 months ago, when he began to become anxious about going to school. He stopped going to school about 12 months ago, and since then his anxiety about dust in the home has increased.

1. What is the diagnosis?
2. What is the management?

Self-assessment: answers

Multiple choice answers

1. a. **True**. Depression is much more common in adults than young people.
   b. **False**. It is commonly associated with anxiety.
   c. **True**.
   d. **False**. Depression is more common in young females.
   e. **True**. It is important, therefore, to carry out a risk assessment in a young person who is suffering from depression.

2. a. **False**. Depression is more common in adults.
   b. **True**. Irritability is particularly common in young people with depression.
   c. **False**. Agitation is more common in elderly people with depression.
   d. **True**. Adolescents commonly withdraw from social interactions when they are depressed.
   e. **False**. Psychotic depression is relatively rare in young people.

3. a. **False**. Psychological treatments are the preferred treatment of choice.
   b. **True**. For all but very mild depression.
   c. **True**.
   d. **False**. Other pharmacological interventions should be considered.
   e. **True**. Young people are very open to social and family influences.

4. a. **False**. Attention deficit hyperkinetic syndrome is associated with excessive excitability and overactivity. Conduct disorder is characterized by disruptive, unruly and aggressive behaviour.
   b. **False**. It is three times more common in boys.
   c. **True**. If it occurs alone, it is suggestive of a poorer long-term outcome.
   d. **False**. It usually starts after the age of 10 years.
   e. **False**. Unruly or aggressive behaviour is a key feature.

5. a. **False**. It is autosomal dominant with partial penetrance.
   b. **False**. Although family therapy and other psychosocial treatments may be of help, the main treatment is haloperidol.
   c. **False**. Stimulants make the symptoms worse.
   d. **True**.
   e. **False**. Tics occur in about 15% of children but Tourette syndrome is much rarer (0.25%).

6. a. **True**. The parents have been the victims of abuse or emotional neglect.
   b. **False**. Young parents rather than elderly parents are associated with non-accidental injury
   c. **True**.
   d. **True**. Support from family or friends is a great asset for stressed parents.
   e. **False**. It occurs across all classes.

7. a. **True**.
   b. **True**.
   c. **True**.
   d. **True**.
   e. **True**. These are all behaviours shown by sexually abused children but none is exclusively seen only in the sexually abused.

8. a. **False**. Begin before the age of 5 years.
   b. **False**. They generally improve with time.
   c. **False**. Most improve without treatment.
   d. **False**. Behavioural treatment is the most appropriate.
   e. **True**. Fears of the dark are also common.

9. a. **True**.
   b. **False**. Occurs in about 4% of children.
   c. **True**. This is often the initiating factor but the condition then continues regardless.
   d. **False**. This usually increases the fear in the long term.
   e. **False**. This would lead to an increase in the severity of the symptoms.

10. a. **False**. Most children are of low intelligence.
    b. **False**. There is no significant impairment in language or cognitive development in Asperger syndrome.
    c. **False**. There is little improvement.
    d. **False**. Children are characteristically aloof and appear distant and detached.
    e. **False**. There is avoidance or poor eye contact.

Case history answers

History 1

This young person needs a detailed assessment. She will be admitted to a young person's adolescent ward in a children's hospital. She will be assessed the next day by a member of the child psychiatry team (either psychiatrist, social worker or specialist nurse).

The assessor will want to assess her risk of future self-harm or suicide. In addition, it will be important to assess whether she is suffering from a depressive illness (evidence of low mood, irritability, social withdrawal) or any other psychiatric disorder (e.g. conduct disorder, although this is less likely).

It will be important to interview her mother. As the young person has taken her mother's antidepressants, it implies that her mother may be suffering from depression herself. Both mother and daughter may need help.

If the young girl's symptoms are relatively recent in onset, they may be a reaction to her mother's depression. If this is the case, the main focus of treatment would be arranging for the mother to have treatment for her illness, and for the young girl to have psychological help to adjust to the change in her mother. This may involve brief individual and family sessions. If she has developed a serious depressive illness, she may require cognitive therapy. If the girl's problems are long standing and precede her mother's illness, she and her family may need longer-term help, depending upon the nature of her problems.

History 2

1. The fact that he has had a period of continence at night for several months suggests his recent problem is psychological. To be certain, you need to establish whether he ever wets himself in the day. If he does not, this implies that he has some bladder control, and is extremely unlikely to have an underlying physical problem.
2. In relation to advice, Mrs King says that she has tried everything. You need to establish what things she has tried, and whether there is any possibility that she may have been inadvertently making the problem worse. She may have been restricting

David's fluid intake for several hours before he goes to sleep, or trying to lift him or wake him at night. She may have passed on to him her anxiety, so he has become worried and preoccupied. It is important to let her know that occasional bed wetting is normal at David's age and that boys more frequently wet the bed than girls. You should advise her not to restrict his fluids before bedtime with the exception of drinks that contain caffeine. She should not try to lift him at night. She should neither praise dry nights nor scold him for wet nights. You advise her to explain to him that he is growing up and is gradually gaining control of his bladder. You tell her to tell him that this takes time, and she and he can tell that his body is gradually gaining control as he has had a period of being dry. You suggest to her that his recent incontinence may be a sign that he is worried about something that has happened and you ask her to reflect on this. Have there been any changes in the family, any upsets, or upheavals? You reassure her that it is very unlikely that there is anything physically wrong, and his problem will settle given time.

History 3

1. This young person developed separation anxiety about 18 months ago. His symptoms have dramatically developed over the ensuing year because of his parents oversolicitous behaviour. He now has a severe anxiety disorder with obsessional features.
2. He will require individual psychological treatment (anxiety management techniques and cognitive behavioural therapy) and the family will require intensive help to enable the parents to re-establish a normal pattern of behaviour at home. The young person will also require help to return to school.

15 Medico-legal issues

Overview

This chapter describes the main medico-legal issues in relation to the practice of psychiatry in England and Wales. Under common law, powers may be used in an emergency situation to detain or briefly treat individuals with mental illness, when no statutory protections or mechanisms are in place. Actions should be performed out of necessity to protect either the individual or others from potential harm. Common law also gives powers to doctors to treat patients medically if their capacity to give consent is impaired and if the medical treatment required is urgent. Capacity and mental illness are not the same, and a patient can be mentally ill, but retain capacity, and, therefore, the right to refuse medical treatment.

The Mental Health Act (1983) gives powers to doctors and mental health professionals to admit and treat patients with mental illness on a compulsory basis. The most commonly used parts of the Mental Health Act (1983) are described in the chapter. All patients have rights of appeal under the Act, which are usually heard by a mental health review tribunal. Homicide by mentally ill patients is very rare, and two thirds of people killed by mentally ill individuals are close relatives. Homicide of a total stranger is very unusual. The assessment of dangerousness in the mentally ill, however, is important and is described in the chapter. Forensic psychiatry is the specialty of psychiatry that deals with the assessment and treatment of mentally ill offenders. There are parts of the Mental Health Act (1983) that deal specifically with the treatment and detention of mentally ill offenders. These are briefly described. Finally, the likely reforms to the Mental Health Act (1983) that have currently been proposed by the government are briefly described.

15.1 Common law

Learning objectives

You should:

- understand the principle of necessity
- understand the principle of duty of care
- be familiar with the common law and the powers for immediate treatment
- be able to assess a patient's capacity for consent.

Common law refers to that body of rights, duties, obligations and liabilities recognized by the courts over the years. It is made up of principles identified by the judges and adapted and changed to meet the needs of particular cases or particular developments in our society. This case law should be distinguished from statute law, which comprises the rules and regulation agreed by the authority of Parliament and implemented by the passing of Parliamentary Acts. The Mental Health Act (1983) is an example of statute law.

Under common law, every adult has the right and capacity to decide whether or not he/she will accept medical treatment, even if refusal may result in deterioration in the individual's physical or mental health. The reasons for the refusal are irrelevant. In relation to the treatment of mentally ill people, powers under common law may be used in an emergency situation when no statutory protections or mechanisms are in place.

Principle of necessity

The courts have recognized the existence of a common law principle of 'necessity'. This power allows members of the public and health professionals to intervene on an emergency basis to temporarily restrain a mentally ill person until appropriate action can be taken.

Duty of care

Common law imposes a 'duty of care' on all professional staff to all persons within a hospital. This means that health professionals are expected to provide proper care for mentally ill people, and this expectation goes beyond the responsibility of ordinary members of the public. Actions involving the use of reasonable restraint and driven by professional responsibility in circumstances of necessity are supported by common law. However, actions performed out of necessity should not continue for an unreasonable length of time, and progress should be made either to a situation of consent or to the use of powers under the Mental Health Act (1983).

In practice, common law gives legal powers to doctors or other health professionals to restrain, and in some circumstances treat, patients who are judged to be mentally ill. These powers only last, however, for a 'short period of time' (the exact time has not been determined in law). In the setting of the A&E department, common law enables staff to detain a patient who is mentally ill for a period of time until the appropriate order under the Mental Health Act (1983) can be implemented.

Capacity for consent

All doctors must be able to assess a patient's capacity to give consent for medical treatment. This is not necessarily a psychiatric issue; however, psychiatrists are often asked for advice in relation to difficult cases or situations. The criteria for capacity for consent are shown in Box 72. Provided a patient can understand and retain medical advice, and can consider the consequences of not proceeding with that advice, he/she is fully entitled to refuse medical treatment, even if it means their medical condition will deteriorate, or he/she may even die. The presence of psychiatric illness does not automatically mean that the capacity to give consent may be impaired. For instance, a patient with schizophrenia who is floridly psychotic will still be able to give consent for medical treatment, if the criteria in Box 72 are met. However, the presence of mental illness can impair a patient's capacity for informed consent, and where there is doubt, a psychiatrist should be asked to provide an assessment.

> **Box 72**
> Criteria for capacity for consent
>
> The patient must be able to:
>
> - comprehend and retain information that is material to the decision to accept or refuse treatment, especially as to the likely consequences of having or not having the particular treatment in question
> - believe the medical advice to be true
> - be able to use the information received and be able to weigh it up as part of the process of coming to a clear decision.

15.2 The Mental Health Act (1983)

> ### Learning objectives
>
> You should:
>
> - understand the legal definition of mental disorder for the purposes of the Act
> - be familiar with specific sections of the Mental Health Act (1983) in relation to the assessment and treatment of patients on a compulsory basis
> - know under which powers patients admitted to medical wards in a hospital can be detained
> - be aware of patient's rights of appeal.

The present law that covers the care and treatment of mentally disordered people in England and Wales is contained in the Mental Health Act 1983. Scotland has a separate legal system. The Mental Health Act (1983) gives powers to doctors and mental health professionals to admit and treat patients with mental illness on a compulsory basis. Whereas the number of formal admissions to NHS facilities was reasonably stable during the 1980s, recent figures show a rise in the number of patients detained under the Act. In 1994–1995, the number of formal admissions under the Act increased by 55%. The number of men admitted increased by 77%. Since then, the number of patients detained under the Act has increased further. At the same time, the overall number of admissions to hospital has decreased.

The reason for this dramatic increase in the use of the Act is unclear. However, closure of psychiatric beds has resulted in greater pressures on inpatient services. It is possible that the threshold for admission has risen, with patients being admitted at later stages of their illnesses, when they have less insight and are more likely to refuse treatment.

Definition of mental disorder and mental illness

In the Mental Health Act (1983), there are two terms that are used to describe psychiatric illness. The first is 'mental disorder' and the second is 'mental illness'. It is important to understand that these are legal not medical terms. Mental disorder for the purposes of the Act is defined as mental illness, arrested or incomplete development of mind, psychopathic disorder and any other disorder or disability of mind. The term 'mental illness' is not defined in the Act and, therefore, can include a broad range of disorders of mind including delirium and dementia, as well as more formal forms of psychiatric disorder such as schizophrenia.

Most compulsory patients are committed to, or detained in, hospital by means of an application made by the patient's nearest relative, or an approved social worker, and supported by one or two doctors. The application is made to the managers of an appropriate hospital. There are three types of application for admission to hospital, which are colloquially known as 'Sections': Section 2, Section 3 and Section 4. There are two types of application for care in the community: Section 7 and Section 25a. There are two applications that cover the detention of a patient already admitted to hospital on a voluntary basis: Section 5.2 and Section 5.4. Details in relation to each of these different procedures are shown in Table 39.

In all cases the patient must be suffering from some form of mental disorder (as defined under the Act) of a degree that warrants the detention of the patient in a hospital for assessment for at least a limited period and that is in the interest of either his/her own health and safety or with a view to the protection of others.

Applications for admission to hospital

Section 2

Under Section 2 of the Act, an application for admission for assessment authorizes the patient's detention for up to 28 days. Treatment can be given without the patient's consent during this time. The application by either the nearest relative or social worker must be supported by recommendations from two doctors, one of whom must be approved under the Act as being a specialist in mental disorder. The other doctor should preferably be the patient's GP. The exact nature of the disorder does not need to be specified, as the patient is being admitted for assessment.

Section 4

Under Section 4 of the Act, an application for admission for assessment may be made in an emergency with the support of only one medical recommendation. The application can again be made by either the nearest relative or an approved social worker, but the doctor need not be an approved specialist. Preferably, the doctor should be either the patient's GP or be a mental health specialist who has had previous acquaintance with the patient. The order lasts for 72 hours and is usually only used in cases where the delay in obtaining the support of two medical recommendations would lead to risk for the patient, other members of staff or the public.

Section 3

Under Section 3 of the Act, an application for admission for treatment can be made by either the nearest relative or by a social worker. The application must again be supported by recommendations from two doctors, one of whom has to be an approved specialist in mental disorder. As the patient is being admitted for treatment, the specific nature of the mental disorder must be specified by the two doctors making the recommendation. In the case of psychopathic disorder or mental impairment, compulsory admission for treatment can only be undertaken if such treatment is likely to alleviate or prevent a deterioration of the patient's 'condition'.

Applications for care in the community

Section 7

Under Section 7 of the Act, an application for the reception of a patient into the guardianship of a local social services authority or private individual may be made in the same way as an application for admission for hospital treatment, but to the local authority rather than the hospital. The nominated guardian can stipulate where the patient is to live, how the patient should spend his or her time and who must be allowed to see the patient. However, under this part of the Act, the guardian cannot insist that the patient accepts treatment.

Section 25a

Section 25a of the Act was introduced from April 1996 by the Mental Health (Patients in the Community) Act

Table 39 Part II of the Mental Health Act (1983); orders relating to civil detention

Order	Duration	Recommendations and applications	Rights of Appeal	Purpose	Location
Section 2	28 days	2 doctors (1 S12 app.) plus 1 SW or NR	Yes	Assessment	Community or hospital
Section 3	6 months	2 doctors (1 S12 app.) plus 1SW or NR	Yes	Treatment	Community or hospital
Section 4	72 hours	1 doctor plus 1 SW or NR	No	Assessment	Community or hospital
Section 5:2	72 hours	1 doctor (in charge of patients' treatment)	No	Holding power	Hospital
Section 5:4	6 hours	1 RMN	No	Holding power	Hospital

SW, social worker; NR, nearest relative; RMN, registered mental nurse; S12 app, approved under Section 12 of the Mental Health Act (1983) as a specialist in mental disorder.

1995. An application, supported by a social worker and one other doctor, can be made by the patient's psychiatrist for the patient to be supervised after the patient is discharged from hospital. This only applies to patients who have been detained for treatment under Section 3 of the Act.

The grounds for implementing a supervision order are as follows:

1. There would be a substantial risk of serious harm to the health and safety of the patient or the safety of others, or of the patient being seriously exploited, if he/she were not to receive the aftercare services
2. The patient being subject to aftercare under supervision is likely to help to secure that he/she receives aftercare services.

Applications to detain a patient in hospital

Section 5.2

Section 5.2 applies to patients who have been admitted to hospital on a voluntary basis but who later need to be detained on a compulsory basis. It is an emergency order that lasts for 72 hours. It requires the signature of one registered medical practitioner, who does not have to be a mental health specialist. The order can apply to patients admitted to psychiatric or general hospitals. This order only applies to patients who have been formally admitted to a hospital and cannot be used to detain patients brought to an A&E department.

Section 5.4

Section 5.4 is referred to as 'the nurses' holding power'. It enables a registered mental nurse to prevent an informal patient from leaving hospital for up to 6 hours, thus enabling time for a doctor to arrive. There are no rights of appeal.

Discharge of a patient

A patient can be discharged from a compulsory order at any time by the medical officer responsible for his/her care. In addition, as soon as patients are discharged from hospital, the order is rescinded.

Before patients are discharged from hospital, a planning meeting, called a 'Section 117' meeting, is held with the intention of coordinating the patient's follow-up care in the community. All relevant staff and health workers are invited to this meeting, including the patient's GP.

Although treatment cannot be given to patients against their will while they are in the community, recent changes to mental health law have enabled psychiatrists to place certain conditions upon patients who are at high risk of relapse through non-compliance.

As discussed above, under Section 25a, the patient can be required to remain resident at an agreed place and also to attend for treatments, although the treatment itself is not compulsory. Patients can be returned to hospital if they fail to comply with these requirements.

Rights of appeal

Under the Mental Health Act (1983), patients have the right to appeal against compulsory detention. Hospital managers have an obligation to inform patients of their rights in regard to this area and to facilitate the patient's ability to make an appeal. The patient makes an appeal to a mental health review tribunal. Each panel has three types of member: legal members appointed by the Lord Chancellor, medical members appointed by the Lord Chancellor after consultation with the Department of Health, and lay members also appointed by the Lord Chancellor after consultation with the Department of Health. Patients admitted for assessment can apply to a mental health review tribunal within 14 days beginning on the day of their admission.

Mental Health Act Commission and Code of Practice

The Mental Health Act Commission is an official Government body that was set up following the 1983 legislation. Its purpose is to monitor the way the Mental Health Act is implemented by health professionals so that good practice is followed and patient's rights are protected.

The Mental Health Act Commission visits all mental hospitals at least once per year, inspects complaints and publishes reports. It is made up of health professionals and lay members.

A Code of Practice has been published that lays out standards for best practice in relation to the Act.

Treatment under the Mental Health Act (1983)

Medical treatment under the Act can only be given for the express purpose of treating the patient's mental disorder. The Act does not give power to give treatment for physical disorders that are unrelated to the patient's mental disorder. In cases where the physical disorder is contributing to, or is a cause of, the patient's mental disorder, treatment for the physical disorder can be given under the Act (for example the treatment of a patient's delirium). Under these criteria as well, in extreme cases, artificial feeding can be given as a treatment for anorexia nervosa.

Section 58

There are special provisions under the Act for the administration of certain kinds of treatment for mental disorder. Electroconvulsive therapy (ECT) can only be given if the patient consents or if an independent doctor certifies that the treatment is required in order to alleviate or prevent deterioration of the patient's condition. Pharmacological treatment can be given against the patient's consent for the first 3 months of a treatment order. If after this time, the patient continues to refuse pharmacological treatment, an assessment from an independent doctor is required to specify that the treatment should continue.

Section 57

Section 57 of the Act covers treatments that involve the destruction of brain tissue by surgical operation or the surgical implantation of hormones for the purpose of reducing male sexual drive. These treatments, unlike ECT and pharmacological treatment, cannot be given even if the patient gives informed consent. They can only be given if:

1. An independent doctor and two other people who are not doctors certify that the patient is capable of understanding the nature, purpose and likely effects of the treatment and has consented to it
2. The independent doctor must also certify that the treatment is likely to alleviate or prevent a deterioration in the patient's condition.

15.3 Assessment of dangerousness

Learning objectives

You should:

- be aware of the true risk of homicide in patients with mental illness
- be able to carry out a brief risk assessment of dangerousness.

Homicide is a relatively rare act carried out by patients with mental illness, and most patients with mental illness are neither threatening nor violent in their behaviour. The high public profile of a small number of individual cases of homicide by mentally ill patients has, however, increased public concern about issues of safety and the mentally ill. In a recent study of 39 cases of homicide by mentally ill patients, two thirds were committed by male patients, and the most common psychiatric diagnosis was schizophrenia. Table 40 provides more details of individual psychiatric diagnoses and the association with homicide for males and females.

Table 40 Psychiatric diagnoses of 39 patients who committed homicide

Psychiatric diagnosis	Number	Males	Females
Schizophrenia	16	15	1
Affective illness	14	5	9
Personality disorder	9	7	2
Total	39	27	12

From Royal College of Psychiatrists, 1996.

For females the most common psychiatric diagnosis in relation to homicide was affective disorder, and there was only one case of a female patient with schizophrenia who committed homicide. The most frequent causes of death were stabbing (17) and asphyxiation (seven). Members of the patient's family were most at risk, and 64% of all the homicides were of family members. Homicide of a total stranger was very unusual; there were only three cases in all.

Dangerousness

One of the key strategies in trying to prevent homicide by mentally ill patients is the regular assessment of dangerousness of the patient. This is not a static condition, as the degree of dangerousness can fluctuate depending on the patient's mental state or other factors. The following key points need to be considered.

1. Current mental state:
   - is the patient showing evidence of aggressive or threatening behaviour?
   - does the patient hold any abnormal beliefs that could potentially result in violence? (For example, does the patient believe he is being persecuted by a specific individual and have plans to harm this individual?)
   - does the patient have extreme feelings of jealousy towards his/her partner and has he/she threatened the patient in any way?
   - is the patient experiencing auditory hallucinations that are telling him/her to be violent?
   - what degree of insight does the patient have into these abnormal experiences?
   - how able is he/she to resist acting upon them?
   - how willing is he/she to accept treatment?
2. Recent act of violence. If the patient has recently committed an act of violence, the nature of this episode should be assessed, with a view to possible repetition:
   - how serious was the episode?
   - how bizarre was the episode?
   - how potentially serious could the episode have been?
   - did the patient give any warning beforehand?

- was the episode provoked or unprovoked?
- was anyone (e.g. staff or relative) able to detect a change in the patient's behaviour before the episode?
- how unpredictable was the episode?
- is the patient able to discuss the episode and tell staff why he/she carried out the episode?
- does the patient have any regrets?
- was the patient mentally unwell at the time?
- if so, was the violence directly related to his illness?

3. Previous history of violence:
   - does the patient have a previous history of violence?
   - how serious was this?
   - how predictable was the violence?
   - was the violence associated with mental illness or did it occur when the patient was well?

4. Alcohol and drug use:
   - did the violence occur when the patient was under the influence of alcohol or drugs?
   - is alcohol or drugs thought to be a serious contributing factor to the risk of violence?
   - how likely is the patient to remain abstinent?

5. Provoking circumstances: is the patient likely to re-experience circumstances or individual people that provoked previous violence?

6. Response to treatment: if violence or the risk of violence is associated with mental illness, what is the likely response to initial treatment and how likely is the patient to comply with treatment in the long term?

15.4 Forensic psychiatry

Learning objectives

You should:

- be aware of the range of services for mentally ill offenders.
- be aware of the position under the Mental Health Act (1983) of offenders with personality disorders.

Forensic psychiatry is the speciality of psychiatry that deals with the assessment and treatment of mentally ill offenders. There are specific forensic sections of the Mental Health Act (1983) that give powers to the courts and specialized hospitals and secure units to detain mentally ill people who have committed criminal offences. It is not necessary for most doctors to be familiar with these specific sections, although it is important to understand that different powers under the Act are used to detain mentally ill patients who commit criminal offences.

In English law, a person is only regarded culpable of a criminal offence if he/she was able, at the time of the offence, to choose whether or not to perform the criminal action. In other words, whether he/she had criminal responsibility for the actions. The presence of mental illness does not necessarily mean that the patient's responsibility was impaired at the time of an offence, and forensic psychiatrists are often asked to make a judgement in relation to this specific point. If the person's ability was deemed to have been impaired at the time of the offence, a plea of diminished responsibility may be entered. In relation to homicide and the important charge of murder, if a plea of diminished responsibility is upheld, the person can only be charged with the lesser offence of manslaughter.

The courts usually take into account psychiatric evidence when sentencing offenders. This often includes the psychiatrist's judgement as to the suitability of treatment, and the dangerousness of the patient, if a violent act has been committed. In most cases, the patient will be treated on an informal basis, as either an inpatient or an outpatient. In cases of violence or serious offences such as murder, arson and rape, treatment is provided in a secure setting, and the appropriate mental health legislation will be used to detain the patient.

There are a range of services for mentally disordered adult offenders, depending upon the level of security that is required. For individuals who require high security there are three special hospitals in the UK: Broadmoor, Rampton and Ashworth. Individuals who require a medium level of security are managed in medium secure units, which are run by regional forensic psychiatry services. There are 15 units in England and Wales. Other offenders who pose less of a risk to the general public may be treated by local district psychiatric services or by the private sector.

Under the terms of the Mental Health Act (1983), patients with personality disorder can only be detained if their condition is considered to be responsive to treatment. As there is little evidence that severe personality disorder is responsive to treatment (Ch. 10), relatively few people who fit this diagnosis are detained using Mental Health legislation. Instead, they are usually dealt with by the courts in the normal way and, if found guilty of an offence, receive sentencing. There has been recent controversy about the management of people with severe personality disorder, as they are regarded by the lay public as being 'mad' although they do not meet medical criteria for recognized forms of psychotic illness. There have been some high profile cases where such individuals have been denied psychiatric treatment and have then gone on to commit serious offences. In reality such people fall into a grey area between madness and badness. Most people who steal, who are aggressive, or who commit sexual offences, are not ill. On the one hand, if personality disorder is considered to be a mental illness, there is a real concern amongst psychiatrists that any aberrant behaviour (such as stealing or common assault) will be construed as illness. On

Table 41 The main parts of the Mental Health Act (1983) in relation to the compulsory detention of mentally ill offenders

	Section 35	Section 36	Section 37 (hospital order)
Grounds for admission/detention	Preparation of report	Remand for medical treatment	Detention in hospital for treatment of mental disorder
Statutory forms required	Court order and one medical recommendation	Court order and two medical recommendations	Court order and two recommendations
Application	Anyone awaiting trial (Crown or Magistrates) for an offence punishable with imprisonment	Anyone in custody awaiting trial (Crown Court) for an offence punishable with imprisonment	Crown court or Magistrates court; alternative to prison sentence at the time of sentencing
Medical recommendation	Reason to suspect the accused is suffering from mental illness	Individual is suffering from mental disorder and requires hospital treatment	Individual is suffering from mental disorder and requires hospital treatment
Treatment	Only with patient's consent or in an emergency under common law	With or without consent	With or without consent
Duration	28 days	28 days with further periods of 28 days for not more than 12 weeks in total	6 months

the other hand, there is public and political anxiety regarding the dangerousness of such individuals and the risk to the public.

Within the current Mental Health Act (1983), there are specific sections that deal with the compulsory detention of mentally ill offenders. The main sections are summarized in Table 41.

As this book is being written, proposals in relation to a new Mental Health Act are being considered by the government. It is likely that the new Act, when it eventually appears, will specifically address the law pertaining to the compulsory detention and treatment of patients with dangerous and severe personality disorder.

15.5 Reform of the Mental Health Act (1983)

Learning objectives

You should:

- be aware of the likely reforms to mental health legislation
- understand which individuals are likely to be affected.

The government is currently in the process of reforming the 1983 Mental Health Act and has produced a Mental Health White Paper entitled 'Reforming the Mental Health Act'. Part 1 deals with 'The New Legal Framework' and Part 2 deals with 'High-risk Patients'. In this proposed new legislation, there will be greater flexibility in the compulsory treatment of patients as there will be a break in the automatic link between compulsory care and treatment and detention in hospital.

The major changes are summarized below. Further changes may occur before the proposals become enshrined in statute.

Definition of mental disorder

The broad definition of mental disorder, as used in the 1983 Act, is unlikely to change.

Criteria for compulsory detention

The criteria used to determine whether patients should be subject to compulsory detention are likely to change, with a greater emphasis placed on the assessment of the capacity of the patient, and the use of the least possible restrictive environment for treatment.

Assessment

Under the new proposals, decisions to begin assessment and initial treatment of a patient under compulsory powers will be based on a preliminary examination by two doctors and a social worker, or another suitably trained mental health professional.

The initial period of assessment will be limited to a maximum of 28 days, as in the 1983 Act, but during this time, a formal care plan must be drawn up that will give details of the patient's health, social care needs and treatment.

Powers of treatment

After 28 days, continuing use of compulsory powers will have to be authorized by a Mental Health Tribunal (a new independent decision-making body). The tribunal will be able to make a care and treatment order that will authorize the care and treatment specified in a care plan recommended by the clinical team. This must be designed to give therapeutic benefit to the patient or to manage behaviour associated with mental disorder that might lead to serious harm to other people. The first two orders will be for up to 6 months each. Subsequent orders may be for periods of up to 12 months.

Community treatment
It is proposed that both compulsory assessment and treatment may be delivered in the community and will not necessarily require admission to hospital. However, there will be no powers for patients to be given medication forcibly except in a clinical setting. This will mean that some patients will be brought back to hospital/clinic premises for their treatment or will be re-admitted.

Advocacy service
Patients who are subject to compulsory powers will be given a new right of access to advice and support from independent specialist advocacy services.

New Commission for Mental Health
There will be a new Commission for Mental Health. It will be responsible for monitoring the use of formal powers, assuring the quality of statutory training provided for practitioners with key responsibilities under the new legislation and for specialist advocacy services.

New criteria for those posing a risk to others
There will be new criteria under Part II of the legislation for the detention and treatment of individuals who present a significant risk to others. This includes individuals whose risk is as a result of a severe personality disorder (dangerous and severe personality disorder (DSPD)). Under the 1983 Act, such individuals could only be detained using compulsory powers if their condition was 'treatable'. Under the proposed new legislation, individuals with mental health problems who present a high risk to the public will be detained either to receive treatment to address the underlying disorder or to manage behaviour associated with the disorder. The government is committed to spend £126 million in 2000–2003 for the development of new specialist services for those with dangerous and severe personality disorder.

Further reading and sources

Department of Health 1994 Report of the Inquiry into the Care and Treatment of Christopher Clunis. HMSO, London
Department of Health and Welsh Office 1999 Code of Practice: Mental Health Act 1983. The Stationery Office, London (www.doh.gov.uk/mhact1983.htm)
General Medical Council 1998 Seeking patient's consent: the ethical considerations. GMC, London (www.gmc-uk.org)
Hoggett B 1996 Mental health law, 4th edn. Sweet and Maxwell, London.
Royal College of Psychiatrists 1996 Report of the Confidential Inquiry into Homicides and Suicides by Mentally Ill People. Royal College of Psychiatrists, London.

Sources

Department of Health. Full details of the proposals regarding changes to Mental Health Law in England and Wales are available at www.doh.gov.uk/mentalhealth.htm

Self-assessment: questions

Multiple choice questions

1. The Mental Health Act (1983):
   a. Is for the treatment of patients with mental disorder
   b. Is for the treatment of patients with physical disorder
   c. Defines mental disorder according to psychiatric classification system
   d. Is the same as common law
   e. Is the same as the Code of Practice

2. Section 2 of the Mental Health Act (1983):
   a. Is a compulsory order that lasts for 6 months
   b. Is a compulsory order for the admission to hospital of a patient with mental disorder for assessment
   c. Requires the recommendation of one doctor
   d. Does not enable staff to treat patients against their will
   e. Is a part of the Mental Health Act (1983) that is rarely used

3. Section 5.2:
   a. Should be used to detain patients who have been brought to the A&E department
   b. Can only be signed by a psychiatrist
   c. Lasts for 3 days
   d. Lasts for 72 hours
   e. Can be used to detain patients on a medical ward of a general hospital

4. The common law:
   a. Is statute law
   b. Gives powers to members of the public and health professionals to restrain mentally ill individuals who are deemed to be at risk to themselves or others
   c. Expects that health professionals have a 'duty of care' towards the mentally ill, which exceeds the care expected from an ordinary member of the public
   d. Does not apply to members of the House of Lords
   e. Is made up of judicial case law

5. Informed consent:
   a. Can never be given by patients who are mentally ill
   b. Requires that the patient can understand and retain medical information concerning his/her condition
   c. Requires that the patient can weigh up the advantages and disadvantages of accepting or refusing treatment
   d. Requires that the patient believes the doctor
   e. Can be given on behalf of the patient by a nearest relative

6. A supervision order:
   a. Applies to any patient who has been detained under the Mental Health Act (1983)
   b. Requires an application by the patient's psychiatrist, supported by a social worker and two other doctors
   c. Can be implemented if there is a substantial risk of harm to others if aftercare services are not implemented
   d. Allows treatment against the patient's wishes in the community
   e. Is the same as a Section 2

7. Patients with psychopathic personality disorder:
   a. Can never been detained under the Act
   b. Can only been detained if their condition is deemed treatable
   c. Can only be treated under the Act in prison
   d. Have to have committed a serious offence before they can be detained under the Act
   e. Are not allowed to appeal against compulsory detention under the Act

8. The following characteristics increase the risk of dangerousness:
   a. Auditory hallucinations commanding the patient to be violent
   b. Good insight and compliance with treatment
   c. Feelings of extreme jealousy towards partner
   d. History of violence
   e. Evidence of current aggression and threatening behaviour

9. The Mental Health Act Commission:
   a. Has a major role in the protection of the rights and welfare of patients detained under the Mental Health Act (1983)
   b. Was set up 50 years ago
   c. Consists only of patients
   d. Is the same thing as the Code of Practice
   e. Visits all mental hospitals in England at least once every 10 years

10. In relation to treatment under the Mental Health Act (1983):
    a. Treatment for any physical disorder can be authorized
    b. A course of ECT (electroconvulsive therapy), without the patient's consent, can only be given following an independent medical opinion
    c. Psychosurgery can be given provided the patient gives consent
    d. Can never be given to a patient detained under Section 2 of the Act
    e. Under Section 3 of the Act, treatment can be given against the patient's wishes for 6 months before any further official action is required

Case history questions

History 1

A 34-year-old man is brought to casualty by the police. He has been found wandering down a busy dual carriageway. He is naked and has been shouting at cars. He is fully orientated and is not confused. He believes that he is the Son of God and talks about proving this by showing people that he can fly. He does not accept that he is ill and requires treatment.

What would be your management?

History 2

A 56-year-old man is admitted to coronary care following a myocardial infarction. After a few hours he becomes hostile and aggressive towards staff. He believes that they are experimenting on him. He begins to interfere with other patients' treatment. He is obviously confused.

What is your management?

History 3

A 61-year-old woman has chronic renal failure. She is confused and refusing continuous ambulatory peritoneal dialysis (CAPD). She keeps wandering off the ward and staff are becoming increasingly concerned about the constant need to restrain her.

What is your management?

Self-assessment: answers

Multiple choice answers

1. a. **True.**
   b. **False.** It is only for the treatment of mental disorder. Treatment for physical conditions can be given under the Act, but only for the purposes of treating mental disorders.
   c. **False.** Defines mental disorder as mental illness, arrested or incomplete development of mind, psychopathic disorder and any other disorder or disability of mind. This is a legal definition, not a medical one.
   d. **False.**
   e. **False.** The Code of Practice is a guide as to how to implement the Act according to best practice.

2. a. **False.** It lasts for 28 days.
   b. **True.**
   c. **False.** Two doctors are required.
   d. **False.**
   e. **False.** This is one of the most frequently used compulsory orders.

3. a. **False.** Patients who have been brought to an A&E department have not been admitted to hospital, so a Section 5(2) is inappropriate.
   b. **False.** Any doctor.
   c. **False.** 72 hours
   d. **True.**
   e. **True.**

4. a. **False.** It is made up of case law.
   b. **True.** But only for a short period of time.
   c. **True.**
   d. **False.** It applies to anyone.
   e. **True.**

5. a. **False.**
   b. **True.**
   c. **True.**
   d. **True.**
   e. **False.** A nearest relative can assent to treatment but cannot give consent for the patient's treatment.

6. a. **False.** It only applies to patients detained using a treatment order (Section 3).
   b. **False.** The application needs support from a social worker and one other doctor.
   c. **True.**
   d. **False.** Patients can be returned to hospital for treatment against their wishes but not treated in the community against their wishes.
   e. **False.**

7. a. **False.** They can be detained if their condition is considered treatable.
   a. **True.**
   b. **False.**
   c. **False.**
   d. **False.** All patients have the right of appeal.

8. a. **True.**
   b. **False.**
   c. **True.**
   d. **True.** This is one of the best predictors of violent behaviour.
   e. **True.**

9. a. **True.** This is its principal remit.
   b. **False.** Was set up in 1983.
   c. **False.** Consists of professionals and lay members.
   d. **False.** The Code of Practice is a written guide.
   e. **False.** It visits each hospital at least once per year.

10. a. **False.** Only treatments which help of alleviate mental disorder.
    b. **True.** An emergency treatment of ECT can be given without a second opinion but not a whole course.
    c. **False.** A second opinion must be sought, even if the patient gives consent.
    d. **False.**
    e. **False.** After 3 months, the responsible medical officer (RMO) has to ascertain whether the patient will consent to treatment. If the patient does not give consent, the RMO must obtain a second opinion.

Case history answers

History 1

This man requires admission to hospital for assessment. A Section 2 would be the most appropriate order.

History 2

This man requires urgent sedation. As this is an emergency situation, he can be treated under the powers of the common law. As he is confused, he does not have the capacity to give consent. Sufficient staff as is necessary should be summoned and he should be sedated with either intramuscular or intravenous medication. Intravenous medication should never be given to sedate a patient unless:

- immediate control is required
- resuscitation equipment is available.

History 3

This situation has been going on for some time. Although staff are entitled to restrain and treat her under common law, the duration of the problem and the concern of staff require that she be assessed by a psychiatrist. In the psychiatrist's opinion, she has a mental illness (a confusional state), which requires physical treatment to alleviate the symptoms. She is placed initially on a Section 5.2, which is then converted to a Section 2. Her CAPD exchanges are restarted and implemented on a regular basis. In 3 to 4 days she is much better. She is fully orientated and is complying with medication. Her Section order is rescinded.

16 Psychological treatment

Overview

Psychological treatments relieve psychological distress and disability by psychological means. This usually occurs through the medium of a therapeutic relationship between a therapist/doctor and patient/client. There are many different forms of psychological treatments, but the three most widely used within the NHS are cognitive-behavioural treatment, interpersonal/relational therapies and counselling. Each of these will be described in detail in this chapter. Most therapies are given on a one-to-one basis (i.e. one therapist and one patient), but other formats exist, including couple therapy, group therapy and family therapy. Each of these can be delivered using one of the three major forms of psychological treatment. Nearly all psychological treatments that are available in the UK on the National Health Service (NHS) are short term, and they vary in length from a few weeks to a few months. Emphasis is placed upon treating symptoms, improving quality of life and returning patients to a premorbid level of functioning. Psychological services are available in the primary and secondary care settings. Demand, however, is high and there is often a waiting list for treatment. Cognitive-behavioural treatments are usually carried out by clinical psychologists, although there are now a small number of consultant psychiatrists who have been trained to deliver this treatment. Interpersonal/relational therapies are conducted by consultant psychotherapists and clinical psychologists. Counselling is usually conducted by individuals who have undergone a training in counselling, but they may not have a recognized training in any of the mental health professions.

16.1 Cognitive-behavioural treatments

Learning objectives

You should:

- understand the theoretical basis of behaviour therapy and cognitive therapy
- be familiar with the different types of behaviour therapy
- be familiar with cognitive therapy
- understand for which psychiatric conditions each treatment is helpful.

Behaviour therapy

Behaviour therapy is an application of experimental psychology to change symptoms and behaviour. It is based upon learning theory and is largely derived from the work of Skinner. Symptoms are regarded as unwanted conditional responses that can be removed by appropriate re-learning. There are several different behavioural treatments, which can either be given separately or in a combined treatment package. All treatments involve three stages. First, a detailed assessment will be carried out by the therapist, which is called a *behavioural analysis*. The patient's inappropriate behaviour will be scrutinized and factors that re-inforce the problem will be identified. Second, the patient will be asked to *monitor behaviour* using a detailed diary to record specific instances of the behaviour and circumstances when it occurred. Third, the patient will begin to *modify behaviour*, overcoming any anxiety attached to this.

Operant conditioning

Operant conditioning involves the modification of the patient's behaviour using rewards for appropriate behaviour and ignoring inappropriate behaviour. The rewards are contingent upon the patient completing specific tasks. Rewards can take many different forms including praise, tokens, financial incentives, treats, etc. The more a behaviour is rewarded (re-inforced),

Rehabilitation programmes for patients with chronic
schizophrenia
Treatment programmes for patients with chronic pain or
somatization
Modification of inappropriate behaviour in adults with
learning difficulties
Treatment of childhood behavioural problems

the more likely the patient is to repeat the behaviour.
The principles of operant behavioural therapy are
used in a wide number of different treatment settings
(Box 73).

Desensitization

Desensitization is used to treat phobic conditions,
either agoraphobia or specific phobias (e.g. fear of spiders). Patients are taught techniques to control and
reduce anxiety. A hierachy of stimuli that provoke a
feared response in the patient is drawn up, with the least
anxiety-provoking object at the bottom of the hierarchy
and the most feared object at the top of the hierarchy. The
patient, either in imagination or real life, starts with
the bottom of the hierarchy and, using relaxation to
counteract anxiety, experiences the feared object. Once
the patient has overcome his/her anxiety, he/she can
then move on to the next stage. It is important, however, that the patient feels completely settled at a particular stage of the hierarchy before moving on to the next
level.

Exposure

Exposure is sometimes combined with desensitization
for the treatment of agoraphobia. Exposure involves the
real-life experience of the feared object. The therapist
usually accompanies the patient to a situation that is
anxiety provoking (e.g. travelling on a bus). As the
patient becomes more anxious, the therapist encourages
him/her to relax. Both patient and therapist stay in the
feared situation until the patient's anxiety subsides. For
the best chance of success, exposure to feared situations
should be conducted in a gradual way. In the past,
patients were sometimes exposed to their most feared
situation with preliminary treatment. This is called *flood-
ing*. Although the patient's anxiety will eventually fall in
such situations, no matter how frightened he/she is initially, this form of treatment is rarely used now. It is distressing for the patient and compliance is likely to be
low.

Response prevention

Response prevention is used for the treatment of
ritualistic behaviour in obsessive-compulsive disorder.
The patient is encouraged not to perform the specific
ritual (e.g. washing the kitchen floor). In obsessive-
compulsive disorder, rituals usually reduce anxiety.
When the patient is prevented from carrying out the ritual, his/her anxiety will increase. With repeated practice, however, the patient's anxiety subsides and the
frequency of ritualistic behaviour diminishes. The
patient is often helped not to perform the ritual by the
presence of the therapist, who may carry out the treatment in the patient's home. The therapist will sometimes 'model' appropriate behaviour (e.g. not washing
his hands after touching an innocuous object), which
may encourage the patient to copy.

Biofeedback

In biofeedback, patients are taught to control physiological responses that are normally outside the patient's
conscious awareness. The patient is connected to physiological equipment that gives the patient specific
information about certain bodily reactions (e.g. blood
pressure) or functions (e.g. anal sphincter control). The
equipment is designed so that the information regarding body status is provided in a simple form (e.g. a tone
of varying pitch or a visual analogue pictorial display).
The individual then tries to alter the displayed measure-
ment by regulating the relevant function (e.g. relaxing in
order to control blood pressure, or increasing tone in a
sphincter muscle by consciously contracting the muscle). Biofeedback is used in the treatment of many medical disorders including hypertension, anal incontinence
and urinary incontinence.

Cognitive therapy

Cognitive therapy produces benefit by changing maladaptive ways of thinking. It is often used in combination with various behavioural techniques. It was
developed in the 1960s by a psychiatrist called Aaron
Beck. It was initially used for the treatment of depression but has been adapted for use in many different psychiatric conditions (Box 74).

Depressive disorders
Anxiety disorders including panic disorder and
generalized anxiety disorder
Eating disorders
Somatization disorders and hypochondriasis
Schizophrenia: for the treatment of hallucinations or
delusions
Post-traumatic stress disorder
Personality disorders

Beck noticed that when people suffered from depression they invariably described low self-esteem and perceived themselves in a negative way. He postulated that if these negative thoughts could be altered, the depression would improve. There are three main components of Beck's cognitive theory of emotional disorders. The first component is the presence of negative automatic thoughts. These are thoughts that come out of the blue, unconnected to everyday life. They are accepted by the person as being realistic and valid. Their effect, however, is to create self-doubt, disrupt mood and cause further negative thoughts to develop, creating a downward spiral. The second component is the presence of systematic logical errors in the thinking of depressed individuals. Examples are listed in Table 42. These inaccurate appraisals and assumptions produce further lowering of mood, self-doubt and low self-esteem. The third component of the cognitive model is the presence of depressogenic schemata or core beliefs. These are strongly held, long-lasting attitudes about the world that shape the way the individual conducts himself/herself and relates to the world.

Cognitive techniques aim first at making patients reconceptualize their thoughts and memories as simply thoughts and memories that are not made out of stone but can be subject to change. The major techniques used to help patients to challenge or change beliefs are shown in Table 43.

In cognitive therapy for depression, a detailed analysis of the patient's thoughts is carried out to identify thoughts that are unreasonably self-deprecating or pessimistic. The therapist studies each thought in detail and the logic behind it. The patient's views are challenged with logical argument and the unreasonably harsh self-deprecatory attitudes are shown to have no rational foundation. The patient is then encouraged to monitor his/her thoughts, challenge negative thoughts on a regular basis and substitute negative thoughts with more positive, realistic ideas. In particular, the patient is taught to identify negative predictors (thoughts about future events) that lead to avoidance or unbearable anxiety, with subsequent poor performance and confirmation of the core belief (Fig. 11). As patient and therapist start to formulate more realistic ideas, helpful alternative strategies can be developed, and eventually core beliefs can be modified. As the process continues, the patient's mood gradually improves and the patient is encouraged to appreciate the links between negative thoughts and low mood. The model, as stated above, has been applied to a wide range of conditions and it has been extensively evaluated. There is little evidence to suggest that it is a more effective treatment than other psychological treatments, as most studies comparing different psychological treatments report equivalent outcomes. However, there are many more studies evaluating this form of treatment than any other psychological treatment approach, and because of this, it has become the recommended first choice of treatment out of the available psychological therapies for most conditions.

Table 42 Examples of systematic logical errors

Systematic logical error	Example
Arbitrary inference	My friend is out, she must be enjoying herself with someone else
Overgeneralization	Everything I do always goes wrong
Selective abstraction	Although she says she likes me a lot, she did once say she didn't like my hair, which means she can't like me as she says she does
Magnification	If I don't get this piece of work finished in time, the teacher will think I'm completely useless
Minimization	The teacher only said well done because she was in a good mood
Personalization	It's all my fault – I'm the one to blame
Dichotonomous thinking	If she turns me down, I might as well give up

Table 43 Core techniques of cognitive therapy

Technique	Explanation of technique
Thought catching	Teach awareness of depressing thoughts as they occur
Task assignment	Encourage activities that the person has been avoiding
Reality testing	Select tasks that help to test out the truth of fixed negative thoughts
Cognitive rehearsal	Go through with the patient all the thoughts and reasons behind why an activity is being avoided
Dealing with underlying fears and assumptions	Investigate the way in which dysfunctional schemata have built up and how they influence day to day thinking

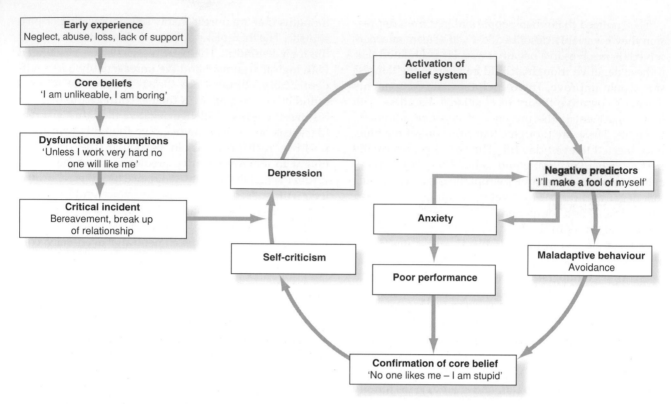

Fig. 11 Diagram showing a cognitive model of depression.

16.2 Interpersonal/relational therapies

Learning objectives

You should:

- have a basic understanding of psychodynamic therapies, interpersonal therapy, psychodynamic-interpersonal therapy and cognitive-analytic therapy
- know the conditions that are treated by these therapies.

The interpersonal therapeutic approaches all share the basic premise that psychological distress is caused by, or exacerbated by, difficulties in making or sustaining interpersonal relationships, and problems in moderating and controlling emotion.

There are several different kinds of therapy with an interpersonal focus: psychodynamic therapy, interpersonal therapy, psychodynamic-interpersonal therapy and cognitive-analytic therapy. Each has a slightly different approach but all try to help the patient to gain greater insight (understanding) of difficulties or problems in relationships, which can then be addressed and improved.

Defence mechanisms

Most of these kinds of therapy will include an evaluation of the patient's defence mechanisms. This term refers to the instinctive way individuals react to and manage frustrating or anxiety-provoking situations. Defence mechanisms are best understood as psychological strategies that help people to maintain self-esteem, contain anger and protect themselves from unpleasant or unbearable feelings.

Certain defence mechanisms are adaptive in that they are likely to invoke beneficial and supportive responses from others, whereas less-adaptive mechanisms often provoke anger and rejection. Defence mechanisms can be classified into mature, immature or primitive categories, according to their tendency to provoke helpful or unhelpful responses from others. Each individual will use a repertoire of different mechanisms to cope with different situations and emotional problems. Individuals who habitually tend to use more mature than immature defence mechanisms are likely to develop close and supportive relationships, be productive at work and be at low risk of both physical and mental disorders. The converse is true of individuals who tend to use more immature than mature defences. Each person's repertoire of defences becomes relatively fixed as he/she enters young adulthood, although longitudinal studies over 30 years have shown that most people develop more mature defences as they get older. Patients with personality difficulties usually employ a range of immature defence mechanisms, which often evoke the opposite behaviour from others that they actually desire. Table 44 lists some of the main kinds of defence mechanism.

Psychodynamic therapy

Psychodynamic therapy has developed from psychoanalysis and the theories of Freud. Central to most therapies derived from psychoanalysis is the concept of conflict (Fig. 12). Individuals have basic drives or instincts (such as aggressive or sexual drives), which cannot always be fulfilled and have to be controlled in order to live within society. Certain drives may result in unacceptable wishes or desires, which may have to be repressed or put out of conscious awareness. This, however, results in inner conflict and the development of symptoms or overt distress, although the individual may not realise the true reason for the distress. Another

Table 44 Defence mechanisms

Defence mechanism	Description	Likely response from others
Mature defences		
Altruism	Channelling one's own needs to be cared for by helping others	Affection, gratitude, high regard
Sublimation	Channelling unacceptable impulses (e.g. aggressive) in a way that is socially acceptable (e.g. sport)	Admiration, camaraderie
Suppression	Being able to put distressing feelings temporarily out of awareness in order to function, but then to be able to acknowledge and share them when it is appropriate	Respect, support, help
Anticipation	Being able to address issues about difficult experiences before they occur (e.g. being able to talk to someone about their imminent death and the pain that it will cause you)	Closeness, expression of affection and the resolution of conflicts
Humour	Dissipating conflict by being able to laugh	Affection, positive response
Immature defences/neurotic		
Displacement	Expressing conflict towards a person or object who is undeserving of it, rather than directing it at person who is really the focus (e.g. kicking the cat)	Rejection
Hypochondriasis	Development of physical symptoms or concerns about physical symptoms as a way of avoiding overt conflict	Initially support but then resentment and frustration from others
Intellectualization	Talking about conflicts in a psychological but emotionally uninvolved way	Unlikely to produce support from others; may keep people at a distance
Acting out	Resolving conflicts by some form of socially unacceptable behaviour (getting drunk or cutting oneself)	Anger and distance from others
Passive aggression	Expressing conflict and anger by some form of inaction, while remaining superficially calm and placid (e.g. restricting food intake)	Anger and frustration in others
Repression	Pushing conflicts out of conscious awareness	No specific positive or negative response
Reaction formation	Forming an opposite conscious opinion to deeply held wishes or desires (e.g. campaigning against homosexuality to ward off 'unacceptable' desires for people of the same sex)	Usually hidden desires become apparent, which leads to alienation from particular social group the individual is part of
Primitive		
Projection	Putting one's own feelings on to some else (e.g. perceiving other people as being angry when you yourself are actually the one who is angry)	Rejection, anger
Splitting	Seeing people as either all good or bad	Anger, frustration and rejection

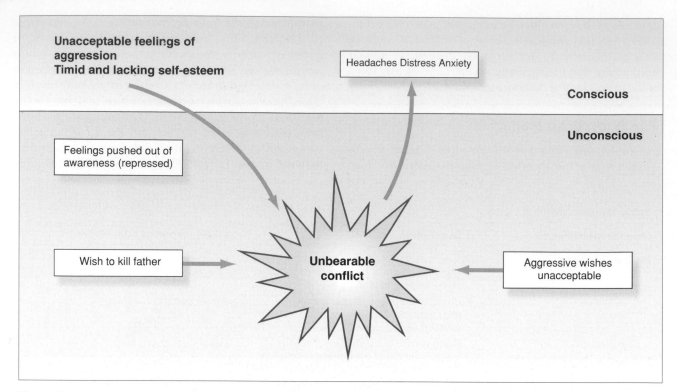

Fig. 12 The concept of conflict illustrated with a 34-year-old man (with violent and alcoholic father) with headaches and anxieties. He is timid and lacking in self-esteem but has underlying unacceptable aggressive feelings, which he feels have to be repressed.

important concept in psychodynamic therapy is *transference*. Transference is the misappraisal and misperception of others based upon previous childhood experiences. The individual is usually unaware of his/her misperceptions and, as a consequence, acts upon them, sometimes with unfortunate consequences.

For example, a 25-year-old woman had been repeatedly sexually abused by her father when a child. She found it difficult to trust people when an adult, and she found it hard to form close and supportive relationships. Her view of the world and relationships was coloured by her childhood traumas, and adult experiences of intimacy felt, to her, as if she was being intruded upon or being violated. Therefore, she perceived others as being abusive towards her, when in reality they were trying to help or offer support. The closer she became to someone else emotionally, the more intense the feeling of being abused. One of the aims of psychological treatment would be to help her to recognize her misperceptions of people, particularly those with whom she felt closely attached, so that she could develop a more realistic and trusting attitude towards others.

In psychodynamic therapy, transference develops in the therapeutic relationship, so the therapist is perceived in a distorted way by the patient. In the above example, the patient may well begin to view the therapist as being abusive were she to embark upon a course

of psychodynamic psychotherapy. However, as treatment occurs in a controlled setting, the therapist should be able to work with the patient, to recognize and understand this process in a direct and immediate way. The therapist may also seek to identify the main repertoire of defensive mechanisms that the patient employs on a regular basis and may try to help the patient to develop more adaptive strategies.

Psychodynamic therapy has been widely practised in the UK, USA and Europe since the 1950s. In the past, treatments were given on a long-term basis (several months to years). Recently, short-term treatments have been developed, but there are relatively few empirical evaluations. Psychodynamic therapy of moderate duration, and carried out in a day hospital setting, is an effective treatment for borderline personality disorder.

Interpersonal therapy

Interpersonal therapy was developed by two psychiatrists called Klerman and Weissman (Klerman et al., 1984). Like cognitive therapy, it was initially developed to treat patients with depression. In interpersonal therapy, there are three phases of development. During the first phase, depression is diagnosed within a medical model and explained to the patient. The major problem associated with the onset of the depression is identified and an explicit treatment contract to work on this problem area is made with the patient. Problem areas are classified into three groups: grief, interpersonal disputes and role transitions. In the second phase of the therapy, the therapist and patient work on the identified problem area, exploring ways of helping the patient to deal with the problem. In the final phase of the therapy, the termination is discussed, progress is reviewed and the remaining work outlined.

Interpersonal therapy has been evaluated in several major empirical studies. It is as effective as cognitive therapy for the treatment of depression and eating disorders. It can be used as a maintenance treatment for patients with chronic symptoms of depression to prevent further relapse. Its effect is additional to the effect of antidepressants. It has also been found to be beneficial for the treatment of depression in patients with physical disease.

Psychodynamic-interpersonal therapy

Psychodynamic-interpersonal therapy was developed by a psychiatrist called Hobson (1985). It has elements of psychodynamic therapy and interpersonal therapy. It places greater emphasis on the patient–therapist relationship as a tool for resolving interpersonal issues than does interpersonal therapy, and there is less emphasis on the interpretation of transference than in psychodynamic therapies.

Key features of the model include (i) the assumption that the patient's problems arise from or are exacerbated by disturbances of significant personal relationships; (ii) a tentative, encouraging, supportive approach from the therapist, who seeks to develop deeper understanding with the patient through negotiation, exploration of feelings and metaphor; (iii) the linkage of the patient's distress to specific interpersonal problems; and (iv) the use of the therapeutic relationship to address problems and to test out solutions in the 'here and now'. Emphasis is placed upon identifying repeated patterns of behaviour within relationships that result in conflict and emotional distress. Support and encouragement is provided to the patient to challenge difficult problem areas in relationships and to develop more adaptive ways of coping.

Psychodynamic-interpersonal therapy has been evaluated in several empirical studies. It is equivalent to cognitive therapy for the treatment of depression. It has been used successfully to treat somatization and is a cost-effective treatment for patients with chronic and enduring symptoms of depression and anxiety. A 1 year treatment has been used to treat borderline personality disorder, with resulting benefits in psychological health and considerable cost savings through reductions in inpatient treatment.

Cognitive-analytic therapy

Cognitive-analytic therapy is a time-limited, integrated psychotherapy that was developed in the UK by Ryle (1995). It incorporates elements of cognitive and psychodynamic approaches. Patients are encouraged to identify repeated difficulties or conflicts that arise in their relationships, so-called 'dilemmas, traps and snags'. Patients' problems are understood in terms of what is called the procedural sequence model (PSM). According to this model, intentional acts or the enactment of roles in relationships are maintained by repetitive sequences of mental, behavioural and environmental processes. During the first few sessions of therapy, patients monitor their relationships and their emotional state to identify target problems and the dilemmas, traps and snags that underlie them (target problem procedures (TPP)). The remaining therapy is spent working on these TPP, trying to identify and revise them so that new ways of handling problems can be developed. The therapist makes use of a variety of different diagrammatic aids to help the patient to make sense of his/her problems. Sequential diagrammatic reformulations are drawn up to help the patient to understand the connection between feelings, past experiences and behaviour (Fig. 13).

There are several evaluations of cognitive-analytic therapy in a clinical setting but, as yet, there are no empirical studies to support its efficacy. It has potential benefits for patients with depression and anxiety disorders, deliberate self-harm and uncontrolled diabetes. A 6 month treatment has been developed for patients with borderline personality disorder.

16.3 Counselling

Learning objectives

You should:

- be aware of the basic principles of counselling
- know for which conditions it is most suitable.

Counselling is widely practised in the primary care setting and in educational institutions (e.g. student counselling services in university or college settings). Those who attend for counselling are usually referred to as clients rather than patients as treatment may take place in a non-NHS setting. There are many different models of counselling (see Further reading), but the most commonly practised form is based on the work of Carl Rogers. Counselling is usually non-directive in that the therapist usually follows the conversation of the client

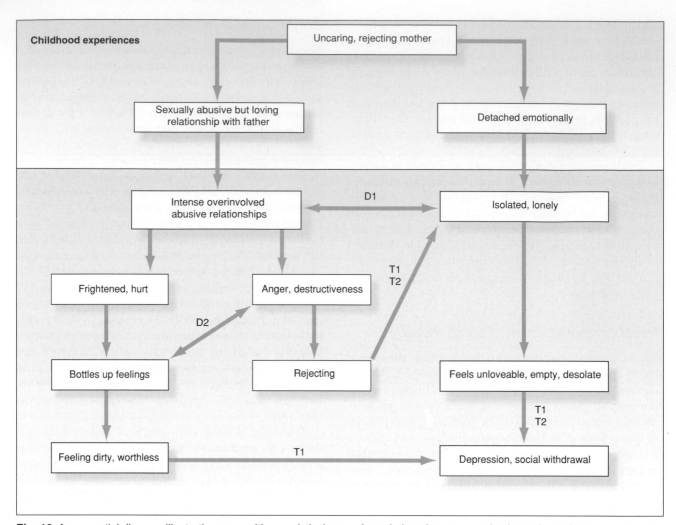

Childhood experiences

Fig. 13 A sequential diagram illustrating a cognitive-analytic therapy formulation. As an example, the pathway for a 32-year-old woman with a previous history of childhood sexual abuse and an uncaring alcoholic mother is given. T1, a repeating trap that produces depression; T2, a repeating trap producing isolation; D1, a dichotomy between feeling either cut-off and lonely or overinvolved and abused; D2, a dichotomy between feeling either destructively angry or emotionally detached.

without trying to impose a specific structure, unlike the other therapies discussed above. The therapist adopts an attitude of unconditional positive regard, which means that no matter what the client discloses, the therapist will remain non-judgemental and try to help. By allowing clients to explore personal difficulties in a supportive and understanding setting, clients themselves are often able to find solutions to their difficulties. The role of the counsellor is to facilitate this process.

The most appropriate use of counselling is for individuals who have stable personalities and a secure social framework but have developed psychological distress in relation to a specific event (such as bereavement). Such individuals can be helped to draw upon their own resources to overcome and adapt to their current difficulties. In these situations, counselling can be

extremely helpful and may prevent long-term problems. Individuals with more complex problems should receive more specific psychological treatments such as cognitive therapy.

Unfortunately, in the primary care setting, GPs refer to counsellors patients with complex and difficult problems, which are unsuitable for such an unstructured intervention. Better education of GPs is required so they can make more appropriate referrals.

There have been relatively few empirical evaluations of counselling in the primary setting. A recent systematic review suggests that it is superior to usual treatment delivered by GPs; however, there are still doubts about its efficacy. Counselling remains popular with patients, and it is a relatively cheap form of treatment compared with most other psychological therapies.

16.4 Other therapeutic approaches

Learning objectives

You should:

- be aware of the basic principles of problem-solving therapy

- be aware of the different forms of therapy involving more than one patient: group, couple, family

- know for which conditions each therapeutic approach is most suitable.

Problem solving

Problem-solving therapy is a fairly simple, psychological treatment approach that has been specifically developed for the treatment of patients with emotional disorders in primary care. There are four main components. First, the patient's symptoms are assessed and any practical or social problems elicited. Second, the patient is given an explanation of the emotional symptoms and how they are caused. Third, the patient is reassured that problem solving is appropriate and effective. Fourth, the treatment is carried out. The patient's problems are clarified in detail, and for each problem one or two achievable goals are identified. The patient is asked to think of as many solutions as he/she can. The patient then chooses the most suitable solution. The patient and therapist devise a plan of action to be carried out before the next treatment session. The progress is then reviewed and evaluated in subsequent treatment sessions. In addition to non-specific emotional disorders in primary care, it has also been used to treat major depressive disorders in a primary care setting.

Family therapy

Family therapy is based upon systems theory. This is the idea that a system or group of people can interact together to produce symptoms unwittingly in one member of the group. For example, in a case of anorexia nervosa, the teenager's symptoms may allow the family as a whole to focus upon the teenager as the 'sick person'. In reality, however, the marital relationship between the parents may be under great strain, but these issues are denied or avoided. The teenager's illness may stabilize the family, as without it, the marriage and the family may split up.

Family therapy is a particularly useful form of treatment for families with children or adolescents who have psychiatric problems. It is also used, however, in the treatment of elderly patients and, where resources permit, it can be useful in schizophrenia and other disorders affecting adults.

Family therapy can be particularly helpful in encouraging family members to stop re-inforcing maladaptive behaviours, and concentrate on encouraging and rewarding positive behaviour.

Families are usually seen altogether with one or two therapists. It is also usual practice for another member of the family therapy team to watch the session via a video link or one-way screen. The way the family interacts with one another during the session often provides the therapist with clues as to how they react with each other at home. One member may be particularly dominant or another member may be silent, or all the family may talk over each other all at once, etc.

The aim of the therapy is to help the family to recognize maladaptive ways of functioning, and help them to develop more fruitful ways of interacting with each other. As the family changes, the symptoms in the member of the family who is the patient often improves.

Couple therapy

Couple therapy is rarely offered in the UK on the NHS in a formal way, although many psychiatrists and clinical psychologists will see couples together for a one-off or a small number of sessions. Couple therapy is usually offered either when conflicts within the marriage/couple relationship are seen as a major cause of the patient's symptoms or when the partner of the patient is

Table 45 The use of group therapy in the NHS

Type of group	Format
Psychoeducational groups	Fixed (1–12 sessions)
Anxiety management groups	Fixed (1–12 sessions)
Alcohol treatment groups	Fixed or slow open
Eating disorder groups	Fixed or slow open
Cognitive-behavioural groups	Fixed
Groups for survivors of sexual abuse	Fixed (1–12 sessions)
Social skills training	Slow open
Psychodynamic groups	Slow open

re-inforcing the patient's maladaptive ways of behaviour and undermining treatment approaches.

Group therapy

Group therapy is widely practised in the NHS. It is obviously more economical than one-to-one therapy but groups themselves also provide particular conditions that can facilitate therapeutic change.

Groups provide support and encouragement. They provide the opportunity to share problems with fellow members and to realise that they are not alone or the only person to suffer such difficulties. Members can experience peer pressure to encourage them to achieve things that otherwise they would not even contemplate. Members can also experience many different types of human relationship within the group. They may experience feelings about authority figures towards the group leader, sibling rivalry with other members of the group or even parental feelings if there is a particularly young person or younger member of the group.

Groups usually meet once or twice per week and consist of 8 to 12 people, with one or two therapists. Group therapy can be time limited (i.e. a specific number of sessions) or open-ended (i.e. continue on a long-term basis), but with members rotating through the group. Table 45 lists some of the ways and conditions for which group therapy is used in the NHS.

Further reading and sources

Clark DM, Fairburn CG (eds) 1996 Science and practice of cognitive behavioural therapy. Oxford University Press, Oxford

Feltham C, Horton I (eds) 2000 Handbook of counselling and psychotherapy. Sage Publications, London

Hobson R 1985 Forms of feeling: the heart of psychotherapy. Tavistock Publications, Tavistock, UK

Klerman E, Weissman M, Rounsaville B, Chevron E 1984 Interpersonal psychotherapy of depression. Basic Books, New York

Ryle A 1995 Cognitive-analytic therapy: active participation in change. A new integration in brief psychotherapy. Wiley, Chichester, UK

Sources

British Association for Counselling and Psychotherapy (BACP). Professional membership association for counsellors and psychotherapists. Provides information about therapies and therapists. http://www.bac.co.uk/

Society for Psychotherapy Research. International organization dedicated to the scientific study of psychotherapy. www.psychotherapyresearch.org

Cognitive Therapy and Research. Good website with information about cognitive therapy and the Beck Institute. www.beckinstitute.org

The cognitive-behaviour therapy (CBT) website. Provides description and explanations of cognitive-behaviour therapy. www.cognitive-behaviour-therapy.org

American Psychological Association. Website provides information about psychological disorders and therapies (e.g. interpersonal therapy). www.apa.org

Relate. A national organization devoted to couple counselling. www.relate.org.uk

The Counselling in Primary Care Trust. Information resource for counsellors, students and anyone interested in counselling in primary care. www.cpct.co.uk

Self-assessment: questions

Multiple choice questions

1. Cognitive therapy:
   a. Is based upon the theories of Freud
   b. Is a recognized treatment for a major depressive disorder
   c. Is superior to antidepressant treatment for major depressive disorder
   d. Is superior to interpersonal therapy for the treatment of major depressive disorder
   e. Is a treatment for bulimia nervosa

2. Psychological treatments that are a proven benefit in schizophrenia include:
   a. Behaviour-based rehabilitation programmes
   b. Cognitive therapy for chronic hallucinations
   c. Psychodynamic therapy for high expressed emotion
   d. Counselling
   e. Marital therapy

3. Counselling:
   a. Is superior to cognitive therapy for the treatment of major depressive disorder
   b. Is widely available in the primary care setting
   c. Is usually non-directive
   d. Aims to help the patient to find solutions to his/her own problems
   e. Requires no skill or training

4. Interpersonal therapies:
   a. Act by changing patient's negative cognitions
   b. Act by rewarding positive behaviour and discouraging negative behaviour
   c. Are as effective as cognitive therapy for the treatment of major depressive disorder
   d. Are better than antidepressants for major depressive disorder
   e. Prevent relapse in patients with chronic depression

5. Useful treatments for somatization include:
   a. Behavioural therapy
   b. Interpersonal therapy
   c. Cognitive therapy
   d. Counselling
   e. Antidepressant treatment

6. Psychological treatments on the NHS:
   a. Are usually short term
   b. Usually involve the patient and therapist meeting five times per week
   c. Are usually conducted on a one-to-one basis
   d. Can never be delivered in a group format
   e. Are only given by clinical psychologist

7. Psychological treatments on the NHS:
   a. Are never given in conjunction with psychotropic drugs
   b. Are only reserved for middle class patients of high intelligence
   c. Are popular with patients
   d. Are not suitable for patients who decline or fail to respond to drug treatment
   e. Are always successful

8. Psychological treatments:
   a. Require no effort or motivation on the part of the patient
   b. Never involve practice or homework between sessions
   c. Should never involve families in the treatment process
   d. Have high drop-out rates
   e. Are sometimes used on a long-term basis for patients with long-standing psychological difficulties or personality disorder

9. Counselling in primary care is usually helpful for the following groups:
   a. Patients with a long history of psychiatric illness
   b. Patients with schizophrenia
   c. Patients who have suffered a bereavement
   d. Patients with a stable premorbid personality and a circumscribed current problem
   e. Patients with a major depressive disorder

10. Cognitive therapy:
    a. Was developed by a psychiatrist named Beck
    b. Is only practised by clinical psychologists
    c. Tries to identify the underlying maladaptive schema that fuel negative thoughts
    d. Involves patients keeping a diary and monitoring their thoughts and behaviour
    e. Is a proven treatment for a wide range of clinical disorders

Case history questions

History 1

A 49-year-old woman visits her GP. She has been feeling low and not sleeping well since the death of her mother, to whom she was very close. The GP has started her on an antidepressant (selective serotonin reuptake inhibitor, SSRI) and she has noticed some improvement. She is still, however, finding it difficult to comes to terms with her mother's death. She has never suffered from psychiatric illness previously. She lived with her mother until her mother's death and has held down a stable job as a librarian for the last 24 years.

What is your further management of this case?

History 2

Miss P is 21 years old and has suffered from bulimia nervosa for the past 18 months. Her GP has referred her to secondary psychiatric services, as counselling did not help and her symptoms are getting worse.

She is assessed by a consultant psychiatrist, who establishes that there is no evidence of any disorder other than an eating disorder.

What is the management?

History 3

Miss X is a 21-year-old woman who has suffered from bulimia nervosa for the last 2 years. She repeatedly cuts herself and has had a series of stormy and unstable relationships. She has one son, who has been placed in care. She was sexually abused as a child and spent many years herself in care as a teenager.

She was referred for cognitive therapy but could not be engaged in treatment and did not comply with any of the homework or specific tasks. She is not suffering from a depressive illness, although at times she can experience very profound dips in her mood. The consultant psychiatrist responsible for her care assesses that her short-term risk of suicide is low, but there is quite a high long-term risk of suicide. Miss X attends the A&E department every time she cuts herself, visits her GP on a frequent basis and makes many demands on psychiatric and social services for help.

What is your management?

History 4

Mr X has suffered from schizophrenia for 6 years. He is helped by medication and has been relatively stable for the last 6 months. He is, however, continuously troubled by auditory hallucinations, which the medication does not affect. He can resist the voices but he finds that they are a continual distraction and he feels very distressed.

What is the management?

History 5

A 51-year-old man has been suffering from a moderately severe depressive illness for the last 6 months. He is opposed to any form of medication and his GP has been struggling to find something that will help. He does not have any current suicidal ideas.

What is the management?

History 6

A 29-year-old woman with type 1 diabetes is referred to the diabetic nurse for counselling. She has had brittle diabetes for 10 years, and her management is chaotic and unpredictable. During the session with the nurse, she admits to having an eating disorder.

What should the management be?

History 7

A 41-year-old man with multiple sclerosis (MS) is being reviewed routinely in the neurology clinic. He lets the doctor know that he has been feeling very low. On closer questioning, he tells the doctor that he has been thinking of killing himself, that he cannot see a future and cannot cope with the illness. He has been unable to sleep for the last few months, has lost 1 stone in weight and appears very low on mental state examination. The doctor refers him to the MS counsellor, who has recently been employed by the neurology unit to help patients adjust to their illness. Unfortunately the man commits suicide 2 weeks later.

What should have been the correct management?

Self-assessment: answers

Multiple choice answers

1. a. **False**. Cognitive therapy is based on the theories of Beck.
   b. **True**. Cognitive therapy is a recognized psychological treatment for major depressive disorder.
   c. **False**. It has equivalent effects to antidepressants for mild-to-moderate depressive disorders. Antidepressants are more effective for severe depressive disorders.
   d. **False**. It has equivalent effects.
   e. **True**. It is an effective treatment for bulimia nervosa.

2. a. **True**. Rehabilitation treatments are based upon behavioural techniques.
   b. **True**. Cognitive therapy is helpful for the treatment of chronic hallucinations in schizophrenia.
   c. **False**. Psychodynamic therapy can intensify the patient's emotional arousal.
   d. **False**. Counselling is not an effective treatment for schizophrenia.
   e. **False**. Marital therapy is not a specific treatment for schizophrenia.

3. a. **False**. Some studies show counselling is inferior or has equivalence to cognitive therapy for the treatment of major depression.
   b. **True**. Counselling is the most commonly available treatment in primary care.
   c. **True**. Counselling is not prescriptive.
   d. **True**. In counselling, the patient's problems are explored and the patient is helped to generate his/her own solutions to the problems he/she faces.
   e. **False**. Counselling requires good interpersonal skills and a recognized training of 1–2 years.

4. a. **False**. Cognitive therapy works by changing the patient's negative cognitions. Negative cognitions may change following interpersonal therapy secondary to other changes the patient makes. They are not, however, the main target of treatment.
   b. **False**. Behavioural therapies work in this way.
   c. **True**. Interpersonal therapy and psychodynamic interpersonal therapy have equivalent effects to cognitive therapy for the treatment of major depressive disorder.
   d. **False**. They are equivalent to antidepressants for mild and moderate states but less effective than antidepressants for severe depressive disorders.
   e. **True**. Interpersonal therapies can help to prevent relapse in patients with chronic depression.

5. a. **True**. Behavioural treatments have been shown to be helpful.
   b. **True**. Psychodynamic interpersonal therapy has been shown to be effective for patients with chronic bowel symptoms.
   c. **True**. Cognitive therapy is effective for patients with chronic fatigue, atypical chest pain and irritable bowel syndrome.
   d. **False**. Counselling has not been demonstrated to be helpful.
   e. **True**. Antidepressants are helpful.

6. a. **True**. Long-term treatment is rarely provided.
   b. **False**. The patient and therapist usually meet once per week.
   c. **True**. Family and group work also occurs, but most treatments are one-to-one.
   d. **False**. Many psychological treatments can be carried out in a group format.
   e. **False**. Although clinical psychologists carry out psychological treatments, many other health professionals, including psychiatrists, specialist nurses and counsellors, also provide treatment.

7. a. **False**. Psychological treatments are often given in conjunction with antidepressant treatment.
   b. **False**. Psychological treatments are available for most people who can speak English.
   c. **True**. Many patients express a preference for psychological treatments over drug treatments.
   d. **False**. Psychological treatments may be especially helpful for patients who decline or fail to respond to drug treatments.
   e. **False**. About 60% of patients are helped by psychological treatment approaches.

8. a. **False**. Psychological treatments require the patient to be an active participant in the treatment.
   b. **False**. Cognitive therapy usually involves homework.
   c. **False**. Many psychological treatments involve the patient's family, particularly family therapy and behavioural treatments.

d. **False**. Studies suggest that over two thirds of patients complete treatment. However, there is a higher attrition rate in the clinical setting.

e. **True**. Long-term treatments are reserved for patients with long-standing psychological difficulties.

9. a. **False**. Counselling is suitable for patients with a brief history of psychological problems.
   b. **False**. It should not be used in schizophrenia.
   c. **True**. Counselling may be very helpful.
   d. **True**. Such patients are very suitable for counselling.
   e. **False**. Other treatments such as cognitive therapy, interpersonal therapy, problem-solving therapy, psychodynamic-interpersonal therapy or antidepressant medication should be used.

10. a. **True**.
    b. **False**. It is predominantly practised by clinical psychologists but other health professionals also practise it. Beck himself was a psychiatrist.
    c. **True**. This is one of the principle components of cognitive therapy.
    d. **True**. This usually occurs.
    e. **True**. Cognitive therapy has been shown to be beneficial for a wide range of disorders.

History 1

This woman has a depressive disorder in the context of a bereavement reaction. She is responding to antidepressants, but the nature of her bereavement is likely to have a severe impact on her life. She has no previous history of psychiatric disorder and has coped well up until the death of her mother. The GP advises counselling with a view to help her to adjust to her mother's death and change in life circumstances.

History 2

The psychiatrist refers her to the clinical psychology service for a course of cognitive-behavioural therapy. The psychiatrist could have referred her for interpersonal therapy but none is available locally.

History 3

This young woman gives a history of lifelong difficulties. There is no recent change in her psychological status; her problems or difficulties can be understood in terms of a borderline personality

disorder. It is unlikely that she will benefit from a very brief psychological intervention. She has already found cognitive-behavioural therapy unhelpful, and she has been difficult to engage in psychological treatment. She is still however symptomatic, very distressed on occasions and a high user of services. Her psychiatrist calls a case conference to see if all health professionals and voluntary agencies can work together to provide:

- a stable place of residence for this young woman
- social support
- long-term psychological treatment.

Her psychiatrist refers her to the local psychotherapy service for psychodynamic-interpersonal therapy. She will see a therapist once per week for 2 years. The initial part of the therapy will focus upon engaging her in psychological treatment, and the therapist will have to work hard to establish a trusting relationship with her. The remainder of the therapy will focus upon the difficulty that she has in establishing and maintaining trusting, stable relationships.

She could also be referred for psychodynamic therapy, delivered in a day hospital setting, or a new variant of cognitive therapy, called 'dialectical behaviour therapy'.

History 4

This man should be referred for a course of cognitive behavioural therapy. The therapy will specifically focus upon teaching Mr X techniques to control and distract himself from the hallucinations.

History 5

This man is referred to the local clinical psychology service for cognitive-behavioural therapy. Interpersonal therapy or psychodynamic interpersonal therapy will be equally helpful but are unavailable.

History 6

The nurse consults with the liaison psychiatry service and she is referred for cognitive therapy. Interpersonal therapy or cognitive-analytic therapy may also be of help.

History 7

The doctor failed to recognize that the patient had a severe depressive illness that required urgent treatment from a liaison psychiatrist.

17 Physical treatments in psychiatry

Overview

Effective drug treatment in psychiatry began to appear in the 1950s with the first antipsychotic drugs (chlorpromazine) and the first true antidepressants (imipramine, amitriptyline). Together they are called psychotropic drugs. There are several classes. Most will not cause dependency, with important exceptions such as the antianxiety drugs benzodiazepines. Psychotropic drugs act on brain neurotransmitter systems. Psychotropic drugs, like other drugs, are evaluated clinically in randomized, controlled trials. Typically, the new drug is tested against placebo or against an existing comparator drug with efficacy already established. There are two main types of drug used in psychiatry: antidepressants, which are used to treat anxiety disorders and depressive disorders, and antipsychotic drugs (neuroleptics), which are used to treat schizophrenia and mania. In addition, there are a variety of other compounds that are used in the treatment of psychiatric conditions including lithium carbonate, benzodiazepines, antidementia drugs and drugs used for the treatment of alcohol or sexual problems.

17.1 Antidepressant drugs

Learning objectives

You should:

- know about the different kinds of antidepressant drug
- know when antidepressant treatment is indicated in psychiatric disorder
- know the main side effects of antidepressant drugs
- be able to explain antidepressant treatment to a patient.

Antidepressants were one of the earliest types of drug used in psychiatry (Table 46). Clinical depression (major depression) involves underactivity of brain 5-hydroxytryptamine (5HT; serotonin) and, to a lesser extent, noradrenaline (norepinephrine). Figure 14 shows how three different classes of antidepressant work towards the final common aim of increasing synaptic 5HT, and Figure 15 shows the 5HT pathways in the brain. The main class are monoamine reuptake inhibitors, which increase 5HT levels in the synapse by blocking its normal reuptake into the presynaptic nerve end. A second class, monoamine oxidase inhibitors (MAOI) increase 5HT by blocking its normal enzymatic breakdown. A third approach, with weak clinical effects only, is to increase 5HT production in the presynaptic neurone by giving a precursor amino acid L-tryptophan.

Antidepressant drugs take 1–3 weeks, sometimes even longer, before mood begins to improve. Sleep is usually first to improve, particularly with more sedative drugs such as amitriptyline, dothiepin or fluvoxamine. Side effects, if they are going to occur, will begin earlier.

Tricyclic antidepressants and selective serotonin reuptake inhibitors
Tricyclic antidepressants block reuptake of 5HT and, to some extent, noradrenline (norepinephrine). They are

effective but have anticholinergic and other side effects and are dangerous in overdose because of their arrhythmic effects. Selective sertonin reuptake inhibitors (SSRIs), with specific 5HT reuptake blockade, were developed in the 1980s and have equivalent efficacy with less anticholinergic, sedative and cardiotoxic effects. Serotonergic noradrenergic reuptake inhibitor (SNRI) drugs block both 5HT and noradrenaline (norepinephrine) reuptake and may be slightly more effective than other drugs in severe depression.

Monoamine oxidase inhibitors

MAOI drugs inhibit the metabolic breakdown of the intracellular monoamines 5HT, noradrenaline (norepinephrine) and dopamine. They are as effective as tricyclic-type or SSRI drugs but have more drug interactions. They block monoamine oxidase in gut and liver as well as in the central nervous system, so causing the rare but important 'cheese reaction', where dietary tyramine (a monoamine) cannot be broken down and causes acute hypertension with headache and palpitations. Pharmacists will give cards warning patients to avoid tyramine-rich foods such as blue cheese, red wine and game. New MAOI drugs selective for blocking only the CNS subtype of the enzyme are available. MAOIs are only used as second-line treatments and are especially effective in depression with marked anxiety symptoms.

Indication for treatment with antidepressants

There are several indications for treatment:

- major depression: the main indication for treatment; 70% of patients will improve (versus 30% on placebo) with antidepressant treatment
- panic disorder: 5HT-specific drugs such as imipramine or SSRIs are most effective.
- obsessive-compulsive disorder
- chronic pain, particularly where depressed mood is present.

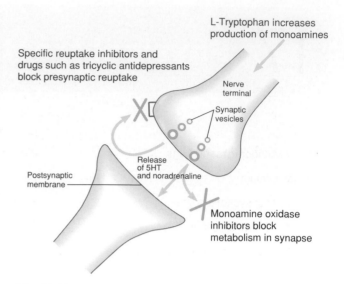

Fig. 14 How antidepressant drugs increase 5-hydroxytryptamine (5HT, serotonin) activity in the synapse.

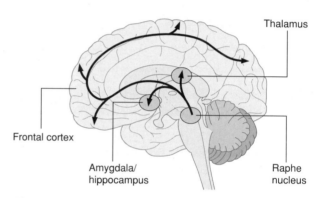

Fig. 15 5-Hydroxytryptamine (5HT, serotonin) pathways in the brain.

Side effects

Side effects are outlined in the Table 47. Anticholinergic side effects are dry mouth and less commonly urinary hesitancy and ejaculatory impotence in men.

Table 46 The main classes of psychotropic drug

Class of drug	Subclasses	Main neurotransmitter involved	Disorders treated
Antipsychotic (alternative name: neuroleptic)	Conventional (typical), atypical	Dopamine	Psychotic disorders such as schizophrenia
Antidepressants	Tricyclic, monoamine reuptake inhibitors, monoamine oxidase inhibitors (MAOI), selective serotonin reupake inhibitors (SSRIs), others	5-Hydroxytryptamine (5HT, serotonin)	Major depression
Mood stabilizers	Lithium, others	Uncertain	Bipolar disorder
Anxiolytics	Benzodiazepines, others	Gamma-aminobutyric acid (GABA)	Anxiety disorders
Hypnotics	Benzodiazepines	GABA	Sleep disorders

Table 47 Side effects of antidepressant drugs

Drug	Anticholinergic effects	Sedation	Cardiovascular effects
Tricyclic antidepressants			
Amitryptiline, imipramine, clomipramine, dosulepin	++	++	++
Lofepramine	+	+	+
Selective serotonin reuptake inhibitors (SSRIs)			
Fluoxetine, fluvoxamine, citalopram, paroxetine, sertraline	−	(+)	(+)
Serotonergic noradrenergic reuptake inhibitors (SNRI)			
Venlafaxine	−	+	+
Monoamine oxidase inhibitors (MAOIs)	+	+	++

Table 48 Common worries about starting antidepressants

Common worries	Your response
What are the side effects?	The most common side effects are dry mouth and sedation with tricyclic-type drugs and nausea and possible sleep disturbance with SSRIs. Postural hypotension with tricyclics important in older patients
Are they addictive?	No. Unlike benzodiazepines, antidepressants do not lead to dependence or withdrawal
Will they work and how quickly?	They are effective in 70% of people with moderate-to-severe depression. They will start to work only after 1–3 weeks, although any side effects will appear straight away
How long do I have to take them for?	It depends if they work. If they do work, they should be continued usually for at least 6 months
What happens if they don't work?	If they haven't worked after 6 weeks at adequate dosage, they should be stopped. Another class of antidepressant, or psychological treatments, should be considered

Cardiovascular effects with tricyclic antidepressants include postural hypotension. Cardiac arrhythmias can occur in patients with a cardiac history or in overdose. Weight gain can occur. Shorter acting SSRIs can result in a discontinuation syndrome if they are stopped suddenly. Some patients experience increased agitation coupled with a variety of somatic complaints on stopping the drug. These symptoms will gradually disappear or will completely stop if the SSRI is restarted. It can then be withdrawn more gradually. SSRIs do not cause psychological craving.

Table 48 shows some of the common worries about antidepressants that should be addressed when explaining their use to patients.

17.2 Lithium

Learning objectives

You should:

- know the main indications for lithium treatment
- know how to prescribe and monitor the drug
- know the important adverse effects of lithium.

The mode of action of lithium is unknown. It interacts with the normal activity of the sodium pump.

Indications

Prophylaxis of bipolar disorder is the main indication. Lithium is usually effective in reducing hypomanic and depressive relapses in bipolar disorder. Because of its potential toxicity, it is usually only given after a person has had two or more hypomanic episodes, or one very severe episode.

Other indications include:

- acute mania: usually used in addition to antipsychotic drugs
- resistant depression, in addition to antidepressant drugs
- prophylaxis of recurrent unipolar depressive disorder: lithium is sometimes used to reduce the frequency of recurrent severe depressive episodes in patients who have no history of mania or hypomania.

Box 75 on page 238 shows how to start and continue with lithium therapy.

Box 75
How to start and continue lithium therapy

Check cardiac, renal and endocrine history
Measure blood pressure, urea and electrolytes, thyroid function
Start low-dose lithium (400 mg daily)
Measure plasma lithium after 4–7 days; adjust dose accordingly
Measuring weekly for 3 weeks

Contraindications

The main contraindications are:

- cardiac failure
- renal disease
- thyroid disease
- pregnancy (fetal anomalies in first trimester).

Side effects

The side effects of lithium occur early and are usually transient:

- nausea and diarrhoea
- fine tremor
- mild diuresis causing thirst and polyuria
- later nephrogenic diabetes insipidus can occur because of inhibition of antidiuretic hormone-induced adenylate cyclase synthesis: occurs in 1–5% and is reversible
- hypothyroidism in 2%.

Alternative to lithium

The anticonvulsants carbamazepine and sodium valproate also have mood-stabilizing properties and can be used if lithium is ineffective or contraindicated. They also require regular monitoring of plasma levels.

17.3 Antipsychotic drugs

Learning objectives

You should:

- know the main types of antipsychotic drug
- know the indications for their use
- know the main adverse effects and drug interactions

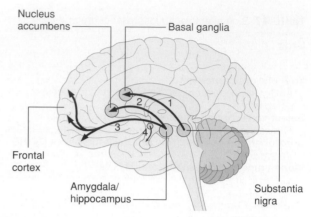

Fig. 16 Dopamine pathways in the brain. 1, Nigrostriatal; 2, mesolimbic; 3, mesocortical; 4, tuberohypophyseal.

Antipsychotic drugs block postsynaptic dopamine receptors. It is thought that the antipsychotic effect for positive symptoms is mediated especially by dopamine D_2 receptor blockade in the mesolimbic pathway, since in vitro affinity of individual drugs to this receptor relates closely to their clinical potency (number of milligrams for a clinical effect). Figure 16 shows the dopamine pathways in the brain.

Different antipsychotic drugs are similar in clinical efficacy, with the exception of clozapine, which is the most effective. They are effective in reducing psychotic symptoms in about 70% of patients, although this effect usually takes 1–4 weeks to start. They are less effective in reducing negative symptoms in schizophrenia.

The two main classes are conventional and atypical antipsychotics. Conventional antipsychotics cause more extrapyramidal side effects (EPS) than atypical drugs, particularly haloperidol and trifluoperazine.

Indications

The main indications for antipsychotic drugs are:

- psychotic symptoms in schizophrenia and when they occur in mania and severe depression
- acutely disturbed behaviour in organic brain disorders such as delirium and dementia
- long-term treatment and prophylaxis in recurrent psychotic disorders, especially schizophrenia.

Side effects

There are a number of side effects:

- extrapyramidal side effects: dopamine receptor blockade in the nigrostriatal pathway causes these side effects (Table 49), some of which resemble the increased muscle tone and bradykinesia (slowness of

Table 49 Extrapyramidal side effects of antipsychotic drugs

Type	Symptoms	Treatment
Early effects Dystonia	Painful, involuntary contraction of a group of muscles, usually in the neck (torticollis) or external ocular muscles (oculogyric crisis); usually occurs shortly after starting drug	Acute treatment with oral or intramuscular anticholinergic (e.g. procyclidine); choice then is to stop or reduce the antipsychotic drug, add regular anticholinergic drug or change to atypical drug
Medium-term effects Parkinsonian side effects	Increased muscle tone, often with superadded tremor, to give cogwheel rigidity; slowness of movement (bradykinesia), mask-like expression, shuffling gait;	Reduce or stop drug; add anticholinergic or change to atypical drug; anticholinergic drugs not effective; change to atypical drug or add beta-blocker
Akathisia	Subjective and objective restlessness of legs	
Late-term effects Tardive dyskinesia	Involuntary movements of face and neck, usually chewing of lips; gradual onset after longer-term treatment	Anticholinergics can make it worse; need to stop or reduce drug or change to atypical drug

movement) of natural Parkinson's disease (which results from reduced dopamine)

- sedation, especially with chlorpromazine, thioridazine, quetiapine, clozapine
- weight gain, especially olanzapine, clozapine
- sexual dysfunction: dopamine blockade in the temporofundibular system raises prolactin, which can cause sexual problems, gynaecomastia in men, amennorrhoea and galactorrhoea in women
- cardiac arrhythmias: if high doses of drug are used
- others: seizures with high doses, anticholinergic effects, antiadrenergic effects causing postural hypotension, skin rashes.

Maintenance treatment in schizophrenia

After acute symptoms have improved, maintenance drug treatment is usually needed to prevent relapse. After a first episode, this should be continued for at least a year. After a second or subsequent episode, treatment should be for at least 2 years and may be indefinite. Data from clinical trials show that the risk of relapse is about 60% in the year after stopping maintenance antipsychotic drugs, compared with 20% if the drug is continued.

Long-acting depot preparations

There are slow-release preparations of antipsychotic drugs such as flupentixol decoanate (Depixol) and fluphenazine decoanate (Modecate). They are given 1–4 times weekly by deep intramuscular injection into the buttock. They are used mainly in the maintenance treatment of schizophrenia in people who are erratic in compliance with oral medication. About one third of patients with chronic schizophrenia will be on depot drug treatment. Compared with oral drug treatment, depot medication has disadvantages of pain and possible infection at the injection site; in addition, emerging side effects cannot easily be reversed while the drug remains in the system. For this reason, a test dose of the preparation to be used is given if the person has not had the depot drug before.

Atypical antipsychotics

Atypical antipsychotics are so-called because they do not cause so many extrapyramidal side effects or raised prolactin as do conventional drugs.

Clozapine

Clozapine is more effective than any other antipsychotic drug. It carries a risk of agranulocytosis of about 0.5%. This makes it a third-line drug, used only after two other antipsychotic drugs have failed. However, 40–60% of such patients will improve with clozapine. It can only be prescribed with regular, initially weekly, white cell counts. It causes no extrapyramidal side effects.

Other atypical antipsychotics

Since 1994, there have been several atypical antipsychotics that act by blocking $5HT_2$ as well as dopamine D_2 receptors. They cause less extrapyramidal side effects than conventional antipsychotics but are probably no more effective. None is as effective as clozapine. They can cause sedation, sexual side effects and weight gain. They are about ten times more expensive than conventional drugs.

17.4 Benzodiazepines

Learning objectives

You should:

- know the main indications for the use of benzopdiazepines in psychiatry
- be aware of the potential for dependency with this class of drugs.

The benzodiazepines increase activity of the inhibitory neurotransmitter GABA (gamma-aminobutyric acid). They were widely used in the 1970s and 1980s for anxiety disorders, but their potential for dependence is high. Use should, therefore, be short term, no more than 2 weeks usually, for reactive anxiety or insomnia. They are relatively safe in overdose. They can be classified according to their half-life into long- (over 24 hours, such as diazepam or chlordiazepoxide), medium- (6–24 hours, such as lorazepam) or short-acting- (less than 6 hours, such as temazepam) drugs.

Indications

The main indications for benzodiazepines are:

- short-term treatment of acute anxiety states (long-acting drugs)
- short-term treatment of insomnia (short-acting drugs)
- treatment of delirium tremens and acute psychotic emergencies (long- or medium-acting drugs)
- premedication for minor medical procedures.

Side effects

The main side effects of the benzodiazepines are:

- drowsiness
- ataxia
- confusion (in the elderly)
- potentiate the effects of alcohol
- dependence: occurs within 2 weeks, with increasing tolerance to the sedative effects and a withdrawal syndrome consisting of anxiety, insomnia, agitation, perceptual disturbances and sometimes seizures.

Other anxiolytic drugs

In anxiety disorders, antidepressant drugs or psychological treatments are better than benzodiazepines. *Beta-blockers* can help by reducing unpleasant autonomic effects such as palpitations if these predominate.

17.5 Other drug treatments in psychiatry

Learning objectives

You should:

- know about new treatments for Alzheimer's disease
- know about drug treatments for different problems associated with substance abuse
- know about drug treatment for erectile dysfunction.

Drug treatments for Alzheimer's disease

The cholinergic system from the basal nucleus of Meynert projecting to the hippocampus and cerebral cortex is central to learning and memory. Loss of cholinergic neurones occurs in Alzheimer's disease. *Cholinesterase inhibitors* slow the metabolism of acetylcholine and have been shown to improve slightly the cognitive deficits in Alzheimer's disease.

Donepezil and rivastigmine are cholinesterase inhibitors that produce modest improvements in the cognitive deficits although the disease continues to progress. They should probably be reserved for patients with early disease. They are mainly for specialist use. Outcome needs to be monitored with rating scales. Rivastigmine causes gastrointestinal disturbances.

Drug treatment of substance use

Self-help and psychological treatments are of most relevance to the treatment of substance use.

Opiate withdrawal (detoxification) is undertaken by using a reducing dose of the synthetic opiate *methadone* and withdrawal symptoms are alleviated with the synthetic opiate antagonist *naltrexone*. Craving following withdrawal is reduced with the SSRI citalopram.

Alcohol detoxification is undertaken by using a benzodiazepine, or the related drug chlomethiazole, in a reducing dose. *Acamprosate* will reduce craving. *Disulfiram* is occasionally used to promote abstinence. It blocks the normal oxidative metabolism of alcohol, causing build up of acetaldehyde and nausea and flushing if a drink is taken.

Erectile dysfunction

Sildafenil (Viagra) inhibits phosphodiasterase type 5 in the corpus cavernosa, increasing smooth muscle relaxation. It augments but cannot initiate an erection. It is effective in 50% of cases of male erectile dysfunction and works well for psychogenic cases and milder organic cases. Side effects are headache and nasal congestion (Ch. 9).

Alternative therapies

St John's wort is an extract from a plant that has been shown to have weak antidepressant properties. Both ginseng and gingko biloba have weak enhancing effects on concentration and memory in normal individuals. Evidence for the effectiveness of other alternative therapies in psychiatric disorder is absent.

17.6 Electroconvulsive therapy and other physical treatments

Learning objectives

You should

- know the main indications for electronconvulsive therapy
- be familiar with how it is administered
- know the main indications for psychosurgery.

Electroconvulsive therapy

Electroconvulsive therapy (ECT) was developed in the 1930s, before the discovery of psychotropic drugs. Once widely used, it is now limited to the treatment of severe major depression that is unresponsive to antidepressant drug treatment. This may include situations that are life threatening because the person is refusing food and drink, depression with psychotic features, and elderly patients sensitive to the side effects of prolonged drug treatment.

In such cases, ECT will often work where other treatments fail. Randomized controlled trials performed comparing it with 'dummy' ECT have shown it to be effective in severe, intractable depression, especially where there are psychotic symptoms. However, relapse can occur especially in the 6 weeks after the course finishes. ECT is often viewed as controversial, for three main reasons: (i) its mode of action is unknown; (ii) it has been used overly widely in the past; (iii) it sounds frightening. Because of this, it is important you see ECT being given in a modern hospital setting and know the advantages and disadvantages.

Modern ECT involves inducing a modified seizure by triggering it with a controlled electric current. The procedure is as follows:

1. Informed, written consent is obtained. (ECT can be given without consent, usually if the person is too ill to consent, under the Mental Health Act after a second medical opinion, but this is rare.)
2. General anaesthetic work-up in consultation with anaesthetist, including physical examination and blood count, electrolytes, chest X-ray and electrocardiograph, if indicated.
3. Nil by mouth prior to procedure.
4. Patient moved to specialized ECT suite with anaesthetist, psychiatrist and nursing staff.
5. Atropinic premedication is given.
6. Induction is instituted with a short-acting anaesthetic agent.
7. A muscle relaxant (suxemethonium [succinylcholine]) is given.
8. Electrodes are applied and the current delivered. The usual procedure is to place the two electrodes, which look like small cardiac resuscitation paddles, at two points over the non-dominant (usually the right) hemisphere: one at the temple and the second above the ear. The current will cause a seizure, which, because of the muscle relaxant, is limited to a slight fluttering of the eyelids. Online electroencephalograph monitoring will confirm a seizure has occurred.
9. The patient is moved to recovery area.

A course of ECT consists of 6–12 treatments spaced at intervals of 3 to 4 days. If it is going to occur, clinical improvement will usually start after the third or fourth treatment.

Side effects

The side effects are those of the general anaesthetic. Headaches can occur for a few hours.

Despite claims, no firm evidence of longer-term memory impairment or brain damage has been shown, even in older patients who have had many treatments.

Neurosurgery for psychiatric disorder

There is evidence that stereotactic surgery to small parts of the white matter in the base of the frontal lobe can alleviate chronic, severe resistant depression if all else fails. This operation is skilled and only very rarely done, needing special consent under the Mental Health Act. Less than 20 patients per year are treated in this way in the UK, usually with few side effects.

Further reading and sources

Bazire S 1997 Psychotropic drug directory: the professionals pocket handbook and aide memoire. Quay Publishing, Lancaster, UK

British Medical Association and the Royal Pharmaceutical Society of Great Britain 2001 British national formulary. BMJ Books, London (Regularly updated versions are published and supplied free to most medical practitioners)

Sources

Useful site with detailed information about antidepressants. www.biopsychiatry.com

Detailed information about all psychotropic drugs. www.psy-web.com

Self-assessment: questions

Multiple choice questions

1. Selective serotonin reuptake inhibitors (SSRI) antidepressants:
   a. Are more effective than tricyclic antidepressants
   b. Are cheaper to prescribe than tricyclic antidepressants
   c. Have a specific action on 5-hydroxytryptamine (5HT)
   d. Can cause weight gain
   e. Are relatively safe if taken in the form of an overdose

2. Lithium carbonate:
   a. Is a tricyclic antidepressant
   b. Is a psychotropic drug
   c. Can be used to treat acute mania
   d. Is safe in overdose
   e. Requires regular monitoring of blood serum levels

3. Clozapine:
   a. Is a neuroleptic
   b. Has marked extrapyramidal side effects
   c. Can cause agranulocytosis
   d. Is the most effective drug treatment for schizophrenia
   e. Is a first-line treatment for schizophrenia

4. Electroconvulsive therapy (ECT):
   a. Is a first-line treatment for depression
   b. Is administered using a muscle relaxant, so the physical signs of a convulsion are modified and barely visible
   c. Is usually given bilaterally, over both hemispheres
   d. Is usually administered to the dominant hemisphere
   e. Is better tolerated than antidepressants by some elderly patients with depressive disorders

5. Benzodiazepines:
   a. Are anxiolytics
   b. Induce dependence
   c. Should not usually be prescribed for more than a 2 week period
   d. Can be used for rapid sedation of severely disturbed patients
   e. Are neuroleptics

Case history questions

History 1

A 30-year-old man attends the clinic complaining of lack of sex drive. He has a history of two episodes of schizophrenia, the last a year previously. He has been taking haloperidol 15 mg daily for most of the past 2 years, although his last relapse occurred a month after he stopped this for a period last year. On examination, he shows mild but definite involuntary chewing movements of his mouth. His mental state is otherwise normal.

1. What might the lack of sex drive be caused by?
2. What are the mouth movements likely to be?
3. What might you advise him?

History 2

A 45-year-old man has been treated with the SSRI citalopram at a dosage of 40 mg daily for a depressive illness. He has been well and functioning normally for over 6 months. He wishes to stop the medication.

What should his GP advise?

History 3

A 39-year-old woman complains of difficulty sleeping. She has had sleeping tablets in the past for similar problems and has asked her GP for a further course. Her GP notes that, in the last 5 years, she has been prescribed sleeping tablets on a fairly regular basis.

1. What should the GP do?
2. What treatment should be given?

Objective structure clinical examination (OSCE)

Topic: Explanation of antidepressant treatment

Mr Murdoch has been feeling low for 6 months. He feels miserable all of the time and is pessimistic about the future. He has had difficulty sleeping, has a poor appetite and has lost 1 stone (6 kg) in weight. He has had thoughts that life is not worth living but has not had active plans to kill himself. You have diagnosed that he has a major depressive disorder and requires treatment with antidepressants. You have 5 minutes to explain to the patient that you want him to start antidepressant treatment.

Please make sure you explain to the patient

- why you think it is required
- how it will work
- how long the patient needs to take it for
- likely side effects and how the patient should manage them
- what positive effects you expect
- when you expect these to occur.

If you have someone who can play the part of the patient, ask them to read the information in the box and then to answer your questions. Also ask them to ask the list of questions. If you are doing this station alone, read the information below and ensure that your information to the patient includes the answers to these questions.

You have been feeling low for 6 months. You feel miserable all of the time and am pessimistic about the future. You have had difficulty sleeping, have a poor appetite and have lost 1 stone in weight. You have had thoughts that life is not worth living but you have not had active plans to kill yourself.

Please allow the candidate to explain to you the reasons for taking antidepressants. If the candidate is unclear or uses words that you do not understand, you can ask the candidate to clarify matters.

Do not object to taking antidepressants or be ideologically opposed to taking medication. You are, however, concerned that antidepressants may be addictive. You should ask the candidate the following questions:

- is the medication addictive?
- can I continue to drive?
- can I drink alcohol?

Self-assessment: answers

Multiple choice answers

1. a. **False**. No evidence of a marked difference between them.
    b. **False**. They are much more expensive.
    c. **True**.
    d. **True**.
    e. **True**. As they do not have the cardiotoxic effects of most tricyclic drugs they are relatively safe, even if taken as an overdose.

2. a. **False**. Lithium has a completely unique biochemical profile and is not a member of any specific drug group.
    b. **True**. The term psychotropic drug is a collective term for drugs that have specific actions on mental state and are used to treat mental illness.
    c. **True**. It can be used in combination with haloperidol to treat acute mania. In these circumstances, a higher serum blood level is usually used. Caution is required as there are reports of severe interactions between lithium and haloperidol.
    d. **False**. Lithium is highly toxic if taken as an overdose and can result in confusion or even coma and death.
    e. **True**.

3. a. **True**.
    b. **False**. It has very few extrapyramidal side effects.
    c. **True**. This severe and dangerous side effect occurs in 0.5% of patients who are prescribed clozapine.
    d. **True**.
    e. **False**. Because of its dangerous side effects, it is not a first-line treatment for schizophrenia.

4. a. **False**.
    b. **True**. In most cases, the signs of an actual convulsion are barely visible, but this is confirmed using electroencephalographic (EEG) monitoring.
    c. **False**. Bilateral ECT is more likely to cause confusion.
    d. **False**. Non-dominant hemisphere.
    e. **True**. The main side effects of ECT are those of the general anaesthetic, rather than the procedure itself.

5. a. **True**.
    b. **True**. They have a high potential for dependence.

c. **True**. Because of problems of dependence if used for longer.
d. **True**. They can be used in combination with a neuroleptic.
e. **False**. Antipsychotic drugs are neuroleptics.

Case history answers

History 1

1. Antipsychotic drug treatment is the most likely cause of his loss of sex drive. It is important to take a brief psychosexual history to clarify the problem, including any other drug treatment he might be taking, and rule out obvious endocrine causes such as hypothyroidism. Check his alcohol history.
2. Early tardive dyskinesia. Check on examination for other extrapyramidal signs. This is also a side effect of his antipsychotic drug treatment.
3. Explain that his drug treatment may be causing his low sex drive and is very likely the cause of his tardive dyskinesia. Options then are to stop the drug, reduce the dose or change to an atypical antipsychotic drug with a lower risk of adverse effects. Stopping the drug is not yet advisable since he relapsed when this was done last year.

History 2

He should be advised to slowly reduce the citalopram over a period of weeks. He should initially reduce the dosage from 40 to 20 mg per day. After 2 weeks, if all is well, it can be reduced to 10 mg for a further 1–2 weeks before stopping the drug. The GP should explain to the patient the reason for this gradual reduction and the possible adverse effects if the drug is stopped too quickly. It is understandable that the patient may be worried about the possibility of the depression recurring once medication has been stopped. He should be reassured that the chances of this are very low and that the GP will re-instate the medication if this happens.

History 3

1. There needs to be a full assessment of her sleep problem. It needs to be established whether there are any obvious causes. It is important to exclude depressive or anxiety disorders, and other physical causes of sleeplessness (e.g. hyperthyroidism).
2. In this case, it becomes clear from a more detailed assessment that the patient has a depressive illness

that has remained undetected and untreated for several months. She is given an explanation of her condition and a rationale for treatment. She is prescribed antidepressant medication (of a more sedative nature) and told that her sleep problem will gradually improve as the depression improves. If there was no underlying cause for her sleep disturbance, it would be unwise for the GP to prescribe further benzodiazepines. In the long term, such prescribing is likely to make her problems worse. She should be encouraged to re-instate a normal pattern of sleeping by the use of a sleep programme. This involves going to bed at a normal time. Not getting out of bed, even if one cannot sleep. Getting up early and not oversleeping in the morning. Keeping active during the day and not resting or taking naps during the daytime. Learning and using relaxation techniques to unwind in the evening. Avoidance of stimulating drinks or foods in the evening hours and restricting fluid intake in the 2–3 hours before sleep.

OSCE answer

Candidates would be marked on this station on whether they made the following points in the explanation and whether they answered the patient's questions clearly.

Information provided to the patient

1. The patient is suffering from depression. Depression is an illness that requires treatment. It is hard to snap out of it. He should consider drug treatment with antidepressants. Psychological treatment may also be helpful but could not be arranged quickly.
2. Antidepressants work by restoring the levels of certain chemicals in the brain that become depleted in depression (or some such explanation).
3. The drug the candidate should recommend should be any selective serotonin reuptake inhibitor (SSRI); a tricyclic antidepressant would also be acceptable. The patient will need to take (*here give the correct dose*

in tablets per day). If you suggested a tricyclic antidepressant, also give now the information for an SSRI (*the remainder of this answer is based on an SSRI*).

4. The patient will need to take antidepressant treatment for at least 6–9 months.
5. It may take 2–3 weeks before the patient notices a beneficial effect.
6. There are relatively few side effects and it is quite safe. The patient may notice nausea or sickness in the first few days which should wear off (award extra marks for knowledge of additional side effects).
7. The candidate should not stop the drug suddenly as he may experience some unpleasant symptoms (this would not be the case if the drug you chose was fluoxetine (Prozac).

In response to the role player's question

1. The drug is not addictive, i.e. the patient will not crave the medication or psychologically feel dependent upon it.
2. The patient should be able to continue driving. The patient would only have to stop driving if the medication made him drowsy (which is unlikely).
3. The patient can drink small amounts of alcohol, strictly in moderation.

An examiner will also be marking communication skills and the following would be considered important:

1. Spoke slowly and used language that the patient understood
2. Adopted a calm and sympathetic manner
3. Made good eye contact
4. Facilitated patient concerns
5. Clarified points the patient did not understand
6. Checked the patient had understood what he had been told
7. Allowed the patient to make an informed choice about treatment.

Index

Q indicates a topic mentioned in a question to which the reader will find more detailed mention in the answer.